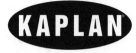

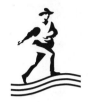

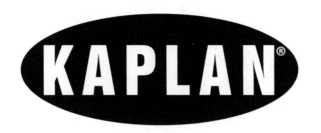

NCLEX-RN*

2002–2003 Edition

Judith A. Burckhardt, M.Ed., R.N.
Barbara J. Irwin, B.S.N., R.N.

Simon & Schuster

NEW YORK · LONDON · SINGAPORE · SYDNEY · TORONTO

*NCLEX is a registered trademark of the National Council of State Boards of Nursing (NCSBN), which is not affiliated with this product.

Kaplan Publishing
Published by Simon & Schuster
1230 Avenue of the Americas
New York, NY 10020

For bulk sales to schools, colleges, and universities, please contact: Order Department, Simon and Schuster, 100 Front Street, Riverside, NJ 08075. Phone: (800) 223-2336. Fax: (800) 943-9831.

Contributing Editor: Rochelle Rothstein, M.D.
Project Editor: Eileen Mager
Cover Design: Cheung Tai
Production Editor: Maude Spekes
Production Manager: Michael Shevlin
Editorial Coordinator: Déa Alessandro
Executive Editor: Del Franz

Manufactured in the United States of America
Published simultaneously in Canada

April 2002

10 9 8 7 6 5 4 3 2 1

ISBN: 0-7432-3295-X

Contents

About the Authors

Judith A. Burckhardt, M.Ed., R.N.

Burckhardt is Executive Director, Nursing and Allied Health for Kaplan, Inc. After graduating from Loyola University in Chicago with a Bachelor of Science in Nursing, she received a Master's in Education from Washington University and is currently enrolled in a doctoral program at the University of Nebraska. Her professional background includes many years of experience as an educator in diploma, A.D.N., and B.S.N. nursing programs. She has developed programs and materials for NCLEX preparation and has presented NCLEX and career development seminars to students, nurses, and health care professionals in the United States and abroad. Burckhardt has also given item-writing workshops for nursing programs. She has written articles for nursing publications and has developed instructor-led continuing education programs for online delivery at Kaplan College School of Nursing.

Barbara J. Irwin, B.S.N., R.N.

Irwin is National Curriculum Director for Nursing programs at Kaplan, Inc. She supervises the development of NCLEX preparation for U.S. nursing students and international nurses, as well as integrated testing programs implemented by nursing schools. While tutoring students that had been unsuccessful on the NCLEX, Irwin developed a series of innovative test-taking strategies that help students achieve success on this high-stakes test. She presents NCLEX and test-taking seminars to nursing school faculties and students nationwide. Irwin received her Bachelor of Science in Nursing from the University of Oklahoma. Her professional background includes experience as a nursing educator and director of a home health agency.

The material in this book is up-to-date at the time of publication. However, the National Council of State Boards of Nursing may have instituted changes after this book was published. Be sure to carefully read the materials you receive when you register for the test.

If there are any important late-breaking developments—or any changes or corrections to the Kaplan test preparation materials in this book—we will post that information online at **kaptest.com/publishing**. Check to see if there is any information posted there regarding this book.

Readers' Comments

Here's what our readers have to say about Kaplan's *NCLEX-RN*:

"After doing all my reviews, I read this book twice and I went to take the test with confidence. I did it— thank you!"
—Elisabeth Boursiquot, Spring Valley, New York

"Out of the 15 NCLEX books I bought, this Kaplan book was the only one that helped. The critical thinking and test-taking skills were very useful in studying for the NCLEX-RN. Thank you so much!"
—Sherrie Corcuera, Barnegat, New Jersey

"I had taken NCLEX twice and failed, I'd taken courses, etc. I didn't need another study book—I needed a book that emphasizes test-taking skills for NCLEX and test anxiety reduction. I took the test for the third time and passed! I have told all my friends about this miraculous book—thank you for the confidence! I did it! I'm an RN!!!"
—Beatrice Ordoñez, O'Fallon, Missouri

"Before I started to prepare for the NCLEX, I started with this book (I'm a foreign nurse from Switzerland), and it really helps me to have a critical thinking strategy and to answer the NCLEX question types. The practice test and the answer key are extremely helpful, the way it explains every single answer. So now, I think I'm ready to start the Kaplan course book. Thank you."
—Celine Cucchia, San Jose, California

"Special thanks to the creators of this wonderful book and others related to NCLEX-RN. It was the best I could ever have gotten. I just feel sorry I didn't take your review class due to [the fact that] I didn't know about you guys until after I took another review class. But I was lucky to find this wonderful book. Thanks! I will recommend this book or anything related to Kaplan to the future generations of my nursing school. You guys are the best! Thank you and keep up with the good work."
—Elvia Manrique, Port Jefferson Station, New York

How to Use This Book

Step One: Read Chapters 1 Through 12

This section contains a comprehensive, detailed strategy guide to approach each type of question on the NCLEX. This information will prepare you for the real thing by teaching you how to analyze each question and use your nursing knowledge to select the correct answer choice.

If you have been educated outside the United States, be sure to also read chapter 13, which contains information, Kaplan strategies, and practice questions exclusively for international nurses.

Step Two: Take the Practice Tests

Kaplan has prepared two different practice tests for your use: the paper-and-pencil test in Part Two of this book and a computer-based exam on the CD-ROM bundled with this book.

If you have access to a computer, you may benefit from taking the electronic test first. (For instructions on how to install and use the software, see the "User's Guide to the CD-ROM" section at the back of this book.) When the test is completed, you will receive immediate feedback on your performance, as the software analyzes your strengths and weaknesses in various content areas. You can then review the areas in which your performance was weak before you tackle the paper-and-pencil test.

If you don't have access to a computer, use the paper-and-pencil test in this book, complete with in-depth answer explanations, to prepare for the real NCLEX.

Step Three: Register for the Exam

When you are prepared to take the NCLEX, use the contact information and licensure requirements provided in Appendix D to initiate the registration process. All of the steps you'll need to follow are contained in chapter 11, "The Licensure Process."

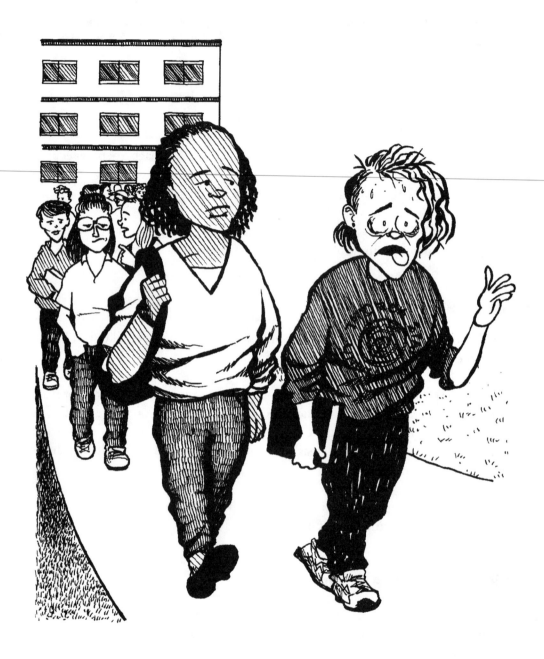

"My assessment of my analysis is that I should have done more planning for the implementation of my NCLEX evaluation."

PART ONE

PREPARING FOR THE NCLEX

CHAPTER ONE

Overview of the NCLEX

LOCATION: Test Center, Anytown, USA.
CANDIDATE: You. You are talking to yourself.
GOAL: To pass the NCLEX.

"O.K., this is it. I've studied for six weeks. I am READY! Come on, come on. Give me the first question. Let's get started!"

A 45-year-old man had a permanent pacemaker implanted one year ago. He returns to the outpatient clinic because he thinks the pacemaker battery is malfunctioning. The nurse would expect the client to exhibit which of the following symptoms?	(1) Abdominal pain, nausea, and vomiting. (2) Wheezing on exertion, cyanosis, and orthopnea. (3) Peripheral edema, shortness of breath, and dizziness. (4) Chest pain radiating to the right arm, headache, and diaphoresis.

Knowledge is Power

The first step in preventing panic is to learn everything you can about the exam.

"Pacemaker battery? PACEMAKER BATTERY? I've studied for six weeks, and they ask me about a PACEMAKER BATTERY? I don't remember reading about pacemaker batteries! I should have rescheduled my test! I should have studied harder. I should have bought that Kaplan book!"

Is this the way you want to begin your professional nursing career? In a panic because you think that you are going to fail the NCLEX exam? Of course not. But if the NCLEX strikes fear into your heart, you need to conquer that fear, and the first step in preventing panic about the NCLEX is to learn everything you can about the exam.

WHAT IS THE NCLEX?

NCLEX stands for *National Council Licensure Examination*, the test administered by the boards of nursing that represent each of the 50 states in the United States, the District of Columbia, and five U.S. territories: American Samoa, Guam, the Northern Mariana Islands, Puerto Rico, and the Virgin Islands. These boards have a mandate to protect the public from unsafe and ineffective nursing care, and each board has been given responsibility to regulate the practice of nursing in its respective state. In fact, the NCLEX is often referred to as "The Boards" or "State Boards."

NCLEX has only one purpose: to determine if it is safe for you to begin practice as an entry-level nurse.

Passing NCLEX = RN

You must pass the NCLEX to be a licensed registered nurse.

Why Must You Take the NCLEX?

The NCLEX is prepared by the National Council of State Boards of Nursing (NCSBN). Each state requires that you pass this exam to obtain a license to practice as a registered nurse. The designation *registered nurse* or *R.N.* indicates that you have proven to your state board of nursing that you can deliver safe and effective nursing care. The NCLEX is a test of minimum competency and is based on the knowledge and behaviors that are needed for the entry-level practice of nursing. This exam tests not only your knowledge, but also your ability to make competent nursing judgments.

What Is Entry-Level Practice of Nursing?

In order to define *entry-level* practice of nursing, the National Council conducts a job analysis study every three years to determine what entry-level nurses do on the job. The kinds of questions they investigate include: In which clinical settings does the beginning nurse work? What types of care do beginning nurses provide to their patients? What are their primary duties and responsibilities? Based on the results of this study, National Council adjusts the content and level of difficulty of the test to accurately reflect what is happening in the workplace.

What NCLEX Is *NOT*

It is not a test of achievement or intelligence. It is not designed for nurses who have years of experience. The questions do not involve high-tech clinical nursing or equipment. It is not predictive of your eventual success in the career of nursing. You will not be tested on all the content that you were taught in nursing school.

What Is a CAT?

CAT stands for *Computer Adaptive Test.* Each test is assembled interactively based on the accuracy of the candidate's response to the questions. This ensures that the questions you are answering are not "too hard" or "too easy" for your skill level. Your first question will be relatively easy; that is, below the level of minimum competency. If you answer that question correctly, the computer selects a slightly more difficult question. If you answer the first question incorrectly, the computer selects a slightly easier question (Figure 1). By continuing to do this as you answer questions, the computer is able to calculate your level of competence.

Correct Answer, Next Question's Harder

Test questions are chosen according to the accuracy of your responses.

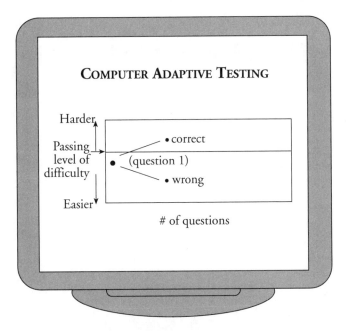

Figure 1

In a CAT, the questions are adapted to your ability level. The computer selects questions that represent all areas of nursing, as defined by the NCLEX test plan and by the level of item difficulty. Each question is self-contained, so that all of the information you need to answer a question is presented on the computer screen with the question and four possible answer choices.

Taking the Exam

There is no time limit for each individual question. You have a maximum of five hours to complete the exam, but that includes the beginning tutorial, a mandatory ten-minute break after the first two hours of testing, and an optional break after an additional 90 minutes of testing. Everyone answers a minimum of 75 questions to a maximum of 265 questions.

Regardless of the number of questions you answer, you are given 15 questions that are experimental. These questions, which are indistinguishable from the other questions on the test, are being tested for future use in NCLEX exams, and your answers do not count for or against you. Your test ends when one of the following occurs:

The Length of Each Test Differs

You answer a minimum of 75 questions to a maximum of 265 questions.

- You have demonstrated minimum competency and answered the minimum number of questions (75)
- You have demonstrated a lack of minimum competency and answered the minimum number of questions (75)
- You have answered the maximum number of questions (265)
- You have used the maximum time allowed (five hours)

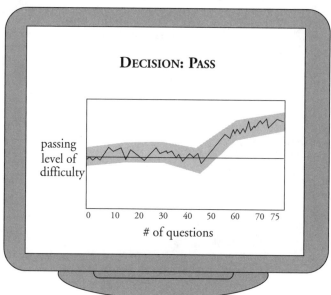

Figure 2

Go the Distance

As long as you are answering questions, you have not failed. Don't lose concentration!

Try not to be concerned with the length of your test. In fact, you should plan on testing for five hours and seeing 265 questions. You are still in the game as long as the computer continues to give you test questions, so focus on answering them to the best of your ability.

Remember, every question counts. There is no warm-up time, so it is important for you to be ready to answer questions correctly from the very beginning. Concentration is also key. You need to give your best to each question because you do not know which will put you over the top.

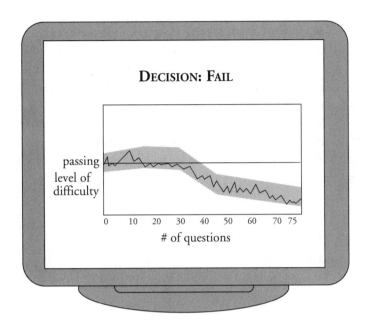

Figure 3

CONTENT OF THE NCLEX

The questions on the NCLEX involve integrated nursing content. Many nursing programs are based on the medical model. Students take separate medical, surgical, pediatric, psychiatric, and obstetric classes. On the NCLEX, all content is integrated.

Look at the following question.

A 23-year-old woman with insulin dependent diabetes mellitus (IDDM) is returned to the recovery room one hour after an uneventful delivery of a 9 lb., 8 oz., baby boy. The nurse would expect the woman's blood sugar to	(1) change from 220 to 180 mg/dL (2) change from 110 to 80 mg/dL (3) change from 90 to 120 mg/dL (4) change from 100 to 140 mg/dL

Is this an obstetrical question or a medical/surgical question? In order to select the correct answer, (2), you must consider the pathophysiology of diabetes along with the principles of labor and delivery. This is an example of an integrated question.

It's All Integrated

The NCLEX is not divided up into separate content areas. The NCLEX tests integrated nursing content.

The NCLEX Test Blueprint

The NCLEX is organized according to the framework "Meeting Client Needs." There are four major categories of Client Needs and ten subcategories. This information is distributed by the developers of the NCLEX, National Council of State Boards of Nursing, Inc.

You're In Charge

Nurses are managers of care.

Client Need #1: Safe and Effective Care Environment

The first subcategory for this client need is **Management of Care** and accounts for **7–13** percent of the questions on the exam. Nursing actions that are covered in this subcategory include:

- Advanced directives
- Advocacy
- Case management
- Client rights
- Concepts of management
- Confidentiality
- Consultation with members of the healthcare team
- Continuity of care
- Continuous quality improvement
- Delegation
- Establishing priorities
- Ethical practice
- Incident/irregular occurrence/variance reports
- Informed consent
- Legal responsibilities
- Organ donation
- Referrals
- Resource management
- Supervision

Here is example of a typical question from this subcategory:

Which of the following assignments, if made by the registered nurse, would be appropriate for a LPN/LVN?	(1) A 56-year-old man with emphysema scheduled to be discharged later today. (2) A 41-year-old woman in traction with a fractured femur. (3) A 34-year-old woman with low back pain scheduled for a myelogram in the afternoon. (4) A newly diagnosed 43-year-old woman with type 1 diabetes mellitus.

The correct answer is (2). This patient is in stable condition and can be cared for by an LPN with supervision of a RN.

Here is another example of a Management of Care question:

After receiving report from the night nurse, which of the following patients should the nurse see FIRST?	(1) A 31-year-old woman refusing Carafate before breakfast. (2) A 40-year-old man with left-sided weakness asking for assistance to the commode. (3) A 52-year-old woman complaining of chills who is scheduled for a cholecystectomy. (4) A 65-year-old man with a nasogastric tube who had a bowel resection yesterday.

The correct answer is (3). This is the least stable patient.

The second subcategory for this client need is **Safety and Infection Control** and accounts for **5–11** percent of the questions on the exam. Nursing actions that are covered in this subcategory include:

- Accident prevention
- Disaster planning
- Error prevention
- Handling hazardous and infectious materials
- Medical and surgical asepsis
- Standard (universal) and other precautions
- Use of restraints

Here is an example of a question from this subcategory:

Prepare for Disaster

Remember your safety and infection control techniques.

The physician orders tobramycin sulfate (Nebcin) 3 mg/kg IV every 8 hours for a 3-year-old boy. The nurse enters the patient's room to administer the medication and discovers that the boy does not have an identification bracelet. What should the nurse do?	(1) Ask the parents at the child's bedside to state their child's name. (2) Ask the child to say his first and last name. (3) Have a co-worker identify the child before giving the medication. (4) Hold the medication until an identification bracelet can be obtained.

The correct answer is (1). This action will allow the nurse to correctly identify the child and enable the nurse to give the medication on time.

Client Need #2: Health Promotion and Maintenance

The first subcategory for this client need is **Growth and Development** and accounts for 7–13 percent of the questions on the exam. Nursing actions that are covered in this subcategory include:

- The aging process
- Ante/intra/postpartum and newborn
- Developmental stages and transitions
- Expected body image changes
- Family planning
- Family systems
- Human sexuality

It is important to understand that not everyone described in the questions will be sick or hospitalized. Some clients may be in a clinic or home-care setting. Some clients may not be sick at all. Wellness is an important concept on the NCLEX. It is necessary for a safe and effective nurse to know how to promote health and prevent disease.

The following is an example of a typical question from this subcategory:

Clients Come in All Shapes and Sizes

Be ready for anything!

A 21-year-old woman in active labor is admitted to the labor suite. An hour later, the membranes rupture spontaneously. The nurse observes a glistening white cord protruding from the vagina. Which of the following actions should be the highest priority of the nurse?	(1) Return to the nurses' station and place an emergency call to the physician. (2) Administer oxygen by mask at 10–12 liters/minute and assess the mother's vital signs. (3) Place a clean towel over the cord and wet it with sterile normal saline. (4) Apply manual pressure to the presenting part and have the mother assume a knee-chest position.

Promote Health

Wellness is the goal.

The correct answer is (4). A prolapsed cord is an emergency situation. The nurse must relieve pressure on the cord to prevent fetal anoxia.

The second subcategory for this client need is **Prevention and Early Detection of Disease** and accounts for **5–11** percent of the questions on the exam. Nursing actions that are covered in this subcategory include:

- Disease prevention
- Health and wellness
- Heath promotion programs
- Health screening
- Immunizations
- Lifestyle choices
- Techniques of physical assessment

Try this question from this subcategory:

The nurse in the out-patient clinic is discussing exercise programs with a group of adults. Which of the following statements, if made to the nurse by one of the participants, indicates the need for further teaching?	(1) "I should individualize my exercise program to meet my needs." (2) "I should incorporate the exercise program into my daily activities." (3) "I should maintain consistent participation in my exercise program." (4) "I should perform vigorous exercise several times a week."

The correct answer is (4). This is a negative question. Exercise does not need to be vigorous, it just needs to increase the client's resting heart rate.

Communication is Important

Communicate therapeutically throughout the exam.

Client Need #3: Psychosocial Integrity

The first subcategory for this client need is **Coping/Adaptation** and accounts for **5–11** percent of the questions on the exam. Nursing actions that are covered in this subcategory include:

- Coping mechanisms
- Counseling techniques
- Grief and loss
- Mental health concepts
- Religious and spiritual influences on health
- Sensory/perceptual alterations
- Situational role changes
- Stress management
- Support systems
- Therapeutic interactions
- Unexpected body image changes

This question is an example of this subcategory:

A 50-year-old male patient comes to the nurses' station and asks the nurse if he can go to the cafeteria to get something to eat. When told that his privileges do not include visiting the cafeteria, the patient becomes verbally abusive. Which of the following approaches by the nurse would be most effective?

(1) Tell the patient to lower his voice because he is disturbing the other patients.
(2) Ask the patient what he wants from the cafeteria and have it delivered to his room.
(3) Calmly but firmly escort the patient back to his room.
(4) Assign a nursing assistant to accompany the patient to the cafeteria.

The correct answer is (3). The nurse should not reinforce abusive behavior. Patients need consistent and clearly defined expectations and limits.

Stop the Violence

Abuse and domestic violence is frequently tested on the NCLEX.

The second subcategory for this client need is **Psychosocial Adaptation** and accounts for **5–11** percent of the questions on the exam. Nursing actions that are covered in this subcategory include:

- Behavioral interventions
- Chemical dependency
- Child abuse/neglect
- Crisis intervention
- Domestic violence
- Elder abuse/neglect
- Psychopathology

- Sexual abuse
- Therapeutic milieu

Questions like this one represent this subcategory:

The nurse in a well-child clinic assesses a 4-year-old girl and observes multiple bruises on her back and buttocks. The parents state they don't know how the girl sustained the injury. It is most important for the nurse to	(1) confront the parents about the suspected abuse. (2) report the suspected abuse to the appropriate authority. (3) refer the family to social services for counseling to prevent abuse. (4) document suspicions about the abuse in the medical record.

The correct answer is (2). According to law, all suspected cases of child abuse must be reported to the appropriate agency or authority. It is not sufficient to just document the suspected abuse in the medical record.

Client Need #4: Physiological Integrity

The first subcategory for this client need is **Basic Care and Comfort** and accounts for **7–13** percent of the questions on the exam. Nursing actions that are covered in this subcategory include:

- Assistive devices
- Elimination
- Mobility/immobility
- Nonpharmacological comfort interventions
- Nutrition and oral hydration
- Palliative/comfort care
- Personal hygiene
- Rest and sleep

Keep Moving

Hazards of immobility are frequently tested.

This question is representative of this question subcategory:

A cast is applied to a 9-month-old girl for the treatment of talipes equinovarus. Which of the following instructions is most essential for the nurse to give to the child's mother regarding her care?	(1) Offer appropriate toys for her age. (2) Make frequent clinic visits for cast adjustment. (3) Provide an analgesic as needed. (4) Do circulatory checks of the casted extremity.

The correct answer is (4). A possible complication that can occur after cast application is impaired circulation. All of these answer choices might be included in family teaching, but checking the child's circulation is the highest priority.

The second subcategory for this client need is **Pharmacological and Parenteral Therapies** and accounts for **5–11** percent of the questions on the exam. Nursing actions that are covered in this subcategory include:

- Adverse effects/contraindications
- Blood and blood products
- Central venous access devices
- Chemotherapy
- Expected effects
- Intravenous therapy
- Medication administration
- Parenteral fluids
- Pharmacological actions
- Pharmacological agents
- Pharmacological interactions
- Pharmacological pain management
- Side effects
- Total parenteral nutrition

Know About Medications

- Actions
- Indications
- Side effects
- Nursing considerations

Try this question from this subcategory:

The home health nurse is going to start an IV with 5% dextrose in water (D_5W) for a 76-year-old woman. To perform the venipuncture the nurse should start the IV using the

(1) veins of the client's wrist on the non dominant side.
(2) veins of the leg so it will not interfere with the client's ability to feed herself.
(3) dorsal veins of the client's forearm on the nondominant side.
(4) dorsal surface of the client's hand on the non dominant side.

The correct answer is (3). This is the best site for the nurse to use for the IV because of its ease of access, availability of elastic veins, and limited use by the client.

The third subcategory for this client need is **Reduction of Risk Potential** and accounts for **12–18** percent of the questions on the exam. Nursing actions that are covered in this subcategory include:

- Diagnostic tests
- Laboratory values
- Pathophysiology
- Potential for alterations in body systems
- Potential for complications of diagnostic tests, procedures, surgery, and health alterations
- Therapeutic procedures

This is a an example of a question from this subcategory:

A 7-year-old girl with type 1 insulin dependent diabetes mellitus (IDDM) has been home sick for several days and is brought to the emergency department by her parents. If the child is experiencing ketoacidosis, the nurse would expect to see which of the following lab results?	(1) Serum glucose 140 mg/dL (2) Serum creatine 5.2 mg/dL (3) Blood pH 7.28 (4) Hematocrit 38%

Procedures Are Important

Procedures are frequently tested on the NCLEX.

The correct answer is (3). Normal blood pH is 7.35–7.45. This indicates diabetic ketoacidosis.

The fourth subcategory for this client need is **Physiological Adaptation**, which accounts for **12–18** percent of the questions on the exam. Nursing actions that are covered in this subcategory include:

- Alterations in body systems
- Fluid and electrolyte imbalances
- Hemodynamics
- Infectious diseases
- Medical emergencies
- Pathophysiology
- Radiation therapy
- Respiratory care
- Unexpected response to therapies

The following question is an example of this subcategory:

Think E.R.

Know what to do in an emergency.

The nurse is delivering external cardiac compressions to a 63-year-old woman while performing cardiopulmonary resuscitation (CPR). It is most important for the nurse to

(1) maintain a position close to the client's side with the nurse's knees apart.
(2) maintain vertical pressure on the client's chest through the heel of the nurse's hand.
(3) re-check the nurse's hand position after every 10 chest compressions.
(4) check for a return of the client's pulse after every 8 breaths by the nurse.

The correct answer is (2). The nurse's elbows should be locked, arms straight, with shoulders directly over hands. Incorrect pressure or improperly placed hands could cause injury to the client.

The Nursing Process

Several concepts are integrated throughout the NCLEX. The most important of these is *the nursing process.*

The nursing process involves the *assessment, analysis, planning, implementation,* and *evaluation* of nursing care. As a graduate nurse, you are very familiar with each step of the nursing process and how to write a care plan using this process. Knowledge of the nursing process is essential to the performance of safe and effective care. It is also essential to answer NCLEX questions correctly.

Now we are going to review the steps of the nursing process and show you how each step is incorporated into test questions. The nursing process is a way of thinking. Using it will help you select correct answers.

First Step

The first step in the nursing process is assessment.

Assessment. Assessment is the process of establishing and verifying a database about the patient. This permits you to identify actual and/or potential health problems. The nurse obtains subjective data (information given to you by the client that can't be observed or measured by others), and objective data (information that is observable and measurable by others). This data is collected by interviewing and observing the client and/or significant others, reviewing the health history, performing a physical examination, evaluating lab results, and interacting with members of the health team.

An example of an assessment test question is:

The nurse obtains a health history from a patient admitted with acute glomerulonephritis that is associated with beta hemolytic *streptococcus*. The nurse would expect which of the following to be significant in the health history?	(1) The patient had a sore throat two weeks earlier. (2) There is a family history of glomerulonephritis. (3) The patient had a renal calculus two years earlier. (4) The patient had an accident involving renal trauma several years ago.

The correct answer is (1). Glomerulonephritis is an immunologic disorder that is caused by beta hemolytic *streptococcus*. It occurs 21 days after a respiratory or skin infection.

Analysis. During the analysis phase of the nursing process, you examine the data that you obtained during the assessment phase. This allows you to analyze and draw conclusions about health problems. During analysis, you should compare the client's findings with what is normal. From the analysis, you establish nursing diagnoses. A nursing diagnosis is an actual or potential health problem that the nurse is licensed to manage.

Here is an analysis question:

The nurse plans care for a patient diagnosed with an acute myocardial infarction. An appropriate nursing diagnosis would be decreased cardiac output secondary to which of the following?	(1) Ventricular dysrhythmias. (2) Congestive heart failure. (3) Recurrent myocardial infarction. (4) Hypertensive crisis.

The correct answer is (1). Ventricular dysrhythmias are common after an MI and reduce the efficiency of the heart.

Planning. During the planning phase of the nursing process, the nursing care plan is formulated. Steps in planning include:

- Assigning priorities to nursing diagnosis
- Specifying goals
- Identifying interventions
- Specifying expected outcomes
- Documenting the nursing care plan

First Things First

You need to establish priorities

Goals are anticipated responses and client behaviors that result from nursing care. Nursing goals are patient centered and measurable, and they have an established time frame. *Expected outcomes* are the interim steps needed to reach a goal and the resolution of a nursing diagnosis. There will be multiple expected outcomes for each goal. Expected outcomes guide the nurse in planning interventions.

This is an example of a planning question:

A 56-year-old man comes to the emergency room complaining of nausea, vomiting, and severe right upper quadrant pain. His temperature is 101.3° F (38.5° C) and an abdominal X-ray reveals an enlarged gall bladder. He is scheduled for surgery. The nurse recognizes that which of the following actions is a priority?	(1) Assessing the patient's need for dietary teaching. (2) Evaluating the patient's fluid and electrolyte status. (3) Examining the patient's health history for allergies to antibiotics. (4) Determining whether the patient has signed consent for surgery.

Consider All Types of Interventions

Nursing interventions can be independent, dependent, or interdependent.

The correct answer is (2). Hypokalemia and hypomagnesemia commonly occur after repeated vomiting.

Implementation. Implementation is the term for the actions that you take in the care of your clients. Implementation includes:

- Assisting in the performance of Activities of Daily Living (ADLs)
- Counseling and educating the patient and family
- Giving care to patients
- Supervising and evaluating the work of other members of the health team

It is important for you to remember that nursing interventions may be:

- *Independent* actions that are within the scope of nursing practice and do not require supervision by others.
- *Dependent* actions based on the written orders of a physician.
- *Interdependent* actions shared with other members of the health team.

The NCLEX includes questions that involve all three types of nursing interventions.

Here is an example of an implementation question:

A 25-year-old man is being treated in the burn unit for second- and third-degree burns over 45% of his body. The physician's orders include the application of silver sulfadiazine (Silvadene cream). The best way for the nurse to apply this medication is to use a sterile	(1) 4 × 4 soaked in saline. (2) tongue depressor. (3) gloved hand. (4) cotton-tipped applicator.

The correct answer is (3). A sterile, gloved hand will cause the least amount of trauma to tissues and will decrease the chances of breaking blisters.

Evaluation. Evaluation measures the patient's response to nursing interventions and indicates the patient's progress toward achieving the goals established in the care plan. You compare the observed results to expected outcomes.

This is an evaluation question:

When caring for a patient with anorexia nervosa, which of the following observations indicate to the nurse that the patient's condition is improving?	(1) The patient eats all the food on her meal tray. (2) The patient asks friends to bring her special foods. (3) The patient weighs herself daily. (4) The patient's weight has increased.

The correct response is (4). The patient's weight is the most objective outcome measure in the evaluation of this client's problem.

Integrated Concepts

Several other important concepts are integrated throughout the NCLEX. They are:

Caring. As you take the NCLEX, remember that the test is about caring for people, not working with high-tech equipment or analyzing lab results.

Communication and Documentation. For this exam, you are required to understand and utilize therapeutic communication skills with all professional contacts, including clients, their families, and other members of

Expected Outcomes

Did it work?

**Who Cares?
YOU Care!**

The NCLEX is about patients.

the health care team. Charting or documenting your care and the client's response is both a legal requirement and a essential method of communication in nursing. On this exam you may be asked to identify appropriate documentation of a client behavior or nursing action.

Cultural Awareness. The clients you care for come from diverse ethnic backgrounds. It is necessary for you to take this into account when planning and implementing safe and effective care.

"I Can Do It Myself!"

That's the goal of self-care.

Self-Care. On the NCLEX the nurse is expected to help the client attain an optimal level of health and independence. The goal is to make the client as independent as is safely permissible.

Teaching/Learning Principles. Nursing frequently involves sharing information with clients and families so optimal functioning can be achieved. You may see questions concerning teaching a client about his diet and/or medications.

You might see some questions on the NCLEX exam that contain graphics (pictures). These questions may include the picture of a patient in traction or it may show the abdomen of a woman who is pregnant. These questions do count, so take them seriously. We have included a question with graphics in the practice test found in this book.

New Test Plan

The National Council evaluates the test plan every three years to determine its relevance to nursing as it is practiced by the beginning nurse. The new test plan, involving the addition of a drop-down calculator and use of a mouse-interface, was voted on by the member boards at the 2000 annual meeting of the National Council of State Boards of Nursing and was implemented April 1, 2001. There are no changes in the subcategories or their assigned percentages. The passing standard also remains unchanged. Though there has been much talk about innovative new item types such as fill-in-the-blank questions, these item types are NOT included in the NCLEX test plan that was implemented in 2001.

Knowledge Is Power

The more knowledgeable you are about the NCLEX exam, the more effective your study will be. As you prepare for the exam, keep the content of the test in mind. Thinking like the test maker will enhance you chance of success on the exam.

Are you still thinking about that pacemaker battery from page 3? What do you think the correct answer is?

A 45-year-old man had a permanent pacemaker implanted one year ago. He returns to the outpatient clinic because he thinks the pacemaker battery is malfunctioning. The nurse would expect the client to exhibit which of the following symptoms?	(1) Abdominal pain, nausea and vomiting. (2) Wheezing on exertion, cyanosis, and orthopnea. (3) Peripheral edema, shortness of breath, and dizziness. (4) Chest pain radiating to the right arm, headache, and diaphoresis.

The correct answer is (3). These are symptoms of decreased cardiac output. These symptoms occur with pacemaker battery failure. Other symptoms include changes in pulse rate, irregular pulse, and palpitations.

GI symptoms (1) are not found with pacemaker malfunction. The items listed in (2) are not symptoms of pacemaker failure. And although chest pain may occur with decreased output (4), chest pain that radiates to the right arm is suggestive of angina. Headache and diaphoresis are not seen with pacemaker failure.

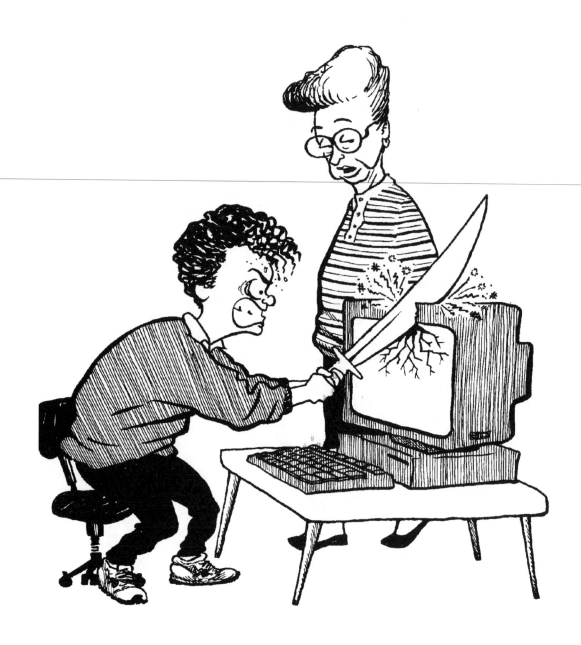

"Trying to whittle a question down to its stem, Sara?"

CHAPTER TWO

Testing, NCLEX-Style

Have you talked to graduate nurses about their experiences taking the NCLEX? They probably told you that the test wasn't like *any* nursing test they had ever taken. How can that be? The NCLEX is a multiple-choice test, and as a nursing student you are used to taking multiple choice tests. In fact, you've taken so many tests by the time you graduate from nursing school, you probably believe that there won't be any more surprises on *any* nursing test. Yet there is one more surprise waiting for you, and it is called NCLEX.

How can the NCLEX seem like a nursing school test, but be so different? NCLEX is a standardized test that is testing a different set of behaviors from those tested in nursing school.

Standardized Exams

Many of you have some experience with standardized exams. You may have been required to take the SAT or ACT to get into nursing school. Remember taking that exam? Was your experience positive or negative?

All standardized exams share the same characteristics:

- Tests are written by content specialists and test construction experts.
- The content of the exam is researched and planned.
- The questions are designed according to test construction methodology (all answer choices are about the same length, the verb tenses all agree, etcetera).
- All the questions are tested before use on the actual exam.

This Isn't Nursing School

NCLEX is a *standardized exam*—very different from many of the tests you took in nursing school.

The NCLEX is similar to other standardized exams in some ways, yet different in others:

- The NCLEX is written by nurse specialists who are experts in a content area of nursing.
- All content is selected to allow the beginning practitioner to prove minimum competency on all areas of the test plan.
- Minimum competency questions are most frequently asked at the application level, not the recognition or recall level. All the responses to a question are similar in length and subject matter, and are grammatically correct.
- All test items have been extensively tested. National Council knows that the questions are valid; all correct responses are documented in two different sources.

What does this mean for you?

- National Council has defined what is minimum-competency, entry-level nursing.
- Questions and answers will be written in such a way that you will not be able predict or recognize the correct answer.
- National Council is knowledgeable about the strategies regarding length of answers, grammar, etcetera. They make sure that you can't use these strategies in order to select correct answers. English majors have no advantage!
- The answer choices have been extensively tested. The people who write the test questions make the incorrect answer choices look attractive to the unwary test taker.

What Behaviors Does NCLEX Test?

Don't Underestimate Yourself

You have a body of knowledge. Use it!

NCLEX does *not* just test your body of nursing knowledge: It assumes that you have a body of knowledge because you have graduated from nursing school. Likewise, NCLEX does *not* just test your understanding of the material: It assumes that you understand the nursing knowledge you learned in nursing school. So what does NCLEX test?

NCLEX primarily tests your nursing judgment and discretion. It tests your ability to think critically and solve problems. NCLEX recognizes that as a beginning practitioner, you will be managing LPN/LVNs and nursing assistants provide care to a group of patients. As the leader of the nursing team, you are expected to make safe and competent judgments about patient care.

Critical Thinking

What does the term *critical thinking* mean? Critical thinking is problem solving that involves thinking creatively. It requires that the nurse:

- Observe
- Decide what is important
- Look for patterns and relationships
- Identify the problem
- Transfer knowledge from one situation to another
- Apply knowledge
- Evaluate according to criteria established

You successfully solve problems every day in the clinical area. You are probably comfortable with this concept when actually caring for patients. While you've had lots of practice critically thinking in the clinical area, you may have had less practice critically thinking your way through test questions. Why is that?

During nursing school, you take exams developed by nursing instructors to test a specific body of content. Many of these questions are at the knowledge level. This involves recognition and recall of ideas or material that you read in your nursing textbooks and discussed in class. This is the most basic level of testing.

The following is an example of a knowledge-based question you might have seen in nursing school.

> Which of the following is a complication that occurs during the first 24 hours after a percutaneous liver biopsy?
>
> (1) Nausea and vomiting.
> (2) Constipation.
> (3) Hemorrhage.
> (4) Pain at the biopsy site.

The question restated is, "What is a common complication of a liver biopsy?" You may or may not remember the answer. So, as you look at the answer choices, you hope to see an item that looks familiar. You do see something that looks familiar: "Hemorrhage." You selected the correct answer based on recall or recognition. NCLEX rarely asks passing questions at the recall/recognition level.

Recall is Just the First Step

How to *apply* what you recall is more important.

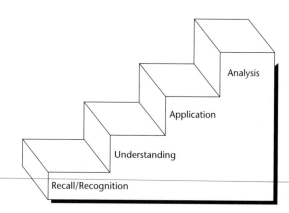

Figure 1: Levels of Questions in Nursing Tests

In nursing school, you are also given test questions written at the comprehension level. These questions require you to understand the meaning of the material. Let's look at this same question written at the comprehension level.

It's the Principle of the Thing

NCLEX is a test that requires application of nursing principles.

> The nurse understands that hemorrhage is a complication of a liver biopsy because
>
> (1) there are several large blood vessels near the liver.
> (2) the liver cells are bathed with a mixture of venous and arterial blood.
> (3) the test is performed on patients with elevated enzymes.
> (4) the procedure requires a large piece of tissue to be removed.

The question restated is, "Why does hemorrhage occur after a liver biopsy?" In order to answer this question, the nurse must understand that the liver is a highly vascular organ. The portal vein and the hepatic artery join in the liver to form the sinusoids that bathe the liver in a mixture of venous and arterial blood.

NCLEX asks few minimum competency questions at the comprehension level. It assumes you know and understand the facts you learned in nursing school.

Minimum competency NCLEX test questions are written at the application and/or analysis level. Remember, NCLEX tests your ability to make safe judgments about patient/client care. Your ability to solve problems is not tested with recall/recognition or comprehension level questions.

Let's look at this same question written at the application level.

Which of the following symptoms, if observed by the nurse during the first 24 hours after a percutaneous liver biopsy, would indicate a complication from the procedure?

(1) Anorexia, nausea, and vomiting.
(2) Abdominal distention and discomfort.
(3) Pulse 112, blood pressure 100/60, respirations 20.
(4) Pain at the biopsy site.

Can you select an answer based on recall or recognition? No. Let's analyze the question and answer choices.

The question is: What is a complication of a liver biopsy? In order to begin to analyze this question, you must *know* that hemorrhage is the major complication. But it's not listed as an answer. Can you find hemorrhage in one of the answer choices?

ANSWERS:
   (1) Anorexia, nausea, and vomiting. Does this indicate that the patient is hemorrhaging? No, these are not symptoms of hemorrhage.
   (2) Abdominal distention and discomfort. Does this indicate that the patient is hemorrhaging? Perhaps. Abdominal distention could indicate internal bleeding.
   (3) Pulse 112, blood pressure 100/60, respiration 20. Does this indicate that the patient is hemorrhaging? Yes. An increased pulse, a decreased blood pressure, and increased respirations indicate shock. Shock is a result of hemorrhage.
   (4) Pain at the biopsy site. Does this indicate the patient is hemorrhaging? No. Pain at the biopsy site is expected due to the procedure.

Ask yourself, "Which is the best indicator of hemorrhage?" Abdominal distention or a change in vital signs? Abdominal distention can be caused by liver disease. The correct answer is (3).

This question tests you at the application level. You were not able to answer the question by recalling or recognizing the word *hemorrhage.* You had to take information you learned (hemorrhage is the major complication of a liver biopsy) and select the answer that best indicates hemorrhage. Application involves taking the facts that you know, and using them to make a nursing judgment. You must be able to answer questions at the application level in order to prove your competence on the NCLEX.

Let's look at a question that is written at the analysis level.

The nurse is caring for a 56-year-old man receiving Haldol 2 mg PO BID. The nurse assists the patient to choose which of the following menus?	(1) 3 oz roast beef, baked potato, salad with dressing, dill pickle, baked apple pie, and milk. (2) 3 oz baked chicken, green beans, steamed rice, 1 slice of bread, banana, and milk. (3) Cheeseburger on a bun, french fries with catsup, chocolate chip cookie, apple, and milk. (4) 3 oz baked fish, 1 slice of bread, broccoli, ice cream, and pineapple drink taken 1/2 –1 hour after the meal.

Sound Familiar?

Analysis questions take the familiar and put it in the unfamiliar.

Many students panic when they read this question because they can't immediately recall any diet restriction required by a patient taking Haldol. Since students can't recall the information, they assume that they didn't learn enough information. Analysis questions are many times written so that a familiar piece of information is put in an unfamiliar setting. Let's think about this question.

What type of diet do you choose for a patient receiving Haldol? In order to begin analyzing this question, you must first recall that Haldol is an antipsychotic medication used to treat psychotic disorders. There are *no* diet restrictions for clients taking Haldol. Since there are no diet restrictions, you must problem-solve to determine what this question is *really* asking. Based on the answer choices, it is obviously a diet question. What kind of diet should you choose for this patient? Since you have been given no other information, there is only one type of diet that can be considered: a regular balanced diet. This is an example of taking the familiar (a regular balanced diet) and putting into the unfamiliar (a patient receiving Haldol). In this question, the critical thinking is deciding what this question is *really* asking.

QUESTION: "What is the most balanced regular diet?"

ANSWERS:

(1) 3 oz roast beef, baked potato, salad with dressing, dill pickle, baked apple pie, and milk. Is this a balanced diet? Yes, it certainly has possibilities.

(2) 3 oz baked chicken, green beans, steamed rice, one slice of bread, banana, and milk. Is this a balanced diet? Yes, this is also a good answer because it contains foods from each of the food groups.

(3) Cheeseburger on a bun, french fries with catsup, chocolate chip cookie, apple, and milk. Is this a balanced diet? No. This diet is high in fat and does not contain all of the food groups. Eliminate this answer.

(4) 3 oz baked fish, 1 slice of bread, broccoli, ice cream, and pineapple drink taken 1/2–1 hour after the meal. Does this sound like a balanced diet? The choice of foods isn't bad, but why would the intake of fluids be delayed? This sounds like a menu to prevent dumping syndrome. Eliminate this answer.

Which is the better answer choice: (1) or (2)? Dill pickles are high in sodium, so the correct answer is (2).

Choosing the menu that best represents a balanced diet is not a difficult question to answer. The challenge lies in determining that a balanced diet is the topic of the question. Note that answer choices (1) and (2) are very similar. Because NCLEX is testing your discretion, you will be making decision between answer choices that are very close in meaning. Don't expect obvious answer choices.

These questions highlight the difference between the knowledge/comprehension-based questions that you may have seen in nursing school, and the application/analysis-based questions that you will see on the NCLEX.

Strategies That Don't Work on the NCLEX

Whether you realize it or not, you developed a set of strategies in nursing school to answer teacher-generated test questions that are written at the knowledge/comprehension level. These strategies include:

- "Cramming" in hundreds of facts about disease processes and nursing care.
- Recognizing and recalling facts rather than understanding the pathophysiology and the needs of a patient with an illness.
- Knowing who wrote the question and what is important to that instructor.

No Need for Caffeine

Cramming won't work on the NCLEX.

- Predicting answers based on what you remember or who wrote the test question.
- Selecting the response that is a different length compared to the other choices.
- Selecting the answer choice that is grammatically correct.
- When in doubt, choosing C.

These strategies will not work on the NCLEX. Remember, NCLEX is testing your ability to make safe, competent decisions.

The first step to becoming a better test taker is to identify:

- What kind of test taker you are.
- What kind of learner you are.

Are You a Successful or Unsuccessful Test Taker?

Successful NCLEX Test Takers:

- Have a good understanding of nursing content.
- Have the ability to tackle each test question with a lot of confidence because they assume that they can figure out the right answer.
- Don't give up if they are unsure of the answer. They are not afraid to think about the question, and the possible choices in order to select the correct answer.
- Possess the know-how to correctly identify the question.
- Stay focused on the question.

Unsuccessful NCLEX Test Takers:

- Assume that they either know or don't know the answer to the question.
- Memorize facts to answer questions by recall or recognition.
- Read the question, read the answers, read the question, and pick an answer.
- Choose answer choices based on a hunch or a feeling instead of thinking carefully.
- Answer questions based on personal experience rather than nursing theory.
- Give up too soon, because they aren't willing to think hard about questions and answers.
- Don't stay focused on the question.

If you are a successful test taker, congratulations! This book will re-enforce your test-taking skills. If you have many of the characteristics of an unsuccessful test taker, don't despair! You can change. If you follow the strategies in this book, you will become a successful test taker.

What Kind of Learner Are You?

It is important for you to identify whether you think predominantly in images or words. Why? This will assist you to develop a study plan that is specific for your learning style. Read the following statement:

A nurse walks into a room and finds the patient lying on the floor.

As you read those words, did you hear yourself reading the words? Or did you see a nurse walking into a room, and see the patient lying on the floor? If you heard yourself reading the sentence, you think in words. If you formed a mental image (saw a picture), you think in images.

Students who think in images sometimes have a difficult time answering nursing test questions. These students say things like:

"I have to study harder than the other students."
"I have to look up the same information over and over again."
"Once I see the procedure (or patient), I don't have any difficulty understanding or remembering the content."
"I have trouble understanding procedures from reading the book. I have to see the procedure to understand it."
"I have trouble answering test questions about patients or procedures I've never seen."

Why is that? For some people, imagery is necessary to understand ideas and concepts. If this is true for you, you need to visualize information that you are learning. As you prepare for the NCLEX exam, try to form mental images of terminology, procedures, and diseases. For example, if you're reviewing information about traction but you have never seen traction, it would be ideal for you to see a patient in traction. If that isn't possible, find a picture of traction and rig up a traction setup with whatever material you have available. As you read about traction, use the photo or model to visualize care of the patient. If you can visualize the theory that you are trying to learn, it will make recall and understanding of concepts much easier for you.

Picture It!

Use imagery when reading test questions.

Remember the *Client* on the NCLEX

Picture yourself caring for a real person.

It is also important that you visualize test questions. As you read the question and possible answer choices, picture yourself going through each suggested action. This will increase your chances of selecting correct answer choices.

Let's look at a test question that requires imagery.

A 16-year-old boy is seen in the emergency room for a fracture of the left femur sustained in a sledding accident. The fracture is reduced and a cast is applied. The patient is taught how to use crutches for ambulating without bearing weight on the left leg. The nurse would expect the patient to learn which of the following crutch-walking gaits?

(1) 2-point gait.
(2) 3-point gait.
(3) 4-point gait.
(4) Swing-through gait.

Don't panic if you can't remember crutch-walking gaits. Instead, visualize!

Step 1. "See" a person (or yourself) walking normally. First the right leg and left arm are extended, and then the left leg and right arm are extended.

Step 2. Put crutches in your hands. Now walk. Each foot and each crutch is a point.

Step 3. "See" a person (or yourself) with a full cast on the left leg, with the foot never touching the ground.

Step 4. Visualize the answers.

(1) 2-point gait. One leg and one crutch would be touching the ground at the same time. Sounds like normal walking. Eliminate this choice because the patient is non-weight-bearing.
(2) 3-point gait. Both crutches and one foot are on the ground. This would be appropriate for a non-weight-bearing patient.

(3) 4-point gait. This would require both legs and crutches to touch the ground. However, in this question the patient is non-weight-bearing. Eliminate this option.

(4) Swing-through gait. This gait means advancing both crutches, then both legs, and requires weight bearing. The gait is not as stable as the other gaits. Eliminate this option: the patient in this question is non-weight-bearing.

The correct answer is (2).

Even if you are unsure of crutch walking gaits, imaging and thinking through the answer choices will enable you to select the correct answer.

Now that you understand what kind of questions NCLEX is going to ask, and you've completed your self-assessment, you probably want to learn more about how you can be successful on the NCLEX. Read on!

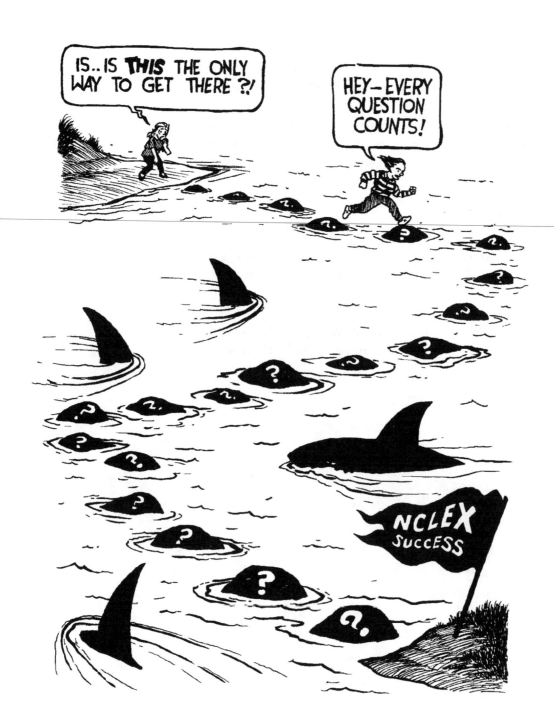

CHAPTER THREE

There's Only One Way to Skin the CAT

The NCLEX is a standardized exam composed of multiple choice test questions written at the application/analysis level. You must think in a specific way to correctly answer questions on the NCLEX exam. This chapter will demonstrate how to:

- Read the question
- Decide what the question is asking
- Evaluate the answer choices
- Select the correct answer

The Multiple-Choice Test Question

To develop an effective set of strategies, it is important that you understand the components of an NCLEX multiple-choice question.

Each NCLEX question is composed of:

- The *stem* of the question. The stem includes the situation that describes the client, his problems or health care needs, and other relevant information. It also includes a question or an incomplete statement. This is the question that you must answer.
- Three incorrect answers, referred to here as *distracters*.
- The correct answer.

The three distracters will probably sound logical to you. They may even be based on information provided in the stem, but they don't really answer the question. Other incorrect answers may be actions that are common nursing practice but not ideal nursing practice.

The correct answer is the only choice that is recognized as correct by NCLEX, so you need to learn to select it. To select a correct response, you must understand the *whys* of nursing care.

You Do the Math

Stem + answer choices = NCLEX question.

Remember that most answer choices are written on the application level: you will not be able to select answers based on recognition or recall. You must understand the whys of nursing actions in order to select the correct response.

Read the following NCLEX-style question. In addition to selecting an answer, identify the components of this question.

The nurse plans care for a 4-year-old girl who has been sexually abused by her father. Play therapy is scheduled. The nurse should know the primary goal of play therapy for a 4-year-old is to	(1) provide her with the opportunity to express anger and hostility by playing with dolls. (2) promote communication since she may lack the emotional and intellectual capacity to express her perceptions verbally. (3) assess whether she is functioning at an age-appropriate developmental level. (4) reveal through direct observation of her at play what type of abuse has been experienced.

The Components

- The stem:
    4-year-old girl
    sexually abused by her father
    play therapy is scheduled
    What is the primary goal of play therapy for a 4-year-old?
- The answer choices:

(1) Opportunity to express anger and hostility. Play therapy will allow children to express anger and hostility if that's what they want to communicate. Some students select this answer because they focus on the treatment of sexual abuse mentioned in the situation. This is a distracter.

(2) Promote communication. Play is the universal language of children. The purpose of play therapy is to give children the opportunity to communicate using their own "language." This is the correct answer.

(3) Assess her developmental level. The nurse might be able to assess whether a child is functioning at an age-appropriate level, but this is not the primary purpose of play therapy. This is a distracter.

(4) Find out what type of abuse she has experienced. The child might communicate the type of abuse she has experienced if that is what she chooses to communicate. The nurse should focus on the purpose of play therapy, not the type of abuse. This is a distracter.

Let's try another question.

A patient is being treated for congestive heart failure (CHF) with diuretic therapy. Which of the following assessments best indicates to the nurse that the patient's condition is improving?	(1) The patient's weight has remained stable since admission. (2) The patient's systolic blood pressure has decreased. (3) There are fewer crackles heard when auscultating the patient's lungs. (4) The patient's urinary output is 1,500 cc per day.

The Components

- The stem:
  congestive heart failure (CHF)
  treatment is diuretic therapy
  How do you know the patient's condition is improving?
- The answer choices:

(1) Weight has remained stable. Patient's weight should decrease since he is taking a diuretic. Weight addresses issues involved with diuretic therapy. However, it is not the best indication of improvement in a patient with congestive heart failure. This is a distracter.

(2) The systolic blood pressure has decreased. Decreased blood pressure may be the result of diuretic therapy, but the reduction could also be due to other causes (change of position, calm rather than an excited state, etcetera). This is not the best indication of an improvement in CHF. This is a distracter.

(3) There are fewer crackles. A patient in congestive heart failure has crackles due to pulmonary edema. Diuretics are given to promote excretion of sodium and water through the kidneys. Decreased crackles would indicate that the pulmonary edema is improving. This is the correct answer.

(4) Output of 1,500 cc in 24 hours. 1,500 cc urinary output is within normal limits. Although a normal output addresses diuretic

therapy, it is not the best indication improvement of CHF. This is a distracter.

Critical Thinking Strategies

- The NCLEX is not a test about recognizing facts.
- You must be able to correctly identify what the question is asking.
- Do not focus on background information that is not needed to answer the question.
- The NCLEX focuses on thinking through a problem or situation.

Now that you are more knowledgeable about the components of a multiple choice test question, let's talk about specific strategies that you can use to problem-solve your way to correct answers on the NCLEX.

The chart on the opposite page illustrates different paths that you must choose from in order to correctly answer NCLEX test questions. The stepping stones between the test taker and the correct answer stand for steps that you must follow in order to find the correct answer for that question type. Nurses who are successful on the NCLEX make deliberate decisions while reading a test question about which path will most likely get them a correct answer. They choose the path; the path does not choose them.

Remember, NCLEX is testing your ability to think critically. Critical thinking for the nurse involves:

- Observation
- Deciding what is important
- Looking for patterns and relationships
- Identifying the problem
- Transferring knowledge from one situation to another
- Applying knowledge
- Discriminating between possible choices and/or courses of action
- Evaluating according to criteria established

Are you feeling overwhelmed as you read these words? Don't be! We are going teach you a step-by-step method to choose the appropriate path.

There are some strategies that you must follow on *every* NCLEX test question. You must *always* figure out what the question is asking, and you must *always* eliminate answer choices.

Critical Thinking Paths to Correct Answers on the NCLEX

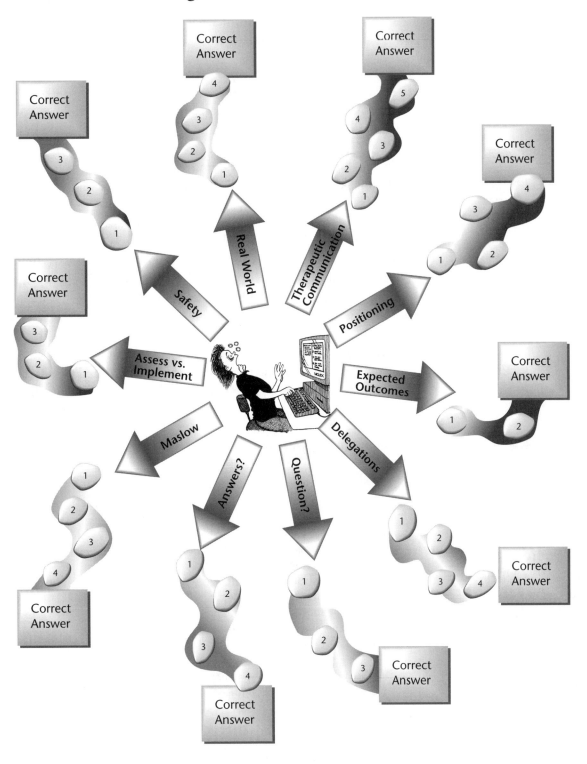

Choosing the right answer often involves choosing the best of several answers that have correct information. This may entail your correct analysis and interpretation of what the question is really asking. So let's talk about how to figure out what the question is asking.

Reword the Question

The first step to correctly answering NCLEX questions is to find out what each question is *really* asking.

Step 1. Read each question carefully from the first word to the last word. Do not skim over the words or read them too quickly.

Step 2. Look for hints in the wording of the question stem. The adjectives *most, first, best,* and *initial* indicate that you must establish priorities. The phrase *further teaching is necessary* indicates that the answer will contain incorrect information. The phrase "client understands the teaching" indicates that the answer will be correct information.

Step 3. Reword the question stem in your own words so that it can be answered with a "yes" or a "no," or with a specific bit of information. Begin your questions with "what," "when," or "why." We will refer to this reworded version as THE REWORDED QUESTION in the examples that follow.

Step 4. If you can't complete step 3, read the answer choices for clues.

Let's practice rewording a question.

Reword!

Reword every question in your own words.

A 6-year-old girl with a fractured femur is brought to the emergency room by her parents. When asked how the injury occurred, her parent state that she fell off the sofa. On examination, the nurse finds several lesions on the child's buttock. Which of the following statements most appropriately reflects how the nurse should document these findings?	(1)
	(2)
	(3)
	(4)

We omitted the answer choices to make you focus on the question stem this time. The answer choices will be provided and discussed later in this chapter.

Step 1. Read the question stem carefully.

Step 2. Pay attention to the adjectives. "Most appropriately" tells you that you need to select the best answer.

Step 3. Reword the question stem in your own words. In this case, it is, "What is the best charting for this situation?"

Step 4. Since you were able to reword the question, the fourth step is unnecessary. You didn't need to read the answer choices for clues.

We have all missed questions on a test because we didn't read accurately. The following question illustrates this point.

A 47-year-old male construction worker is admitted to the hospital for treatment of active tuberculosis. The nurse teaches the patient about tuberculosis. Which statement, if made by the patient, would indicate to the nurse that further teaching is necessary?	(1) (2) (3) (4)

Again, just the question stem is given to encourage you to focus on rewording the question. We will discuss the answer choices for this question later in this chapter.

Step 1. Read the question stem carefully.

Step 2. Look for hints. Pay particular attention to the statement "further teaching is necessary." You are looking for negative information.

Step 3. Reword the question stem in your own words. In this case, it is, "What is incorrect information about tuberculosis?"

Step 4. Since you were able to reword the question, the fourth step is unnecessary. You didn't need to read the answer choices for clues to determine what the question is asking.

Try rewording this test question.

A 20-year-old woman admitted to the hospital in premature labor has been treated successfully. The patient is to be sent home on an oral regimen of terbutaline (Brethine). Which of the following statements, if made by the patient, would indicate to the nurse that the patient understands the discharge teaching about the medication?	(1) (2) (3) (4)

Again, just the question stem is given to encourage you to focus on rewording the question. We will discuss the answer choices for this question later in this chapter.

Step 1. Read the question stem carefully.

Step 2. Look for hints. Pay attention to the words *patient understands*. You are looking for true information.

Step 3. Reword the question stem. This question is asking, "What is true about Brethine?'

Step 4. Since you were able to reword this question, the fourth step is unnecessary. You didn't need to obtain clues about what the question is asking from the answer choices.

Sixth Senses Don't Work

Do not answer questions based on feelings or hunches.

Eliminate Wrong Answers

Now that you've mastered rewording the question, let's examine how to select the correct answer.

Remember the characteristics of unsuccessful test takers? One of their major problems is that they do not thoughtfully consider each answer choice. They react to questions using feelings and hunches. Unsuccessful test takers look for a specific answer choice. The following strategy will enable you to consider each answer choice in a thoughtful way.

Step 1. Cover all answer choices except (1).

KAPLAN

Step 2. Read answer choice (1). Then repeat THE REWORDED QUESTION after reading the answer choice. Ask yourself, "Does this answer THE REWORDED QUESTION?" If you know the answer choice is wrong, eliminate it. If you aren't sure, leave the answer choice in for consideration.

Step 3. Repeat the above process with each remaining answer choice.

Step 4. Note which answer choices remain.

Step 5. Reread the question to make sure you have correctly identified THE REWORDED QUESTION.

Step 6. Ask yourself, "Which answer choice best answers the question?" That is your answer.

Let's practice the elimination strategy using the same questions.

> A 6-year-old girl with a fractured femur is brought to the emergency room by her parents. When asked how the injury occurred, her parent stated that she fell off the sofa. On examination, the nurse finds old and new lesions on the child's buttock. Which of the following statements most appropriately reflects how the nurse should document these findings?
>
> (1) "Six lesions noted on buttocks at various stages of healing."
> (2) "Multiple lesions on buttocks due to child abuse."
> (3) "Lesions on buttocks due to unknown causes."
> (4) "Several lesions on buttocks caused by cigarettes."

THE REWORDED QUESTION is "What is good charting?"

Step 1. Cover all of the answer choices except for (1). Thoughtfully consider each answer choice individually.

Step 2. Read answer choice (1). Does it answer the question, "What is good charting for this situation?"

   (1) "Six lesions noted on buttocks at various stages of healing." Is this good charting? Maybe. Leave it in for consideration.

Step 3. Repeat the process with each remaining answer choice.

Stay Focused

Stay focused on THE REWORDED QUESTION.

(2) "Multiple lesions on buttocks due to child abuse." Is this good charting? No, because the nurse is making a judgment about child abuse.

(3) "Lesions on buttocks due to unknown causes." Is this good charting? Maybe. Leave it in for consideration.

(4) "Several lesions on buttocks caused by cigarettes." Is this good charting? No. The question does not include information about how the burns occurred.

Step 4. Answer choices (1) and (3) remain.

Step 5. Reread the question. This question asks you to identify good charting.

What's Left Is the Answer

If you eliminate three answers choices, the fourth answer choice must be the correct answer.

Step 6. Which is the best charting? "Six lesions noted on buttocks at various stages of healing," or "Lesions due to unknown causes"? Good charting is accurate, objective, concise, and complete. It must reflect the patient's current status. The correct answer is (1).

Some students will select answer (3), thinking, "How can I be sure about the stages of healing?" But the purpose of this question is to test your ability to select good charting. Select the answer choice that shows you are a safe and effective nurse. Remember, questions on the NCLEX are not designed to trick you. Stay focused on the question.

Let's select the correct answer for the second question.

A 47-year-old male construction worker is admitted to the hospital for treatment of active tuberculosis. The nurse teaches the patient about tuberculosis. Which statement, if made by the patient, would indicate to the nurse that further teaching is necessary?	(1) "I will have to take medication for six months." (2) "I should cover my nose and mouth when coughing or sneezing." (3) "I will remain in isolation for at least six weeks." (4) "I will always have a positive skin test for tuberculosis."

THE REWORDED QUESTION: What is incorrect information about tuberculosis?

Step 1. Cover all answer choices except (1).

Step 2. Read answer choice (1). Does it answer the reworded question, "What is incorrect (or wrong) information about tuberculosis?"

(1) "I will have to take medication for six months." Is this wrong information? No, it is a true statement. The patient will need to take a medication, such as INH, for six months or longer. Eliminate this choice.

Step 3. Repeat the process with each remaining answer choice.

(2) "I should cover my nose and mouth when coughing or sneezing." Is this wrong information about TB? No, this is a true statement. TB is transmitted by droplet contamination. Eliminate it.

(3) "I will remain in isolation for at least six weeks." Is this wrong information about TB? Maybe. Leave it in for consideration.

(4) "I will always have a positive skin test for tuberculosis." Is this a wrong statement about TB? No, this is true. A positive skin test indicates that the patient has developed antibodies to the tuberculosis bacillus. Eliminate this choice.

Step 4. Only answer choice (3) remains.

Step 5. Reread the question. The question is, "What is wrong information about TB?"

Step 6. The correct answer is (3). You "know" this is the correct answer because you've eliminated the other three answer choices. The patient does not need to be isolated for six weeks. The patient's activities will be restricted for about two to three weeks after medication therapy is initiated.

A couple of things to remember when using this strategy:

- Eliminate only what you know is wrong. However, once you eliminate an answer choice, do not retrieve it for consideration. You may be tempted to do this if you do not feel comfortable with the one answer choice that is left. Resist the impulse!
- Stay focused on THE REWORDED QUESTION. How many of you have missed a question that asked for negative information because you selected the answer choice that contained correct information?

No Second Chances

Eliminate only what you know is wrong. Once a choice has been eliminated, put it out of your mind.

Here's the last question.

<table>
<tr>
<td>

A 20-year-old woman admitted to the hospital in premature labor has been treated successfully. The patient is to be sent home on an oral regimen of terbutaline (Brethine). Which of the following statements, if made by the patient, would indicate to the nurse that the patient understands the discharge teaching about the medication?

</td>
<td>

(1) "As long as I take my medication, I can be sure I will not deliver prematurely."

(2) "It is important that I count the fetal movements for one hour, twice a day."

(3) "I may feel a rapid heartbeat and some muscle tremors while on this medication."

(4) "Bedrest is necessary in order for the medication to work properly."

</td>
</tr>
</table>

THE REWORDED QUESTION: What is true about Brethine?

Step 1. Cover all answer choices except (1).

Step 2. Read answer choice (1). Does it answer the question, "What is true about Brethine?"

> (1) "As long as I take my medication, I won't deliver prematurely." Is this true about Brethine? No. Brethine will inhibit uterine cotractions, but there is no guarantee that there won't be a premature delivery. Eliminate it.

Step 3. Repeat the process with each remaining answer choice.

> (2) "It is important that I count the fetal movements for one hour, twice a day." Is this true about Brethine? Maybe. Patients are told to be aware of fetal movement. Keep it as a possibility.
>
> (3) "I may feel a rapid heartbeat and some muscle tremors while on this medication." Is this true of Brethine? Yes. Brethine is a smooth muscle relaxant. Side effects include increased maternal heart rate, palpitations, and muscle tremors. Leave this choice in for consideration.
>
> (4) "Bedrest is necessary in order for the medication to work properly." Is this true about Brethine? No. Brethine will work whether the patient is on bedrest or not. Eliminate it.

Step 4. Note that only answer choices (2) and (3) remain.

Step 5. Reread the question to make sure you are answering the right question. The question is, "What is true about Brethine?"

Step 6. Which choice best answers the question, (2) or (3)? If you are focused on the question, you will select (3). Some students focus on the background information (pregnancy). This question has nothing to do with pregnancy. If you chose (2), you fell for a distracter.

Remember: Focus on the question, and not the background information. If you can answer the question—"What is true about Brethine?"—without considering the background information (pregnancy), do it. Many students answer a question incorrectly because they don't focus on THE REWORDED QUESTION. Don't fall for the distracters.

At this point you're probably thinking, "Will I have enough time to finish the test using these strategies?" or "How will I ever remember how to answer questions using these steps?" Yes, you will have time to finish the test. Unsuccessful test takers spend time agonizing over test questions. By using these strategies, you will be using your time productively. You will remember the steps because you are going to practice, practice, practice with test questions. You will not be able to absorb this strategy by osmosis; the process must be practiced repeatedly.

Don't Predict Answers

On the NCLEX, you are asked to select the best answer from the four choices that you are given. Many times, the "ideal" answer choice is not there. Don't sit and moan because the answer that you think should be there isn't provided. Remember:

- Identify THE REWORDED QUESTION.
- Select the best answer from the choices given.

Look at this question.

Decide What's Important

Do not focus on unnecessary information.

You're Not the Weatherman

Do not predict answers.

(1) "The urinary meatus is cleansed with an iodine solution and then a urinary drainage catheter is inserted to obtain urine."

(2) "You will be asked to empty your bladder one half hour before the test; you will then be asked to void into a container."

(3) "Before voiding, the urinary meatus is cleansed with an iodine solution and urine is voided into a sterile container; the container must not touch the penis."

(4) "You must void a few drips of urine, then stop; then void the remaining urine into a clean container, which should be immediately covered."

The nurse describes the procedure for collecting a clean-catch urine for culture and sensitivity to a male patient. Which of the following explanations, if made by the nurse, would be most accurate?

Step 1. Read the question stem.

Step 2. Focus on the adjectives. "Most accurate" should tell you that more than one answer will sound good.

Step 3. Reword the question stem. What is true about a clean-catch urine specimen for culture and sensitivity?

Step 4. Read each answer choice and ask yourself, "Is this true about a clean-catch urine specimen for culture and sensitivity?"

(1) This choice describes how to obtain a catheterized urine specimen. Urine isn't usually collected by catheterization due to the increased risk of infection. This answer does not answer the question about a clean-catch urine specimen. Eliminate.

(2) This describes a double-voided specimen. This action is usually done when testing urine for glucose and ketones. It is not relevant to a clean-catch urine specimen. Eliminate.

(3) This is true of a clean-catch urine specimen for culture and sensitivity. The urinary meatus is cleansed, a sterile container is used, and the penis must not touch the container. Leave it in for consideration.

(4) This does describe a clean-catch urine specimen. The patient does void a few drops of urine, stops, and then continues void-

ing into the container. There is only one problem. For a culture and sensitivity, the container must be sterile. Eliminate.

The correct answer is (3). Many students will select answer choice (4) because they see the expected words: "Void a few drops; stop; continue voiding." Be careful. This question is a good example of why scanning for expected words could get you into trouble. You may see expected words in an answer choice that is not correct.

O.K. You've practiced how to identify the topic of the question and how to eliminate answer choices. You know that predicting answers does not work on the NCLEX. You are well on your way to correctly answering NCLEX test questions. Unfortunately, this is just the starting point. Let's talk about specific paths and how you can correctly decide which paths to use on the NCLEX. Remember, the *correct* answer is at the end of the path!

Practice Makes Perfect

Practice answering test questions.

Recognizing Expected Outcomes

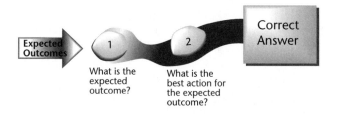

You spent much of your time in nursing school learning about what might go wrong with patients and their care. This makes sense; after all, nurses need to deal with problems and illnesses. Many test questions that your nursing school faculty wrote focused on what was wrong with patients and their care. In order to prove minimum competence, the beginning practitioner must demonstrate the ability to make appropriate nursing judgments. Competent nursing judgments include recognizing both expected and unexpected behaviors, so it is important for you to recognize expected outcomes on the NCLEX. Expected outcomes are the behaviors and changes you think are going to occur as a result of nursing care. These outcomes allow the nurse to evaluate whether goals have been met.

Look at this question:

Is That Normal?

You need to be able to recognize *normal*. Not all questions involve fixing a problem—the problem may not exist, or may have been fixed already.

The physician orders an arterial blood gas (ABG) for a 50-year-old man receiving oxygen at 6 L/min. Results show pH 7.37, HCO_3 26 mmHg, pCO_2 42 mmHg, pO_2 90 mmHg. The nurse should

(1) increase the rate of oxygen flow the patient is receiving.
(2) elevate the head of the bed.
(3) document the results in the chart.
(4) instruct the patient to cough and deep breathe.

If this question were included on one of your medical/surgical tests, you would assume that a problem was being described. So you would choose an answer choice that involved "fixing" the problem. Let's look at this question.

THE REWORDED QUESTION: What should you do with a patient with these ABGs?

Step 1. Recognize normal. Interpret the ABGs. All are within normal limits.

Step 2. Decide how you should use this information. Because they are all normal, let's reword the question again using this information.

Now THE REWORDED QUESTION is: What should you do for a patient with normal ABGs?

ANSWERS:
 (1) "Increase the rate of oxygen the patient is receiving." This is unnecessary since his O_2 is within normal limits. Eliminate.
 (2) "Elevate the head of the bed." This is unnecessary since the ABGs are within normal limits. Eliminate.
 (3) "Document the results in the chart." This action should be done since the ABGs are normal.
 (4) "Instruct the patient to cough and deep breathe." This is usually recommended in a situation in which there is some limitation of respiratory function, e.g., immobility, postoperatively. The only information you are given in this question is the patient's ABGs, which are within normal limits. While this could be done, you are given no indication that it is necessary. Eliminate.

The correct answer is: (3) Document the results. The ABGs are within normal limits. Some students select answer choice (2) because they think there's something they missed, or it must be a trick question. The "trick" is deciding whether the information that you are given is normal or abnormal, and then answering the question accordingly.

Try this question.

A 62-year old woman is brought to the emergency room complaining of pressure in her chest. Her blood pressure is 150/90, pulse 88, respirations 20. The nurse administers nitroglycerine 0.4 mg sublingually as ordered. After 5 minutes her blood pressure is 100/60, pulse 96, respirations 20. The nurse should	(1) notify the physician that the patient has become hypotensive, and obtain an order to administer IV fluids. (2) place the patient in semi-Fowler's position, and administer O₂ at 4 liters. (3) administer a second dose of nitroglycerine. (4) document the results, and continue to monitor the patient.

THE REWORDED QUESTION: What should you do for this patient? To answer this question you need to know what these vital signs indicate.

Step 1. Recognize normal. Nitroglycerine is a potent vasodilator with anti-anginal, anti-ischemic and antihypertensive actions. It increases blood flow through the coronary arteries. Side effects include orthostatic hypotension, tachycardia, dizziness, and palpitations. A decreased blood pressure, increased pulse, and stable respirations after administration of a potent vasodilator is normal and expected.

Step 2. Decide how you should use this information. The question should be reworded as, "What should you do for a patient who has responded as expected to a dose of nitroglycerin?"

ANSWERS:
   (1) Notify the physician that the patient has become hypotensive and obtain an order to administer IV fluids. The blood pressure has decreased due to vasodilatation. Decreased blood pressure is expected. Eliminate.
   (2) Place the patient in semi-Fowler's position and administer O₂ at 4 liters. Respirations are stable and there is no indication of respiratory distress. Eliminate.
   (3) Administer a second dose of nitroglycerine. The nurse should assess the patient for chest pain first, and administer a second dose of the medication only if patient continues to complain of chest pain. Eliminate.
   (4) Document the results and continue to monitor the patient. This is the correct choice because you recognized the patient's response as normal, thus eliminating the other three answer choices.

The correct answer is (4). You would expect a patient's blood pressure to decrease after administration of nitroglycerine. The key to this question is understanding how the medication works, and correctly identifying the expected outcome.

Read Answer Choices to Obtain Clues

Since NCLEX is testing your critical thinking, the topic of the questions may be unstated. You may see a question that concerns a disease process or procedure with which you unfamiliar. Most test takers who are "clueless" about a question will read the question and answer choices over and over again. They do this because they hope that:

- They will remember seeing the topic in their notes or on a textbook page.
- The light will dawn and they will remember something about the topic.
- They believe there is some clue in the question that will point them toward the correct answer.

What usually happens? Absolutely nothing! The student then randomly selects an answer choice. When you randomly select an answer, you have 1 chance in 4 of getting it right. You can better those odds, and here's how: When you encounter a question that deals with unfamiliar nursing content, look for clues in the answer choices instead of in the question stem.

If you find yourself "clueless" after you carefully read a question, follow these steps:

Step 1. Resist the impulse to read and reread the question. Read the question only once. Identify the topic of the question. It is often unstated.

Step 2. Read the answer choices, not to select the correct answer, but to figure out, "What is the topic of the question", or "What should I be thinking?" You are looking for clues from the answer choices.

Step 3. After reading the answer choices, reword the question using the clues that you have obtained.

Step 4. Then use the strategies previously discussed to answer the question you have formulated.

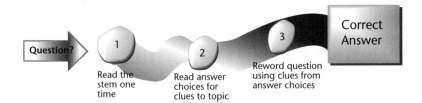

Question? 1 Read the stem one time 2 Read answer choices for clues to topic 3 Reword question using clues from answer choices Correct Answer

Let's try this strategy with a question.

> A 26-year-old man contacts his home care nurse with complaints of nausea and abdominal pain. He has type I insulin dependent diabetes mellitus (IDDM). The nurse should adivse the client to
>
> (1) hold his regular dose of insulin.
> (2) check his blood glucose level every 3–4 hours.
> (3) increase his consumption of foods containing simple sugars.
> (4) increase his activity level.

Clueless?

If you are "clueless," look for clues in the answer choices. Stay calm and focused.

Step 1. Read the stem of the question. Can you identify the topic of the question? No, you can't. The nurse is telling the client to do something, but about what topic? The topic is unstated in the question.

Step 2. Read the answer choices to obtain clues about the topic of the question. Each answer choice deals with ways to maintain a normal blood sugar.

Step 3. Reword the question. "What does the nurse tell the client about "sick day rules?"

ANSWERS:

(1) Hold his regular dose of insulin. This is an implementation that would increase the blood glucose level. The nurse should assess first. Eliminate.

(2) Check his blood glucose level every 3–4 hours. This is an assessment. Before you can advise the client, you must identify whether the client is hypoglycemic or hyperglycemic. Keep this answer for consideration.

(3) Increase his consumption of foods containing simple sugars. This is an implementation and would increase the client's blood glucose level. The nurse should assess first. Eliminate.

(4) Increase his activity level. This is an implementation that would decrease the client's blood glucose level. The nurse should assess first. Eliminate.

The nurse should always assess before implementing nursing care. The correct answer is (2).

No matter how much you prepare for NCLEX, there may be topics you see on your test with which you are unfamiliar. Reading the answer choices for clues will increase your chances of selecting a correct answer. Remember, you *do* have a body of knowledge. You just have to calm down and access this knowledge.

Read this question.

A 54-year-old man is being treated for Addison's disease. The physician orders cortisone 25 mg. PO daily. The nurse should explain to the patient that adjustment of the dosage may be required in which of the following situations?	(1) Dosage is increased when the blood glucose level increases. (2) Dosage is decreased when dietary intake is increased. (3) Dosage is decreased when infection stimulates endogenous steroid secretion. (4) Dosage is increased relative to an increase in the level of stress.

Not sure what Addison's disease is? Not sure how to adjust the dose of cortisone?

Step 1. Read the question once. Resist the impulse to reread the question.

Step 2. Read the answer choices. What should you be thinking? The question concerns cortisone. If the patient is receiving cortisone, Addison's disease must be something that requires cortisone, a hormone from the adrenal glands. You notice that dosages are both increased and decreased.

Step 3. Use these clues to find the answer to THE REWORDED QUESTION, "What is true about adjusting cortisone dosage?"

(1) Dosage is increased when the blood glucose level increases. Is this true about cortisone? No. This sounds like the insulin. Eliminate.
(2) Dosage is decreased when dietary intake is increased. Is this true about cortisone? No. Cortisone requirements are not related to diet. Eliminate.
(3) Dosage is decreased when infection stimulates endogenous steroid secretion. Endogenous means "within the patient." If the patient is receiving cortisone for Addison's disease, he must have

adrenal insufficiency. Therefore, infection can't stimulate steroid secretion. Eliminate.

Step 4. (4) is the correct answer since it is the only choice remaining. Even if you are not confident that cortisone is increased during periods of stress, you can conclude that this is the correct answer because the other choices have been eliminated.

If you're not sure about the topic of the question, read the answer choices for clues.

Let's look at another path.

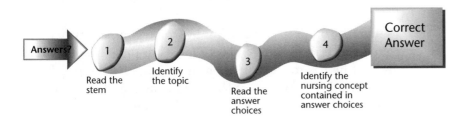

In some questions, NCLEX asks you to figure out what is the topic of the question. In other questions you are required to use critical thinking skills to figure out what the answer choices REALLY mean. NCLEX can take a concept with which you are very familiar, and make it difficult to recognize. The following question illustrates this point.

A 68-year-old man with a history of congestive heart failure (CHF) visits the clinic. He states, "I have not been feeling like my old self for about two weeks." It would be MOST important for the nurse to ask which of the following questions?	(1) "Do your ankles swell at the end of the day?" (2) "Where do you sleep at night?" (3) "How do you feel after you eat dinner?" (4) "Do you have chest pain when you inhale?"

It is not difficult to identify the topic of this question, "What is a priority for a patient with CHF?" Many students get tripped up on this question by not thinking through the answers as carefully as they should. In some questions, you have to figure out the topic of the question. In this question, you have to figure out what the answer choices mean.

Step 1: Read the stem of the question.
Step 2: Reword the question in your own words.
Step 3: Read the answer choices.
Step 4: Think: "What nursing concept should I identify in the answer choices?"

THE REWORDED QUESTION: What is a priority for a patient with CHF?

ANSWERS:

(1) "Do your ankles swell at the end of the day?" Why would you ask a patient this question? Because edema is a symptom of right-sided heart failure. Is right-sided failure your priority? No, left-sided failure takes priority because it affects the lungs. Eliminate this answer.

(2) "Where do you sleep at night?" Why would you ask a patient this question? If he is sleeping in his bed, his breathing is not compromised. If he has to sleep in his recliner, he is having orthopnea. Orthopnea is a symptom of left-sided failure, and this would be a priority. Keep this answer for consideration.

(3) "How do you feel after you eat dinner?" Why would you ask a patient this question? Bloating after meals is a symptom of right-sided failure. This is not as important as breathing problems. Eliminate this answer.

(4) "Do you have chest pain when you inhale?" Why would you ask a patient this question? It does indicate a breathing problem. The student who reacts rather than thinks may select this answer. Pain on inspiration may indicate irritation of the parietal pleura of the lung, and is not associated with CHF. Eliminate this answer.

What Does This Mean?

Figure out what the words are really saying.

The correct answer is (2). In order to select this answer, you must recognize that "Where do you sleep at night?" represents orthopnea. NCLEX will take important concepts such as this, and "hide" the concept in some fairly simple behaviors.

Let's try another question where you have to figure out, "What do the answer choices really mean?"

The nurse is caring for a 41-year-old woman immediately after a paracentesis. It is MOST important for the nurse to ask which of the following questions?	(1) "Do your clothes still feel tight?" (2) "Do you need to void?" (3) "Are you feeling dizzy?" (4) "Do you have any pain?"

Step 1: Read the stem of the question.

Step 2: Reword the question in your own words.

Step 3: Read the answer choices.

Step 4: Think: "What nursing concept should I identify in the answer choices?"

THE REWORDED QUESTION: What is the highest priority for a patient after a paracentesis?

ANSWERS:

(1) "Do your clothes still feel tight?" Why would you ask a patient this question? Clothes should fit looser because the abdominal girth has decreased after fluid has been removed with a paracentesis. This is an expected outcome. Eliminate.

(2) "Do you need to void?" Why would you ask a patient this question? It is imperative to empty the bladder prior to the procedure, not after the procedure. There is no compelling reason to ask the patient this question. Eliminate.

(3) "Are you feeling dizzy?" What makes a patient dizzy? One of the causes is a decrease in cerebral perfusion due to a fall in blood pressure. Could this patient have a decreased blood pressure? Yes. Hypotension and hypovolemic shock are complications of a paracentesis due to removal of a large volume of fluid. Keep this answer for consideration.

(4) "Do you have any pain?" You ask this question to assess pain level. This patient may have discomfort where the paracentesis was performed, but this is an expected outcome. Eliminate.

The correct answer is (3).

These questions illustrate why knowing nursing content is not enough to answer application/analysis level questions. You must be able to effectively use the information you learned in nursing school to answer NCLEX-style test questions. Review the lessons that you learned in this chapter:

- Reword the question
- Eliminate answer choices you know to be incorrect
- Don't predict answers
- Recognize expected outcomes
- Read answer choices to obtain clues

Remember, there is only ONE way to skin the CAT!

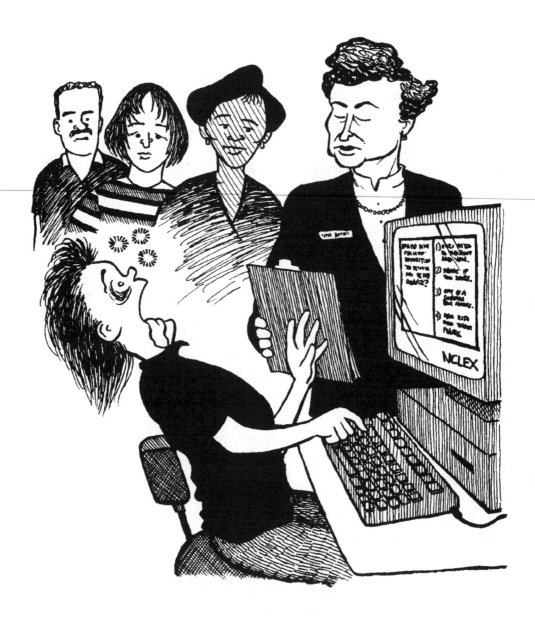

This 22-year-old has lost consciousness. What is the first action you should take?
1) Immobilize her keyboard.
2) Make an assessment of the circumstances surrounding her studying habits.
3) Put her in semi-Fowler's position to facilitate guessing.
4) Have her roommate check her pedal pulse.

CHAPTER FOUR

Maslow Is a Verb

An hour after admission to the nursery, the nurse observes a newborn baby having spontaneous jerky movements of the limbs. The infant's mother had gestational diabetes mellitus (GDM) during pregnancy. Which of the following actions should the nurse take FIRST?

(1) Give dextrose water.
(2) Call the physician immediately.
(3) Determine the blood glucose level.
(4) Observe closely for other symptoms.

Verify!

When assessing a patient, the nurse must verify the assessment with objective data.

As you read this question you are probably thinking, "All of these look right!" or "How can I decide what I will do first?" The panic sets in as you decide what is the best answer from four answer choices that you think are all correct. Don't panic. You can answer these questions correctly! One of the biggest challenges facing you as a candidate for nursing licensure is to correctly answer the priority questions. You will recognize these questions because they will ask you, "What is the best, most important, first, or initial response by the nurse?"

The correct answer is (3). You probably recognized the baby's jerky movements as an indication of hypoglycemia. Don't forget that an important part of the assessment process is *validating* what you observe. You must complete an assessment before you analyze, plan, and implement nursing care.

As a registered professional nurse, you will be caring for patients who have multiple problems and needs. As a part of your professional role, you will interact with all members of the health care team. How do you manage all of the needs and problems that you deal with daily? You must be able to establish priorities by deciding which needs take precedence over the other needs.

The following situation might sound familiar: You are called to a patient's room by a family member and find the patient lying on the floor. He is bleeding from a wound on the forehead, and his indwelling catheter is dislodged and hanging from the side of the bed. Where do you begin? Do you call for help? Do you return him to bed? Do you apply pressure to the cut? Do you reinsert the catheter? Do you call the doctor? What do you do first? This is why establishing priorities is so important.

Don't Give Up

Saying "This is too hard" won't help you.

Your nursing faculty recognized the importance of teaching you how to establish priorities. They required you to establish priorities both in clinical situations and when answering test questions. These are the type of questions that nursing students find most controversial.

Here is an example of a nursing school test question:

Which of the following would most concern the nurse during a patient's recovery from surgery?	(1) Safety. (2) Hemorrhage. (3) Infection. (4) Pain control.

Don't Raise Your Voice

You can't argue with NCLEX.

Instructor: "The correct answer is (2)."

Student: "Why isn't infection the correct answer? It says right here *[pointing to textbook]* that infection is a major complication after surgery!"

Instructor: "Yes, infection is an important concern after surgery. But, if the patient has a life-threatening hemorrhage, then the fact that the wound is infected is immaterial."

Student: "But it says here on page 106 that infection is a major complication after surgery. You can't count this answer wrong!"

In some situations, the faculty member will give you partial credit for your answer, or will "throw the question out" because there is more than one right answer. But you won't get the opportunity to argue about questions on the NCLEX. The NCLEX test makers don't throw questions out because you don't like them. You either select the answer they are looking

KAPLAN

for, or you get the question wrong. In the question above, all of the answers listed are important when caring for a postoperative patient, but only one answer is the best.

The critical thinking required for priority questions is for you to recognize patterns in the answer choices. By recognizing these patterns, you will know which path you need to choose to correctly answer the question. This chapter will present several strategies to help you establish priorities on the NCLEX: the Maslow strategy, the nursing process strategy, and the safety strategy. We will outline each strategy, describe how and when it should be used, and show you how to apply these strategies to NCLEX-style questions. By using these strategies, you will be able to eliminate the second-best answer and correctly identify the highest priority.

Strategy One: Maslow

"Oh, no," you're probably thinking. "Not Maslow! Isn't he the guy that talks about self-actualization? What is self-actualization, anyway?" You may have discounted Maslow when you were in nursing school, but now that it's time to establish priorities on the NCLEX, Maslow should become your best friend.

Maslow's hierarchy of needs is crucial to establishing priorities on the NCLEX exam. Maslow identifies five levels of human needs: physiological, safety or security, love and belonging, esteem, and self-actualization.

Maslow's Hierarchy

Self-actualization
Self-esteem
Love and belonging
Safety and security
Physiological needs

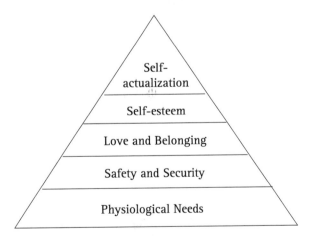

Because *physiological needs* are necessary for survival, they have highest priority and must be met first. Physiological needs include oxygen, fluid, nutrition, temperature, elimination, shelter, rest, and sex. If you don't have oxygen to breathe or food to eat, you really don't care if you have stable psychosocial relationships!

Safety needs can be both physical and psychosocial. Physical safety includes decreasing what is threatening to the patient. The threat may be an illness (myocardial infarction), accidents (a parent transporting a newborn in a car without using a car seat), or environmental threats (the client with COPD that insists on walking outside in 10° F temperatures).

To attain psychological safety, the client must have the knowledge and understanding about what to expect from others in his environment. For example, it is important to teach the client and his family what to expect after a CVA. It is also important that you allow a woman preparing for a mastectomy to verbalize her concerns about changes that might occur in her relationship with her partner.

To achieve love and belonging, the client needs to feel loved by family and accepted by others. When a client feels self-confident and useful, he will achieve the need of esteem as described by Maslow.

The highest level of Maslow's hierarchy of needs is self-actualization. To achieve this level the client must experience fulfillment and recognize his or her potential. In order for self-actualization to occur, all of the lower-level needs must be met. Because of the stresses of life, lower-level needs are not always met, and many people never achieve this high level of functioning.

Use Maslow's Needs to Establish Priorities

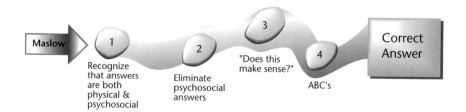

The first strategy to use in establishing priorities is a four-step process, beginning with Maslow's hierarchy. To use the Maslow strategy, you must first recognize the pattern in the answer choices.

Step 1. Look at your answer choices.

If answer choices are both physical and psychosocial, it's time to "Maslow" the answer choices.

Step 2. Eliminate all psychosocial answer choices. If an answer choice is physiological don't eliminate it yet. Remember, Maslow states that physiological needs must be met first. While pain certainly has a physiological component, reactions to pain are considered "psychosocial" on this exam and will become a lower priority.

Step 3. Ask yourself: Does this choice make sense?

Next, consider each of the remaining answer choices. Take the time to read each choice carefully and ask yourself, "Does this answer make sense with regard to the disease or situation as described in the question?" If it makes sense as an answer choice, keep it for consideration and go on to the next choice.

Step 4. Can you apply the ABCs?

Look at the remaining answer choices. Can you apply the ABCs? The ABCs mean airway, breathing, and circulation. If there is an answer that involves maintaining a patent airway, it will be correct. If not, is there a choice that involves breathing problems? It will be correct. If not, go on with the ABCs. Is there an answer pertaining to the cardiovascular system? It will be correct. What if the ABCs don't apply? Compare the remaining answer choices and ask yourself, "What is the highest priority?" This is your answer.

Let's apply this technique to a couple of sample NCLEX-style test questions.

A woman is admitted to the hospital with a ruptured ectopic pregnancy. A laparotomy is scheduled. Preoperatively, which of the following goals is most important for the nurse to include on the patient's plan of care?	(1) Fluid replacement. (2) Pain relief. (3) Emotional support. (4) Respiratory therapy.

Look at the stem of the question. The words *most important* mean:

- This is a priority question.

Think ABCs

Airway
Breathing
Circulation

- There probably will be more than one answer choice that is a correct nursing action, but it will not be the most important or highest priority action.

Step 1. Look at the answer choices. You will see that both physical and psychosocial interventions are included. It is time to "Maslow."

Step 2. Eliminate the answer choices that are psychosocial interventions. Answer choice (2), which is pain relief, should be discarded. Remember, pain is considered a psychosocial problem on the NCLEX. Answer choice (3), emotional support, is also a psychosocial concern. Eliminate this answer.

You have now eliminated two of the possible choices. You are halfway there!

Step 3. Ask yourself the question, "Does this make sense?"

(1)　Fluid replacement makes sense, because this patient has a ruptured ectopic pregnancy. An ectopic pregnancy is implantation of the fertilized ovum in a site other than the endometrial lining, usually the fallopian tube. Initially, the pregnancy is normal, but as the embryo outgrows the fallopian tube, the tube ruptures, causing extensive bleeding into the abdominal cavity.

(2)　Respiratory therapy does not make sense with a ruptured ectopic pregnancy. The obstetrical patient is not likely to need respiratory care prior to surgery. Eliminate this answer choice.

You are left with the correct answer, (1). After reading this question, many students select answer choices (2) or (3) as the correct answer. They justify this by emphasizing the importance of managing this woman's pain, or addressing her grief about losing the pregnancy. Neither answer choice takes priority over the physiological demand of fluid replacement prior to surgery.

Ready for another question? Try this one.

The nurse obtains a diet history from a pregnant 16-year-old girl. The girl tells the nurse that her typical daily diet includes cereal and milk for breakfast, pizza and soda for lunch, and a cheeseburger, milkshake, fries, and salad for dinner. The most accurate nursing diagnosis based on this data is	(1) altered nutrition: more than body requirements related to high-fat intake. (2) knowledge deficit: nutrition in pregnancy. (3) altered nutrition: less than body requirements related to increased nutritional demands of pregnancy. (4) risk for injury: fetal malnutrition related to poor maternal diet.

Step 1. Look at the answer choices. You will see that both physical and psychosocial interventions are included. It is time to "Maslow."

Step 2. Eliminate all answer choices that are psychosocial concerns. In this case, that means (2). Knowledge deficit is a psychosocial need.

Step 3. Ask yourself the question, "Does this make sense?"

(1) "More than body requirements related to high fat intake" does make sense. This diet is high in fat.

(3) "Less than body requirements related to increased nutritional demands of pregnancy" also makes sense. This diet has an adequate number of calories, but it is deficient in the needed vitamins and minerals.

(4) "Fetal malnutrition related to poor maternal diet" does not make sense. There is an adequate number of calories to support fetal growth. Eliminate it.

You have now eliminated two of the choices. Let's go on.

Step 4. Read answer choices (1) and (3) and compare. Which is higher priority: the fact that this pregnant 16-year-old's diet contains too much fat, or that the diet does not have enough nutrients? Insufficient nutrients is a higher priority so the correct answer is (3).

Many students, when they first read this question, choose (2), knowledge deficit. According to Maslow, physiological needs always take priority over psychosocial needs. Using this strategy on the NCLEX will enable you to choose the correct answer.

Physical Needs First

Eliminate psychosocial needs.

Now, let's try another question.

The nurse plans care for a 14-year-old girl admitted with an eating disorder. On admission, the girl weighs 82 lbs. and is 5'4" tall. Lab test indicate severe hypokalemia, anemia, and dehydration. The nurse should give which of the following nursing diagnoses the highest priority?	(1) Body image disturbance related to weight loss. (2) Self-esteem disturbance related to feelings of inadequacy. (3) Altered nutrition: less than body requirements related to decreased intake. (4) Decreased cardiac output related to the potential for dysrhythmias.

Remember to Breathe

Physiological needs are most important. Psychosocial needs can be eliminated.

The first thing you notice in this question stem is the phrase "highest priority." This alerts you that there may be more than one answer that could be considered correct.

Step 1. Look at the answer choices. Both physical and psychosocial interventions are included. It is time to "Maslow."

Step 2. Eliminate any answer choices that are psychosocial. This includes (1) and (2). It is easy to see that body image disturbance is a psychosocial concern. The same is true of answer choice (2), self-esteem disturbance. Answer choices (3) and (4) are physiological.

You have now eliminated all but two answer choices:

Step 3. Ask yourself: Does "altered nutrition: less than body requirements related to decreased intake" make sense? Remember, the patient has anorexia and is 5'4" tall and weighs 82 lbs. Yes, it does make sense.

Does "decreased cardiac output related to the potential for dysrhythmias" make sense? Dysrhythmias are a concern for a patient with severe hypokalemia, which often occurs with anorexia. Yes, it does make sense.

You still have work to do.

Step 4. Now use the ABCs to establish priorities. Decreased cardiac output is a higher priority than altered nutrition. One answer choice remains: (4).

When you first read this question, you probably identified each of the answers choices as appropriate for a patient with anorexia. Only one nursing diagnosis can be the highest priority. By using strategies involving Maslow and the ABCs, you will choose the correct answer on your NCLEX.

Strategy Two: Assessment vs. Implementation

A second strategy that will assist you to establish priorities involves the assessment and implementation steps of the nursing process. As a nursing student you have been drilled so that you can recite the steps of the nursing process in your sleep—assessment, analysis, planning, implementation, and evaluation. In nursing school, you did have some test questions about the nursing process, but you probably did not use the nursing process to assist you in selecting a correct answer on an exam. On the NCLEX, you will be given a clinical situation and asked to establish priorities. The possible answer choices will include both the correct assessment and implementation for this clinical situation. How do you choose the correct answer when both the correct assessment and implementation are given? Think about these two steps of the nursing process.

Assessment is the process of establishing a data profile about the patient and his or her health problems. The nurse obtains subjective and objective data in a number of ways: talking to clients, observing clients and/or significant others, taking a health history, performing a physical examination, evaluating lab results, and collaborating with other members of the health care team.

Once you collect the data you compare it to the client's baseline or normal values. On the NCLEX, the client's baseline may not be given, but as a nursing student you have acquired a body of knowledge. On this exam you are expected to compare the client information you are given to the "normal" values learned from your nursing textbooks.

Assessment is the first step of the nursing process and takes priority over all other steps. It is essential that you complete the assessment phase of the nursing process before you implement nursing activities. This is a common mistake made by NCLEX test takers: don't implement before you assess. For example, when performing CPR, if you don't access the airway before performing mouth to mouth resuscitation, your actions may be harmful!

Nursing Process

Assess
Analyze
Plan
Implement
Evaluate

Assess First

Always assess before you implement.

Implementation is the care you provide to your patients. Implementation includes: assisting in the performance of activities of daily living (ADL); counseling and educating the client and the client's family; giving care to patients and clients; supervising and evaluating the work of other members of the health team. Nursing interventions may be independent, dependent, or interdependent. Independent interventions are within the scope of nursing practice, and do not require supervision by others. Instructing the client to turn cough and deep breathe after surgery is an example of an independent nursing intervention. Dependent interventions are based on the written orders of a physician. On the NCLEX, you should assume that you have an order for all dependent interventions that are included in the answer choices.

You've Got the Power

On the NCLEX, always assume that you have a physician's order to intervene.

This may be a different way of thinking from the way you were taught in nursing school. Many students select an answer on a nursing school test (that is later counted wrong) because the intervention requires a physician's order. Everyone walks away from the test review muttering "trick question." It is important for you to remember that there are no trick questions on the NCLEX. You should base your answer on an understanding that you have a physician's order for any nursing intervention described.

Interdependent interventions are shared with other members of the health team. For instance, nutrition education may be shared with the dietitian. Chest physiotherapy may be shared with a respiratory therapist.

The following strategy, utilizing the assessment and implementation phases of the nursing process, will assist you in selecting correct answers to questions that ask you to identify priorities.

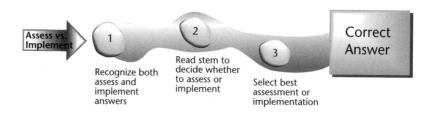

Try this strategy on the following question.

The mother of a 10-year-old boy with IDDM (insulin dependent diabetes mellitus) calls the physician's office to discuss the child's self-monitoring blood glucose (SMBG) home reading. He is being tightly regulated with a combination of NPH and regular insulin before breakfast and supper. The past two mornings his blood sugar reading were 220 mg/dL and 210 mg/dL. The nurse should advise the mother to

(1) continue with his medication regimen.
(2) check his blood sugar during the night.
(3) give his NPH insulin later in the evening.
(4) serve his bedtime snack earlier in the evening.

REWORDED QUESTION: "What advice should the nurse give the mother about her diabetic child that is hyperglycemic in the morning?"

Step 1. Read the answer choices to establish a pattern. There is one assessment answer (2) and three implementation answers (1), (3), and (4). You can use the assessment/validation vs. implementation strategy.

Step 2. Refer to the question to determine if you should be assessing or implementing. The child's mother tells you that blood sugars have been elevated the last two mornings. This indicates that there is a problem. According to the nursing process, you should assess first. Eliminate answers (1), (3), and (4).

Step 3. The correct answer is (2). This question is about the Somogyi effect, which is rebound hyperglycemia that occurs in response to a rapid decrease in blood glucose during the night. Treatment includes adjusting the evening diet, changing the insulin dose, and altering the amount of exercise to prevent nocturnal hypoglycemia. Even if you've never heard of the Somogyi effect, you are still able to correctly answer this question using the assessment versus implementation strategy.

Let's look at another question.

A 12-year-old boy was riding his bike to school when he hit the curb. He fell and hurt his leg. The school nurse was called and found him alert, conscious but in severe pain with a possible fracture of the right femur. What is the first action that the nurse should take?	(1) Immobilize the affected limb with a splint and ask him not to move. (2) Make a thorough assessment of the circumstances surrounding the accident. (3) Put him in semi-Fowler's position for comfort. (4) Check the pedal pulse and blanching sign in both legs.

The words *first action* tell you that this is a "priority" question.

Think Before You Act

Action doesn't always mean *implementation*.

REWORDED QUESTION: What is the highest priority for a fractured femur?

Step 1. Read answer choices to establish a pattern. The answer choices are a mix of assessment/validation and implementation. This is the strategy to use.

Step 2. Determine whether you should be assessing or implementing. According to the question, the nurse has determined that the boy has a possible fracture. This implies that the nurse has completed the assessment step. It is now time to implement.

Step 3. Eliminate answers (2) and (4) because they are assessments. This leaves you with choices (1) and (3). Which takes priority, immobilizing the affected limb, or placing the boy in a semi-Fowlers's position to facilitate breathing? The question does not indicate any respiratory distress.

The correct answer is (1), immobilize the affected limb.

Some students will choose an answer involving the ABCs without thinking it through. Students, beware. Use the ABCs to establish priorities, but make sure that the answer is appropriate to the situation. In this question, breathing was mentioned in one of the answer choices. If you thought of the ABCs immediately without looking at the context of the question, you would have answered this question incorrectly.

Look at this question in another form.

A 12-year-old sixth grade boy was riding his bike to school when he hit the curb. The boy tells the school nurse, "I think my leg is broken." What is the first action the nurse should take?	(1) Immobilize the affected limb with a splint and ask the client not to move. (2) Ask the client to explain what happened. (3) Put the client in semi-Fowler's position to facilitate breathing. (4) Check the appearance of the client's leg.

Step 1. Determine whether you should be assessing or implementing. In this question, the client has stated "my leg is broken." This statement is not the nurse's assessment. This alerts the nurse that there is a problem, and the nurse should begin the steps of the nursing process. The first step is assessment.

Step 2. Eliminate answers (1) and (3). These are implementations.

Step 3. What takes priority? Assessment of the leg takes priority over an assessment of what happened to cause the accident. The correct answer is (4).

Strategy Three: Safety

Nurses have the primary responsibility of ensuring the safety of clients. This includes clients in health care facilities, in the home, at work, and in the community. Safety includes: meeting basic needs (oxygen, food, fluids, etcetera), reducing hazards that cause injury to patient (accidents, obstacles in the home), and decreasing the transmission of pathogens (immunizations, sanitation).

Remember that the NCLEX is a test of minimum competency to determine that you are able to practice safe and effective nursing care. Always think safety when selecting correct answers on the exam. When answering questions about procedures, this strategy will help you to establish priorities.

Do No Harm

Decide what will cause the least amount of harm.

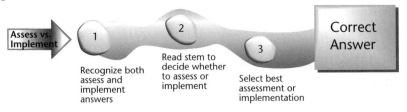

Apply this strategy to the following question.

A 4-year-old child undergoes a tonsillectomy for treatment of chronic tonsillitis unresponsive to antibiotic therapy. After surgery, the child is brought to the recovery room. Which of the following actions should the nurse include in his plan of care?	(1) Institute measures to minimize crying. (2) Perform postural drainage every two hours. (3) Cough and deep breathe every hour. (4) Give ice cream as tolerated.

Reworded Question: What should you do after a tonsillectomy?

Step 1. Are all the answer choices implementations? Yes.

Step 2. Can you answer the question based on your knowledge of a tonsillectomy? If not, continue to Step 3.

Step 3. Ask yourself, "What will cause my patient the least amount of harm?" Minimizing crying (1) will help prevent bleeding. Keep in consideration. Postural drainage (2) may cause bleeding. Eliminate. Coughing and deep breathing (3) may cause bleeding. Eliminate. Give ice cream (4) may cause the child to clear his throat causing bleeding. Eliminate.

The correct answer is (1). The nurse must prevent postoperative hemorrhage, a complication seen after this type of surgery. Crying would irritate the child's throat and increase the chance of hemorrhage.

Let's try another question.

A 52-year-old man is receiving intravenous cimetidine (Tagamet). After 20 minutes of the infusion, the patient complains of a headache and dizziness. Which of the following actions should the nurse take FIRST?	(1) Stop the infusion. (2) Call the physician. (3) Reposition the patient. (4) Call the pharmacist.

REWORDED QUESTION: What should you do if patient is having side effects to a medication being administered?

Step 1. Are all answers implementations? Yes.

Step 2. Can you answer this question based on your knowledge? If not, proceed to step 3.

Step 3. Ask yourself the question, "What will cause my patient the least amount of harm?"

(1) Stopping the infusion would not harm the patient. If the symptoms described are due to a side effect of the medication, this action would help the patient. Leave this choice in for consideration.

(2) Calling the physician would not harm the patient. Leave it in for consideration.

(3) Repositioning the patient would not harm the patient, but would not help the patient. Eliminate.

(4) Calling the pharmacist would not harm the patient, but would not help him. Eliminate.

Choices (1) and (2) are left to consider. Choice (1) is the correct answer. NCLEX wants to know what decision you are going to make, not what decision the physician will make.

Let's look at one more question.

An 84-year-old man is admitted with a diagnosis of dementia. He attempts several times to pull out his nasogastric tube. An order for cloth wrist restraints is received by the nurse. Which of the following actions by the nurse is most appropriate?	(1) Attach the ties of the restraint to the bed frame. (2) Perform range of motion to the restrained extremities once a shift. (3) Remove the restraints when the patient is up in a wheelchair. (4) Explain the need for restraints only to the family since the patient is confused.

Reworded Question: "What is the safest way to apply restraints?"

Step 1. Are all answers implementations? Yes.

Step 2. Can you answer this based on your knowledge? If not, proceed to step 3.

Step 3. Ask yourself, "What will cause the least amount of harm to the patient?"

(1) Attaching the ties of the restraint to the bed frame will not harm the patient. Retain this answer.

(2) Performing range of motion once a shift will not harm the patient. However, it should be performed more frequently. Retain this answer.

(3) Removing the restraints when the patient is up in a wheelchair will be harmful to the patient. Restraints should not be removed when the patient is unattended. Eliminate it.

(4) Explaining the need for restraints only to the family can cause harm to the patient. Restraints can increase the confusion or combativeness of the patient. Even though the patient is confused, he needs to receive an explanation. Eliminate it.

You are now considering answer choices (1) and (2). What will cause the least amount of harm to the patient? Attaching the ties of the restraint to the bed frame or performing range of motion to the extremities once a shift? Range of motion should be performed every two to four hours to prevent loss of joint mobility. Eliminate (2).

The correct answer is (1). Attaching the ties of the restraint to the bed frame will allow the nurse to raise and lower the side rail without injury to the patient.

Priorities are an important component of the NCLEX. To help you select correct answers, think:

- Maslow
- The Nursing Process
- Safety

Answer these three questions using the appropriate priority strategy. The explanations follow the questions.

KAPLAN

Question 1

The nurse cares for a 72-year-old man with a diagnosis of cerebral vascular accident (CVA). The nurse is feeding the patient in a chair when he suddenly begins to choke. Which of the following actions should the nurse take FIRST?

(1) Check for breathlessness by placing an ear over the patient's mouth and observing the chest.
(2) Leave the patient in the chair and apply vigorous abdominal or chest thrusts from behind the patient.
(3) Ask the patient, "Are you choking?"
(4) Return the patient to the bed and apply vigorous abdominal or chest thrusts while straddling the patient's thighs.

It's As Easy As 1, 2, 3

Always prioritize:

Maslow
Nursing process
Safety

Question 2

A 35-year-old woman with a history of bipolar disorder is admitted to the psychiatric hospital. She was found by the police attempting to climb onto the wing of a plane at the airport. Her husband reports that she has not eaten or slept in two days, and he suspects she has stopped taking lithium. On admission, the nurse should place the highest priority on which of the following patient care needs?

(1) Teaching the patient about the importance of taking lithium as prescribed.
(2) Providing the patient with a safe environment with few distractions.
(3) Arranging for food and rest for the patient.
(4) Setting limits on the patient's behavior.

Question 3

The physician orders a nasogastric tube inserted and connected to low intermittent suction for a patient with an intestinal obstruction. Two hours after the insertion of the nasogastric tube, the patient vomits 200 cc. While irrigating the nasogastric tube, the nurse notes resistance. The nurse should

(1) replace the nasogastric tube with a larger one.
(2) turn the client on his left side.
(3) change the suction from intermittent to continuous.
(4) continue the irrigation.

Let's see if you were able to correctly determine which strategy you should use to determine priorities.

Question 1

"What action should the nurse take first" tells you this is a priority question. Look at your answer choices to determine a pattern. (1) and (3) are assessments. (2) and (4) are implementations. Use the nursing process to select the correct answer.

Step 1. Determine whether you should be assessing or implementing. According to the situation, the patient has begun to choke. This alerts the nurse that there is a problem. The first step of the nursing process is to assess.

Step 2. Eliminate (2) and (4) because they are implementations.

Step 3. What takes priority? Assessing for breathlessness by placing an ear over the patient's mouth or assessing the patient by asking, "Are you choking?" Inability to speak or cough indicates the airway is obstructed. Breathlessness should be checked only in an unconscious patient. The correct answer is (3).

Question 2

Look at the answer choices. They include both physiological and psychosocial interventions. It's time to Maslow.

Step 1. Eliminate all answer choices that are psychosocial—(1) and (4).

Step 2. Answer the question, "Does this make sense?"

(2) Providing the patient with a safe environment does make sense. Retain this answer.
(3) Arranging for food and rest also makes sense. Retain this answer.

Step 3. Answer the question, "What takes highest priority?" Providing for a safe environment or providing for food and rest? According to Maslow, food and rest take highest priority. The correct answer is (3).

Question 3

This question is about a procedure. Read the answer choices to establish a pattern. All of the answers are interventions. If you are unsure about a procedure, think safety.

Step 1. What is the question? What should the nurse do when resistance is met while irrigating an NG tube? If you're not sure, think safety.

Step 2. Answer this question: "What will cause the patient the least amount of harm?"

(1) Replacing the nasogastric tube with a larger one could harm the patient by damaging the mucosa. Eliminate it.
(2) Turn the client to his left side. That would not hurt the patient. Retain this answer.
(3) Changing the suction from intermittent to continuous is never done because it will erode the mucosa. Eliminate it.
(4) Continuing the irrigation when there is resistance might be harmful. Never force an irrigation. Eliminate it.

The correct answer is (2). The tip of the tube may be against the stomach wall. Repositioning the patient might allow the tip to lay unobstructed in the stomach.

Don't you think that these critical thinking strategies have unlocked the secrets of answering priority questions? Read on for more critical thinking strategies.

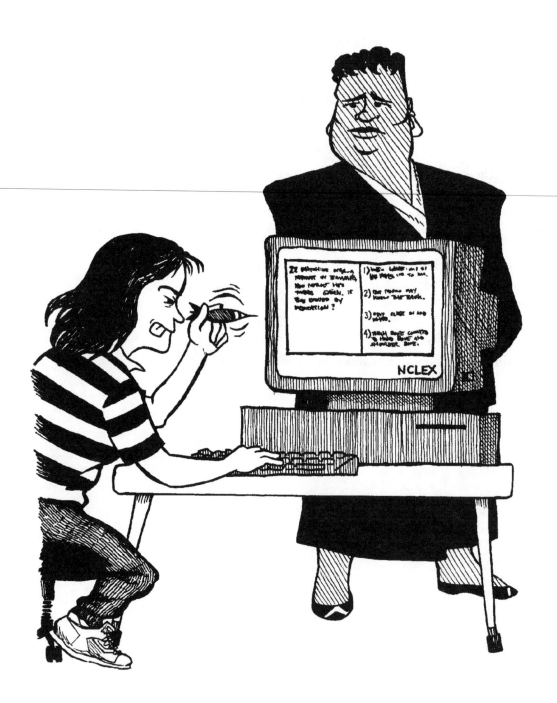

"That's not going to work on the NCLEX, Kerri."

CHAPTER FIVE

The NCLEX Isn't the Real World

One of the biggest obstacles that graduate nurses face when answering NCLEX questions is that more than one answer choice appears correct. Your "real world" experience often makes more than one answer choice seem right. Some of you are LPNs or LVNs completing your RN studies, while others are EMTs. Some of you worked during school as student techs. All of you, however, spent time in clinical during your nursing education. All of this adds up to a lot of experience. Experience will help you get a job, but answering questions based on your experience can be dangerous on the NCLEX.

Look at the following question:

> On admission to the hospital an 84-year-old man appears disheveled and is restless and confused. During the patient's second day on the unit, a nurse approaches the patient to administer medication. The nurse is unable to identify the patient because his arm band is missing. Which of the following actions by the nurse is the best?
>
> (1) Have the patient's roommate identify him.
> (2) Ask the patient to state his full name.
> (3) Ask one of the other nurses to identify the patient.
> (4) Look in the chart at the picture of the patient.

Do Everything By the Book

Be careful about using your "real world" experience. All correct answers are based on textbook nursing practices.

Let's see how someone using his or her real world experience would approach this question:

(1) "The roommate is never involved in identification of a patient."
(2) "A confused patient cannot be relied on for an accurate identification."

(3) "Sounds reasonable. I have seen this done in some circumstances."

(4) "A picture? What picture? I've never seen a picture of a patient in a chart!"

Possible conclusions drawn by this person would include: *"OK, I've seen one nurse ask another for information so (3) must be the answer,"* or *"Well, maybe the patient isn't all that confused, so I'll select (2)."*

According to nursing textbooks, asking another health care professional is not the correct way to identify a patient. Many acute care settings now include a photo of the patient in the chart for just this type of situation. The correct answer to this question is (4). Many students reject this answer because there are rarely pictures of patients in the charts. Real world experience doesn't count, though; in this case, the patient does have a picture in his chart.

The NCLEX is a standardized exam administered by the National Council of State Boards of Nursing, Inc. Because the NCLEX test is a national exam, students should be aware that in some parts of the country, nursing is practiced slightly differently. But to assure that the test is reflective of national trends, questions and answers are all carefully documented. The test makers make sure that the correct answers are documented in at least two standard nursing textbooks or one textbook and one nursing journal.

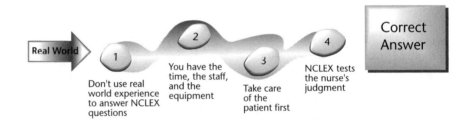

Real World

1 Don't use real world experience to answer NCLEX questions

2 You have the time, the staff, and the equipment

3 Take care of the patient first

4 NCLEX tests the nurse's judgment

Correct Answer

When you are unsure of an answer choice, don't ask yourself, "What do they do on my floor?" but "What does the medical/surgical textbook writer Brunner say?" or "What do Potter and Perry say to do?" This test does not necessarily reflect what happens in the "real world," but is based on textbook nursing.

Some examples to remember when taking the NCLEX:

- You have all of the time and resources you need to provide appropriate care to your client. (Checking for bowel sounds for five minutes in all four quadrants, no problem!)
- You have all of the equipment you need. (Remember the bath thermometer you learned to use in the nursing lab? For the NCLEX you will have one available to test the temperature of bath water.)
- There are *no* staffing problems on the NCLEX. You are caring only for the client described in the question, and that person is your only concern.
- All care given to clients is "by the book." No shortcuts are used. (You would not turn off an IV solution, flush the line, give another IV solution, flush the line, and then restart the original IV solution that was ordered to be run continuously.)

Time Is On Your Side

On the NCLEX, don't worry about "real world" concerns, such as limited time and resources.

Answer the following question.

> A 45-year-old man is treated in the emergency room for acute alcohol intoxication. He has a five-year history of alcohol abuse. He is agitated and verbally abusive. His admission orders include chlordiazepoxide (Librium) 50 mg IM or PO every 4–6 hours for agitation. The nurse should take which of the following precautions after Librium is administered?
>
> (1) Place the patient in restraints.
> (2) Leave the patient in a room by himself until the tranquilizer takes effect.
> (3) Assign a practical nurse to stay with the patient and assess his condition.
> (4) Ask the security guard to stay with the patient.

Let's look at this using "real world" logic.

(1) Place the patient in restraints. Yes, that is done in the "real world."

(2) Leave the patient in a room by himself. Yes, that is done in the "real world," but most students recognize that it is not the best answer.

(3) Assign a practical nurse to stay with the patient. Sounds good, but what if you don't have enough staffing to assign an LPN/LVN to sit with this patient?

(4) Ask the security guard to stay with the patient. Yes, in the "real world" security is called when patients are agitated.

According to "real world" logic, the correct answer must be (1) or (4). However, textbook theoretical nursing practice states that this patient should not be left alone while in an agitated state. A professional should remain with the patient. Therefore, the correct answer is (3).

Yes, I Have It in Writing

The correct answer choices can be documented in at least two sources.

Use your real world experience to help you visualize the patient described in the test question, but select your answers based on what is found in nursing textbooks.

Your nursing faculty has probably been very conscientious about instructing you in the most up-to-date nursing practice. According to the National Council, the primary source for documenting correct answers is in nursing textbooks, and the most up-to-date practice might not always agree with the textbooks. When in doubt, always select the textbook answer!

The next question illustrates this point.

A 22-year-old woman is admitted to the hospital and delivers a healthy 7 lb, 2 oz girl. The mother decides to bottle feed her infant. Which of the following statements, if made by the mother after a teaching session, indicates to the nurse that the patient needs further instruction?

(1) "I'll pump my breasts and use warm packs to relieve breast pain."
(2) "I'll use a tight bra and ice packs to relieve engorgement discomfort."
(3) "I'll take the medication prescribed by the doctor for pain."
(4) "I'll take the pills ordered by my doctor to help stop the production of milk."

Let's look at these answers more closely.

(1) Pumping the breasts will stimulate milk production. This is clearly wrong.

(2) Wearing a tight bra and using ice packs are appropriate interventions for a nonbreastfeeding mother.

(3) Taking a medication (mild analgesic) is an appropriate intervention for a nonbreastfeeding mother.

(4) Taking medication to prevent lactation: According to the most current theory, medications are not used as frequently to prevent lactation because of the dangerous side effects. But a medication may be prescribed to prevent lactation. This would be considered an appropriate intervention.

The correct answer is (1).

First Take Care of the Patient, Then the Equipment

The NCLEX tests your ability to use critical thinking skills to make nursing judgments. It is very important that you remember to:

- Take care of the patient first
- Take care of the equipment second

A 36-year-old woman sustains a fractured left femur in a car accident. She is placed in balanced suspension skeletal traction using a Thomas splint and a Pearson attachment. The patient tells the nurse that she has "terrible" pain in her left thigh. Initially the nurse should

(1) determine that all the weights and ropes from the traction apparatus are in line and hanging free.
(2) ask the patient for more information about the location and characteristics of her pain.
(3) check the Thomas splint and Pearson attachment to make sure they are appropriately positioned.
(4) explain to the patient that pain she is experiencing in the affected leg is a common occurrence.

Put That Down and Help Me!

Always take care of the patient first before the equipment.

Let's review the answers:

(1) All weights should be hanging free in balanced suspension skeletal traction. This answer choice has you checking the equipment, not the patient. Your first concern should be the patient, not the traction.

(2) The nurse should focus on assessing the patient and her problem before assessing the function of the equipment. All complaints of pain should be thoroughly investigated by the nurse.

(3) This answer choice has you checking the equipment, not the patient. Your first concern should be the patient, not the traction.

(4) Any complaints of pain are considered abnormal and should be thoroughly investigated by the nurse.

The correct answer is (2).

Laboratory Values

Answering questions about lab values is another example of how the "real world" does not work on the NCLEX. In nursing school, you learned lab values for a specific test and you may not have remembered them after the test. While you were in the clinical setting, the emphasis was on interpretation of lab values. Since most lab slips contained a listing of normal values, you were able to compare the patient's results to the normal levels. Questions on the NCLEX will not provide you with a listing of normal lab values.

Know What's Normal

Memorize normal lab values and be able to interpret them.

To answer questions on the NCLEX, you must:

- Know normal lab test results
- Correctly interpret normal or abnormal lab test results

Compare the following two questions.

A 66-year-old woman is admitted to the hospital with flulike symptoms. When taking the history the nurse learns that the patient has been taking Lanoxin (Digoxin) 0.125 mg PO daily and furosemide (Lasix) 40 mg PO daily for three years. Last month her physician changed the prescription for Digoxin to 0.25 mg qd. The nurse would expect the physician to order which of the following laboratory tests?

(1) Serum electrolytes and digoxin level.
(2) White blood cell count and hemoglobin and hematocrit.
(3) Cardiac enzymes and an arterial blood gas.
(4) Blood cultures and urinalysis.

Most of you are probably familiar with the concepts presented in this question. The physician has increased the patient's dose of digoxin. Lasix is a potassium-wasting diuretic. The patient will likely develop digitalis toxicity if she has a low potassium level. Serum electrolytes and digoxin level (1) is the correct answer.

Now look at this question.

The nurse plans care for a 15-year-old girl admitted with complaints of fever, vomiting, and diarrhea. The nurse writes the following nursing diagnosis on the patient's care plan: "fluid volume deficit." Which of the following changes in laboratory values would demonstrate an improvement in the patient's condition?	(1) Urine specific gravity, 1.015; hematocrit, 37%. (2) Urine specific gravity, 1.030; hematocrit, 47%. (3) Urine specific gravity, 1.015; hematocrit, 46%. (4) Urine specific gravity, 1.025; hematocrit, 35%.

In order to correctly answer this question, you must know:

- The normal levels of hematocrit (male 42–50%, female 40–48%) and the specific gravity of urine (1.010–1.030).
- How the hematocrit and specific gravity levels are affected by a fluid volume deficit.

Fluid volume deficit occurs when water and electrolytes are lost in the same proportion as they exist in the body. When a patient is dehydrated, both the specific gravity of urine and the hematocrit become elevated. The correct answer is (2).

Answer this question:

A 64-year-old woman is hospitalized with a diagnosis of atrial fibrillation. Heparin 5,000 units is ordered every 12 hours to be given subcutaneously. The physician orders daily partial thromboplastin times (PTT). The result of the patient's most recent PTT is 55. Which of the following actions should be taken by the nurse?	(1) Document the results and administer the Heparin. (2) Withhold the Heparin. (3) Notify the physician. (4) Have the test repeated.

In order to answer this question you need to know:

- The normal range for a PTT is 20–45 seconds.
- The therapeutic range for a patient receiving heparin, an antico-

agulant, is one-and-a-half to two times the control or normal level.

Evaluate the answer choices.

(1) "Document the results and give the heparin." The patient's most recent PTT is 55. This is not 1 1/2–2 times the control or normal so the medication should be given.

(2) "Withhold the heparin." The PTT level is not yet within what is considered an effective therapeutic level. This patient needs the anticoagulant.

(3) "Notify the physician." There is no reason to notify the physician. The patient has not reached the therapeutic level of heparin.

(4) "Have the test repeated." There is no reason to have the test repeated. The patient has not achieved the therapeutic level.

The correct answer is (1).

Know Your Rights

Remember the "five rights" of medication administration.

Medication Administration

An important function in providing safe and effective care to patients is the administration of medications. Much of your clinical preparation time was involved in preparing drug cards, learning about medications, and administering medications safely. Because this is one of the responsibilities of a beginning practitioner, questions about medications are often an important part the NCLEX. The nurse who is minimally competent is knowledgeable about medications and uses the "five rights" when administering medication.

In nursing school, most questions about medication followed the same pattern. You were told the patient's diagnosis, the name of the medication, and then are asked a question. Even if you didn't know the information about the medication, sometimes you were able to select the correct answer by knowing the diagnosis.

NCLEX does not give you any clues from the context of the question. The questions on this exam include the name of the medication, almost always identifying it by both trade and generic names. Most of the time, you will not be given the reason the patient is receiving the medication.

Let's look at some medication questions.

The physician orders furosemide (Lasix) and spironolactone (Aldactone) for a patient. Prior to administering the medication, the nurse determines that the patient's potassium is 3.2 mEq/L. In addition to notifying the physician, the nurse should anticipate taking which of the following actions?	(1) Do not administer the Lasix or Aldactone. (2) Administer the Aldactone only. (3) Administer the Lasix only. (4) Administer the Lasix and Aldactone.

Anything Out of the Ordinary?

Know side effects and nursing implications of medications.

This is a typical NCLEX-style medication question. The question concerns the side effects and nursing implications of Lasix and Aldactone.

(1) The potassium level is below normal (3.5–5.0 mEq/L). Lasix is a potassium-wasting diuretic. Aldactone is a potassium-sparing diuretic. There is no reason to hold the Aldactone because the patient has a low potassium level. Eliminate this answer.

(2) The Aldactone should be administered.

(3) Do not administer the Lasix since it is a potassium-wasting diuretic. The patient's potassium level is already low. Eliminate.

(4) Do not administer the Lasix. Eliminate.

The correct answer is (2).

Let's try this next question.

A 45-year-old man returns to the clinic two weeks after being started on allopurinol (Zyloprim) 200 mg PO daily. The nurse reviews information about this medication with the patient. Which statement by the patient indicates that the teaching was effective?

(1) "I should take my medication on an empty stomach."
(2) "I should take my medication with orange juice."
(3) "I should increase my intake of protein."
(4) "I should drink at least eight glasses of water every day."

To answer this question you need to know information about Zyloprim, an antigout agent that reduces uric acid.

(1) Zyloprim is best tolerated with or immediately after meals to reduce GI irritation. Eliminate.

(2) Orange juice makes the urine acidic. Zyloprim is more soluble in alkaline urine. Eliminate.

(3) It is not necessary to increase the intake of protein when taking Zyloprim. Eliminate.

(4) Zyloprim can cause renal calculi. The patient should drink 3,000 ml/day to reduce the risk of kidney stone formation.

The correct answer is (4). You must know medications for the NCLEX.

Notify the Physician

The Buck Stops Here

Don't pass the buck on the NCLEX.

Another behavior that commonly occurs in the real world is calling the physician. In nursing school you were encouraged to notify your instructor of changes in your patient's condition. Be very careful how you handle this on the NCLEX. More often than not, the answer choice that states "call the physician, contact the social worker, or refer to the chaplain" is the WRONG answer. Usually there is something you need to do first before you make that call. NCLEX does not want to know what the physician is going to do. NCLEX wants to know what you, the registered professional nurse, will do in a given situation.

Answer this question.

A 53-year-old man is receiving packed red blood cells. Several minutes after the infusion is started, he complains of itching and develops hives on his chest and abdomen. Which of the following actions should the nurse take first?	(1) Slow down the rate of the transfusion. (2) Call the physician for an order for an antihistamine. (3) Mix IV fluid with the blood to dilute it. (4) Stop the transfusion.

THE REWORDED QUESTION: What should you do first for this patient? It sounds like the patient is having an allergic reaction to the transfusion. If this is what's going on, what should you do?

(1) If the patient is having a transfusion reaction, slowing down the rate of the transfusion is not the right action.

(2) Antihistamines are given for allergic reactions. The doctor needs to be notified. This answer might be a possibility, but is there something you should do first?

(3) Mixing IV fluids with blood is done to decrease the viscosity of RBCs. This doesn't have anything to do with an allergic transfusion reaction. Eliminate.

(4) If the patient was having a transfusion reaction, the best action is to stop the transfusion. This is the correct action to take first, before the physician is called.

The correct answer is (4). After the transfusion is stopped, you will contact the physician and antihistamines will probably be ordered.

Before you want to choose the answer choice that involves "call the physician," look at the other answer choices very carefully. Make sure that there isn't an answer that contains an assessment or action you should do before making the phone call.

Here is one last "real world" question:

Hold the Phone

Think before calling the physician in an NCLEX answer. The test-makers want to know what *you* would do in a situation, not what the doctor would do!

> Upon returning from lunch the nurse is approached in the elevator by a hospital employee from another unit. The employee states that her close friend is a patient on the nurse's unit. The employee asks how her friend is doing and if all of her tests were normal. The nurse should
>
> (1) answer the employee's questions softly so other people on the elevator will not hear.
> (2) refuse to discuss her friend's medical condition. Suggest that she visit her friend.
> (3) give the employee the name of the patient's physician to call for this information.
> (4) tell the employee about the results of the patient's tests since they were within normal limits.

THE QUESTION: What should a nurse do when asked about a patient by a hospital employee?

(1) Discussing patient information in a public place is a breach of confidentiality. Eliminate.

(2) This does not violate the patient's right to privacy and confidentiality. Keep in consideration.

(3) Providing any information about a patient to someone not directly involved in the patient's care is a breach of privacy. Eliminate.

(4) It is a breach in the patient's right to privacy to share information with others without the patient's permission. Eliminate.

The correct answer is (2).

Expect to see real-world situations on your NCLEX, but make sure that you do not choose real world answers! These strategies should help you use your previous nursing experience without encountering any pitfalls.

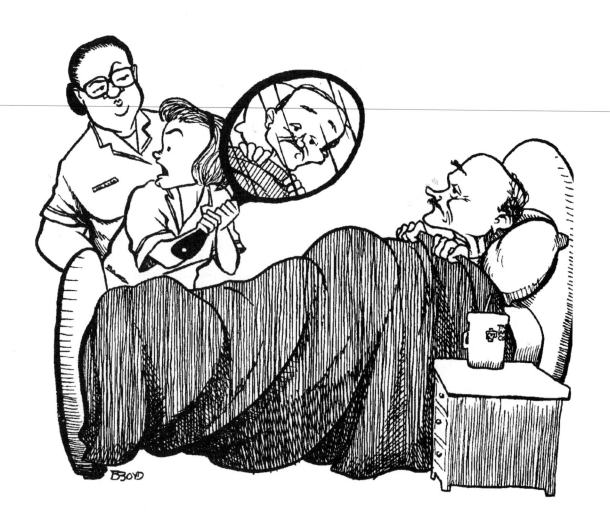

"You SAID 'reflect their feelings!'"

CHAPTER SIX

Therapeutic Communication

What kind of thoughts do you have when you read the words, *therapeutic communication*? Are they: *"No big deal. Those questions are really easy for me,"* or *"Yuck! Not therapeutic communication. I hate those questions!"*

No matter what your response is to therapeutic communication, you are familiar with the topic. After all, you were drilled in therapeutic communication throughout nursing school because communication is essential in order to be a safe and effective nurse. On the job, you must be able to communicate effectively with your clients, family members, significant others, and other members of the health care team. Communicating therapeutically is emphasized on the NCLEX because it is critical to your success as a beginning practitioner.

Therapeutic communication means listening to and understanding the client while promoting clarification and insight. It enables the nurse to form a working relationship with both the patient and peers, using both verbal and nonverbal communication. Remember that nonverbal communication is the most accurate reflection of attitude.

Therapeutic responses include those found on the next page.

RESPONSE	GOAL/PURPOSE
Using silence	Allows the client time to think and reflect; conveys acceptance. Allows the client to take the lead in conversation.
Using general leads or broad opening	Encourages the client to talk. Indicates your interest in the client. Allows the client to choose the subject.
Clarification	Encourages recall and details of a particular experience. Encourages description of feelings. Seeks explanation; pinpoints specifics.
Reflecting	Paraphrases what client says. Reflects on what client says, especially the feelings conveyed.

There are many questions on the NCLEX that require you to select the correct therapeutic communication response. As with other answer choices on the NCLEX, you must select the BEST answer from:

- Four answer choices that you believe all are correct.

- Four answer choices that you believe all are wrong.

Using the following strategies will help you select the correct answers.

HOW TO SELECT THE CORRECT THERAPEUTIC COMMUNICATION ANSWER

Eliminate!

Do not look for the correct response. Instead, eliminate the wrong answers.

Use this strategy:

Step 1. Use the following strategies to eliminate answer choices.

Step 2. If there is more than one response left, identify the answer choice that reflects feelings and provides information.

Strategies for Therapeutic Communication

As with other NCLEX questions, one of the biggest errors that students commit when trying to answer therapeutic communication is to *look for the correct answer*. Remember, you are selecting the *best* answer from the four possible answers that you are given. To select the *best* answer, you must eliminate responses.

Use these strategies to eliminate answer choices:

Authoritarian Answers

Eliminate answer choices in which the nurse is telling the patient what to do without regard to the patient's desires or feelings. Examples include:

- Insisting that the patient follow unit rules.
- Insisting that the patient do what you command, immediately.

Close-Ended Questions

Eliminate close-ended questions that can be answered with the words *yes, no,* or another monosyllabic response. Close-ended questions discourage the client from sharing thoughts and feelings. Examples include:

- "Are you feeling guilty about what happened?"
- "How many children do you have?"

"Why" Questions

Eliminate responses that are "why" questions: ones that seek reasons or justification. "Why" questions imply disapproval of the patient who may become defensive. A "why" question can come in many forms and need not always begin with "why." Any response that puts the patient on the defensive is nontherapeutic and therefore incorrect. Some examples of "why" responses:

- "What makes you think that?"
- "Why do you feel this way?"

"Let's Explore" Questions

Another incorrect answer choice that many graduate nurses select is the choice that includes the word "explore." On the NCLEX, avoid being a junior psychiatrist. It isn't the nurse's role to delve into the reasons why the patient is feeling a particular way. The patient must be allowed to

Why Ask Why?

Remember, don't ask why!

verbalize the fact that he or she is sad, angry, fearful, or overwhelmed. Some examples of "let's explore" responses:

- "Let's talk about why you didn't take your medication."
- "Tell me why you *really* injured yourself."

"Don't Worry" Questions

Eliminate answer choices that offer false reassurance. These responses would discourage communication between the nurse and the patient by not allowing the patient to explore his or her own ideas and feelings. False reassurance also discounts what the patient is feeling. Some examples:

- "It is going to be OK."
- "Don't worry. Your doctors will do everything necessary for your care."

Nurse-Focused Answers

Eliminate all answer choices if the focus of the comment is on the nurse. Be careful, because these answer choices may sound very empathetic. The focus of your communication should always be on the patient. Examples of responses to avoid:

- "That happened to me once."
- "I know from experience this is hard for you."

Using these types of nontherapeutic responses to eliminate possible answer choices is a very effective way of answering therapeutic communication questions. Don't simply look for the specific words that you see here; you may need to "translate" the answer choices into the above errors of therapeutic communication.

Using the Process of Elimination

How do you select the correct response? By choosing whatever response is left! The correct response will usually contain one or both of the following elements:

Give correct information. Offering information encourages further communication from the client. Examples of giving correct information include:

- "You are experiencing acute alcohol withdrawal; you may see and feel things that aren't real."
- "There are many reasons for memory loss; tell me more about what you have noticed."

This Isn't About You

Focus on the *client*, not on the nurse.

Be empathetic and reflect the patient's feelings. *Empathy* is the ability to perceive what another person experiences using that person's frame of reference. Reflection communicates to the patient that the nurse has heard and understands what the patient is trying to communicate. When reflecting feelings, the nurse focuses on the feelings and not the content of what is said. Examples of empathetic, reflective statements:

- "I can see that you are frightened about being here, but I'm a nurse in a hospital."
- "You seem very upset. Tell me how you're feeling."

Let's practice these strategies on NCLEX-style test questions.

A 50-year-old woman is admitted to the emergency room with a diagnosis of acute myocardial infarction. She tells the nurse, "I'm scared, I think I'm going to die." Which of the following responses by the nurse would be MOST appropriate?	(1) "Everything is going to be fine. We'll take good care of you." (2) "I know what you mean. I thought I was having a heart attack once." (3) "I'll call your doctor, so you can discuss it." (4) "It's normal to feel frightened. We're doing everything we can for you."

Step 1. Eliminate incorrect answer choices using the strategies.

(1) This is a "don't worry" response. There is no acknowledgment of the patient's fears. Eliminate it.

(2) The focus of this response is on the nurse, not the patient. Eliminate it.

(3) It is within the scope of nursing practice for the nurse to respond to the patient's feelings. Don't pass the buck. Eliminate it.

(4) Responds to feeling and provides information.

Step 2. One answer was not eliminated: (4). This is the correct answer. The nurse acknowledges that the patient feels frightened and provides information.

A Word from Harry Truman

Don't pass the buck. Know what is within the scope of the RN's responsibilities.

That wasn't so bad, right? Let's try another question.

A 28-year-old mother of two children is to undergo a breast biopsy. She tells the nurse, "If lose my breast, I know my husband will no longer find me attractive." Which of the following responses, by the nurse, would be MOST appropriate?	(1) "You don't know if you are going to lose your breast. They are just doing the biopsy now." (2) "You should focus on your children. They are young and they need you." (3) "You seem to be concerned that your relationship with your husband might change." (4) "Why don't you wait and see what your husband's reaction is before you get upset."

This Isn't the Army

Don't be authoritarian.

Step 1. Eliminate answers.

(1) This response gives false reassurance and discounts the patient's feelings. Eliminate it.

(2) This response is authoritarian: the nurse tells the patient what to do. Eliminate it.

(3) This response reflects the fears of the patient. The response is open-ended and allows the patient to express what she is feeling. Keep it in for consideration.

(4) This response dismisses the feelings that the patient is experiencing and gives advice. Eliminate it.

Step 2. You have eliminated 3 answer choices. The correct answer is (3).

Try one more question.

A patient in the psychiatric unit asks the nurse, "Am I in a special radioactive shelter? When was it last checked for radioactivity?" Which of the following responses, if made by the nurse, would be MOST appropriate?	(1) "This is a hospital, and we do not have a nuclear medicine department here." (2) "Don't worry, you're safe. There's no radioactivity here." (3) "I'm sure your safety is of concern to you, but this is a hospital." (4) "Please share with me what makes you think there is radioactivity here."

KAPLAN

Step 1. Eliminate answer choices.

(1) This response provides information. Leave it in for consideration.

(2) This response offers false reassurances. Eliminate it.

(3) This response reflects the patient's concern about safety and provides information. Keep it in for consideration.

(4) This response allows the patient to verbalize, but you don't want to encourage a patient with psych problems to talk about hallucinations or delusions. Rather, you want your discussion to focus on the feelings that accompany them. Eliminate it.

Step 2. You still have more than one response. Go on to Step 3.

Step 3. Reread (1) and (3). Look for the answer choice that reflects feelings and gives information.

The correct answer is (3).

Some things to remember about selecting correct responses to therapeutic communication questions are:

- No matter how confident you are about an answer choice, read all of the choices before selecting a response.
- Even if you would never say any of the responses given, choose the "textbook" answer.
- When you first read the responses, don't look for the correct response. Always eliminate answers first.

If you follow the Kaplan strategies for therapeutic communication, you will be able to select the correct answers to this question type on the NCLEX.

Treat It Like a Contract

Read *all* choices before selecting the correct answer.

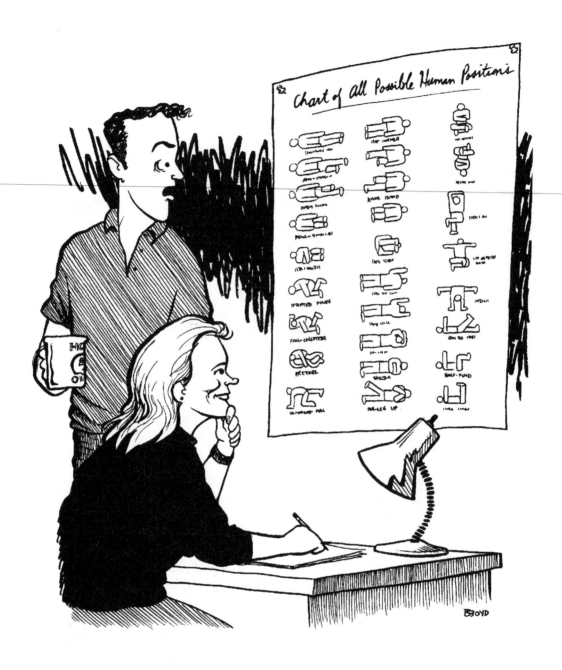

"'PROMOTE'!? I'd think you would want to PREVENT some of these!!"

CHAPTER SEVEN

Questions on Positioning

The nurse cares for a 38-year old-man after an appendectomy. The patient continues to complain of discomfort to the nurse shortly after receiving an analgesic. Which of the following measures, if taken by the nurse, would be MOST appropriate?

(1) Notify the physician.
(2) Place him in Fowler's position.
(3) Massage his abdomen.
(4) Provide him with reading material.

How do you feel about answer choices that involve positioning? Many graduate nurses are not comfortable answering these questions because:

- They don't understand the "whys" of positioning
- They don't know the terminology
- They have difficulty imaging the various positions

Since many illnesses affect body alignment and mobility, you must be able to safely care for these patients in order to be an effective nurse. Correspondingly, these topics are also important on the NCLEX. The successful test taker must correctly answer questions about impaired mobility and positioning.

Immobility occurs when a patient is unable to move about freely and independently. To answer questions on positioning, you need to know the hazards of immobility, normal anatomy and physiology, and the terminology for positioning.

Assume the Position, Please

Positioning is important for the NCLEX.

Strategies for Positioning Questions

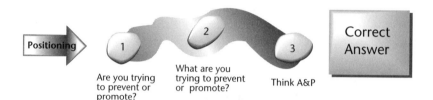

What's That Word Again?

Know your terminology.

If you have difficulty answering positioning questions, the following strategy with assist you in selecting the correct answer.

Step 1. Decide if the position for the patient is designed to prevent something or promote something.

Step 2. Identify what it is that you are trying to prevent or promote.

Step 3. Think about anatomy, physiology, and pathophysiology.

Step 4. Which position best accomplishes what you are trying to prevent or promote?

Prevent or Promote?

When positioning a patient, decide what you are trying to *prevent* or *promote*.

Does this sound a little confusing? Hang in there. Let's walk through a question using this strategy.

Immediately after a percutaneous liver biopsy, the nurse should place the patient in which of the following positions?	(1) Supine. (2) Right side-lying. (3) Left side-lying. (4) Semi-Fowler's.

Before you read the answers, let's go through the four steps outlined above.

Step 1. By positioning the patient after a liver biopsy, are you trying to prevent something or promote something? Answer: You position a patient after this procedure to prevent something.

Step 2. What are you trying to prevent? Answer: The most serious and important complication after a percutaneous liver biopsy is hemorrhage. How did you know that you are trying to prevent hemorrhage? You accessed what you know about a liver biopsy.

Step 3. Think about principles of anatomy, physiology, and pathophysiology. What do you do to prevent hemorrhage? Answer: You apply pressure. Where would you apply pressure? On the liver. Where is the liver? On the right side of the abdomen under the ribs.

Step 4. How should the patient be positioned to prevent hemorrhage from the liver, which is on the right side of the body?

Now look at your answer choices.

(1) "Supine." If you lay the patient flat on his back, no pressure will be applied to the right side. Eliminate.
(2) "Right side-lying." If you lay the patient in a right side-lying position, will pressure be applied to the right side? Yes. Keep it in for consideration.
(3) "Left side-lying." No pressure is applied to the right side. Eliminate.
(4) "Semi-Fowler's." If you lay the patient on his back with head partially elevated, no pressure is applied to the right side. Eliminate.

The correct answer is (2). Some students select (3) because they don't know normal anatomy and physiology. Some students select (4) because semi-Fowler's position is used for a lot of reasons.

Things to Remember

- Even if you didn't memorize what position to use before, during, and after a procedure, *think about the question for a moment.* You can figure out what position is needed.
- You cannot figure out the correct position if you do not know what the terms mean (supine, Trendelenburg, Fowler's).
- You cannot figure out a correct position if you do not know anatomy and physiology. If you think the liver is on the left side of the body, you are in trouble!
- You cannot figure out a correct position if you do not know what you are trying to accomplish. If you couldn't remember that a complication after a liver biopsy is hemorrhage, your best hope of selecting the correct answer would be to throw a dart.
- To those students who think in images, you should form a mental image of each position. Picture yourself placing the patient in each position, and then see if the position makes sense.

Picture It

Visualize the position!

Let's try another question using the strategies for positioning.

An angiogram is scheduled for a 52-year-old woman with decreased circulation in her right leg. After the angiogram, the nurse should place the patient in which of the following positions?	(1) Semi-Fowler's with right leg bent at the knee. (2) Side-lying with a pillow between her knees. (3) Supine with her right leg extended. (4) High-Fowler's with her right leg elevated.

Let's go through the steps.

Step 1. By positioning the patient after an angiogram, are you trying to prevent something or promote something? Answer: You are trying to promote something.

Step 2. What are you trying to promote? Answer: Adequate circulation of right leg.

Step 3. Think about your principles of anatomy, physiology, and pathophysiology. What promotes adequate circulation in the right leg? Answer: Don't constrict blood flow. Keep the leg at or below the level of the heart.

Step 4. How will the patient be positioned after an angiography to prevent constriction of vessels and keep the right leg at or below the level of the heart?

Look at the answer choices.

(1) "Semi-Fowler's with the right leg bent at knee." The head of the bed is elevated 30° to 45° in this position. The leg is lower than the heart. If the right leg is bent at the knee, this could constrict arterial blood flow. Eliminate.

(2) "Side-lying with a pillow between her knees." Use of a pillow in this position could create pressure points in the right leg. You don't want the knees bent. Eliminate.

(3) "Supine with leg extended." In this position, the leg is at the level of the heart. Circulation will not be constricted because the leg is straight. Keep this answer in for consideration.

(4) "High-Fowler's with her right leg elevated." The head of the bed is elevated 60° to 90° in this position. Elevating the leg promotes venous return. Eliminate.

The correct answer is (3). The patient is on bedrest for eight to twelve hours in a supine position after an angiogram.

Wasn't that easy? If you didn't know the specific positioning needed after an arteriogram, you can apply your knowledge to select the correct answer *by just thinking about it.*

Are you ready for another question?

The nurse cares for a 36-year-old woman after a lumbar laminectomy. Which of the following statements BEST describes the method of turning a patient following a lumbar laminectomy?	(1) The head of the bed is elevated 30°; the patient locks her knees when turning. (2) A pillow is placed between the patient's legs; her body is turned as a unit. (3) The patient straightens her back and grasps the side rail on the opposite side of the bed. (4) The head of the bed is flat; the patient bends her knees and rolls to the side.

O.K. Lumbar laminectomy. This question isn't about positioning after a procedure. It asks how to turn the patient after surgery. Let's see if the strategy for positioning works.

Step 1. When turning the patient after a laminectomy, are you trying to prevent or promote something? Answer: promote.

Step 2. What are you trying to promote? Answer: a straight back. The patient can't bend or twist the torso.

Step 3. Think about the principles of anatomy, physiology, and pathophysiology. A laminectomy is removal of one or more vertebral laminae. After a laminectomy, the back should be kept straight.

Step 4. How should the patient be turned in order to keep the back straight?

(1) If the head of the bed is elevated 30°, the back will not be straight. Eliminate.

(2) If a pillow is placed between the legs and the body is rolled as a unit, the patient's back will be kept straight. Keep in for consideration.

(3) If the patient grabs the opposite side rail, the patient's torso will twist. The back will not be straight even though the patient straightened her back before turning and twisting. Eliminate.

(4) If the head of the bed is flat, patient's back will be straight. If the patient bends her knees and rolls to her side, her back will not be kept straight. Eliminate.

The correct answer is (2). That is a textbook description of log rolling. But, if you didn't recall log rolling, you were able to select the correct answers by thoughtfully considering each answer choice.

Practice this strategy on positioning questions. Positioning is an important part of the NCLEX. You must be able to correctly answer these questions in order to prove your competence. If you use this strategy, you will be thinking about your nursing principles and you will select correct answers!

Would you like to know the answer to the first question?

The nurse cares for a 38-year-old man after an appendectomy. The patient continues to complain of discomfort to the nurse shortly after receiving an analgesic. Which of the following measures, if taken by the nurse, would be MOST appropriate?	(1) Notify the physician. (2) Place him in Fowler's position. (3) Massage his abdomen. (4) Provide him with reading material.

As you can see, not all of the answer choices involve positioning. Use strategies that are appropriate to other answer choices.

THE REWORDED QUESTION: What should the nurse do to help this patient with pain relief?

(1) Calling the doctor is passing the buck. See if there isn't another answer choice that is more appropriate.

(2) Fowler's position. Why change this patient's position? To promote pain relief. Will Fowler's position decrease the patient's pain? Yes, by relieving pressure on the patient's abdomen. This answer is a possibility.

(3) Massaging his abdomen will increase the patient's pain. Eliminate.

(4) Providing him with reading materials might distract him from his discomfort, but this is not an appropriate intervention for a patient in pain. Eliminate.

The correct answer is (2).

Practice the positioning strategy and you will select more right answers!

Essential Positions to Know for the NCLEX

Don't Just Play Twister

Know when and why certain positions are used.

Position	Therapeutic Function
Flat (supine)	Avoids hip flexion, which can compress arterial flow.
Dorsal recumbent	Supine with knees flexed; more comfortable.
Side lateral	Allows drainage of oral secretions.
Side with leg bent (Sim's)	Allows drainage of oral secretions; decreases abdominal tension.
Head elevated (Fowler's)	Increases venous return; allows maximal lung expansion. High Fowler's: 60 to 90 degrees Fowler's: 45 to 60 degrees Semi-Fowler's: 30 to 45 degrees Low Fowler's: 15 to 30 degrees
Feet and legs elevated	Increases blood return to heart; relieves pressure on lumbrosacral area.

Feet elevated and head lowered (Trendelenburg's)	Used to insert CVP line, or for treatment of umbilical cord compression.
Feet elevated 20 degrees, knees straight, trunk flat, and head slightly elevated (modified Trendelenburg's)	Increases venous return; used for shock.
Elevation of extremity	Increases venous return. Increases blood volume to extremity.
Flat on back, thighs flexed, legs abducted (lithotomy)	Increases vaginal opening for examination.
Prone	Promotes extension of hip joint. Not well tolerated by persons with respiratory or cardiovascular difficulties.
Knee-chest	Provides maximal visualization of rectal area.

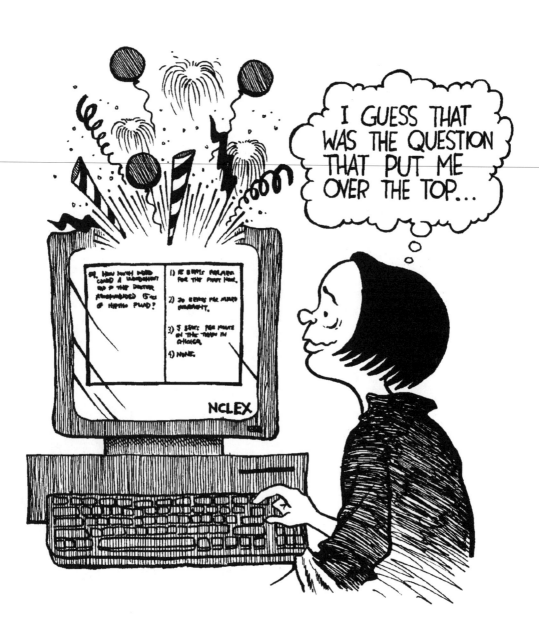

CHAPTER EIGHT

Management of Care

A 7-year-old boy with a compound fracture of the left femur is being admitted to a pediatric unit. Which of the following actions is best for the nurse to take?	(1) Ask the nursing assistant to obtain the child's vital signs while the nurse obtains a history from the parents. (2) Ask the LPN/LVN to assess the peripheral pulses of the child's left leg while the nurse completes the admission forms. (3) Ask the LPN/LVN to stay with the child and his parents while the nurse obtains phone orders from the physician. (4) Ask the nursing assistant to obtain equipment for the child's care while the nurse talks with the child and his parents.

You may be thinking, "Why are they asking me this? I've never had the opportunity to ask the LPN/LVN or nursing assistant to do anything!"

Every three years, the National Council of State Boards of Nursing conducts a job analysis study to determine the activities required of a newly licensed registered nurse. Based on this study, National Council adjusts the content of the test to accurately reflect what is happening in the workplace. This ensures that the NCLEX tests what is needed to be a safe and effective nurse.

With the recent changes in health care, the role of the nurse has expanded. In addition to providing quality patient care, the nurse is also responsible for coordination and supervision of care provided by other health care workers. Many health care settings are staffed by registered nurses, licensed vocational nurses/licensed practical nurses (LVN/LPN), and

Who's In Charge Here?

The NCLEX contains questions about delegation and supervision. Even if you have no direct experience in these areas, the Rules of Management will get you through the test.

unlicensed assistive personnel (UAP) such as nursing assistants and support staff. It is the responsibility of the registered nurse to coordinate the efforts of these health care workers to provide affordable quality patient care. Appropriate supervision of LPN/LVN and/or unlicensed assistive personnel by the registered professional nurse is essential for safe and effective patient care. To reflect these changes, the NCLEX test plan now contains questions about delegation and assignment of patient care.

There are several reasons why you may find these questions difficult to correctly answer on the NCLEX. You might not have any practice answering multiple-choice test questions about management. Many nursing schools test the content presented in the management course with essay questions rather than multiple-choice questions. You have received lectures regarding management of care, but your clinical rotation in management may have been less than ideal. Your experience may have been restricted to caring for one or two patients without any opportunity to supervise others, or you may have spent time on a hospital unit providing patient care under the supervision of a preceptor. These experiences don't necessarily prepare you to answer the management of care questions you will see on the NCLEX.

Don't despair! Here are some rules of management that will help you choose more right answers when answering management of care questions on the NCLEX.

The Rules of Management

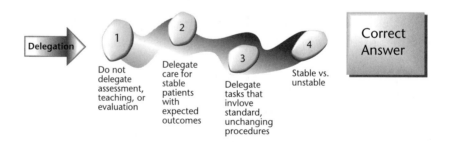

Rule #1: *Do not delegate the functions of assessment, evaluation, and nursing judgment.* During your nursing education, you learned that assessment, evaluation, and nursing judgment are the responsibility of the registered professional nurse. You *cannot* give this responsibility to someone else.

Rule #2: *This is not the real world.* Do not make decisions regarding management of care issues based on decisions you may have observed during your clinical experience in the hospital or clinic setting. Remember, the NCLEX is ivory-tower nursing. The answers to the questions are found in nursing textbooks or journals. Always ask yourself, "Is this textbook nursing care?"

Rule #3: *Delegate activities for stable patients with predictable outcomes.* If the patient is unstable, or the outcome of an activity not assured, it should not be delegated.

Rule #4: *Delegate activities that involve standard, unchanging procedures.* Activities that frequently reoccur in daily patient care can be delegated. Bathing, feeding, dressing, and transferring patients are examples. Activities that are complex or complicated should *not* be delegated.

Rule #5: *Remember priorities!* Remember Maslow, the ABCs, and stable versus unstable when determining which patient the RN should attend to first. Keep in the mind that you can see only *one* patient or perform *one* activity when answering questions that require you to establish priorities.

Let's take a closer look at the question above and use these rules to eliminate answer choices.

A 7-year-old boy with a compound fracture of the left femur is being admitted to a pediatric unit. Which of the following actions is best for the nurse to take?	(1) Ask the nursing assistant to obtain the child's vital signs while the nurse obtains a history from the parents.
	(2) Ask the LPN/LVN to assess the peripheral pulses of the child's left leg while the nurse completes the admission forms.
	(3) Ask the LPN/LVN to stay with the child and his parents while the nurse obtains phone orders from the physician.
	(4) Ask the nursing assistant to obtain equipment for the child's care while the nurse talks with the child and his parents.

On first glance, all the answers seem possible. Let's look at this question using the steps outlined in this book.

Step 1. Reword the question in your own words. It asks what the nurse should do when a child with a fractured femur is first admitted. That question is very broad. To establish *exactly* what is being asked, you must read the answer choices. In each answer, the RN is delegating tasks to the LPN/LVN or nursing assistant. The real question is, "What is appropriate delegation?"

Step 2. Eliminate answer choices based on the Rules of Management.

It's Your Job

Do not delegate assessment. Assessing the patient is *your* job!

(1) Ask the nursing assistant to obtain the child's vital signs while the nurse obtains a history from the parents. Obtaining vital signs is an important part of assessment. According to Rule #1, the registered nurse cannot delegate assessment. Eliminate this answer choice.

(2) Ask the LPN/LVN to assess the peripheral pulses of the child's left leg while the nurse completes the admission forms. Checking the peripheral pulses is an important assessment for this patient because of the diagnosis of a fractured left femur. The nurse needs to assess the patient before delegating activities to someone else. Assessment of the patient is much more important than completing paperwork. Eliminate it.

(3) Ask the LPN/LVN to stay with the child and his parents while the nurse obtains phone orders from the physician. There is no assessment, evaluation or nursing judgment involved in this option so leave it in for consideration.

(4) Ask the nursing assistant to obtain equipment for the child's care while the nurse talks with the child and his parents. The nurse is with the child and his parents while the nursing assistant obtains needed equipment. There is no assessment, evaluation, or nursing judgment when gathering equipment, so leave this choice in for consideration.

You are left with answer choices (3) and (4). You are halfway to the correct answer. Can you apply Rule #2—this is not the real world—to eliminate another answer choice?

Remember, you shouldn't make decisions on management of care issues based on what you may have seen done in the hospital or clinic setting. Answer #3 indicates that the nurse is on the phone and the LPN/LVN is with the patient. Have you seen this done in the real world? Probably. Is this what nursing textbooks and journals say should be done in this situation? Probably not. Eliminate it.

The correct answer is (4). The nurse is caring for the child and his parents while the nursing assistant goes to get something. Remember, the emphasis on the NCLEX is placed on providing care to patients according to how nursing care is defined in textbooks and journals.

Here is another management of care question.

Which of the following tasks is appropriate for the nurse to delegate to an experienced nursing assistant?	(1) Obtain a 24-hour diet recall from a patient recently admitted with anorexia nervosa. (2) Obtain a clean catch urine specimen from a patient suspected of having a urinary tract infection. (3) Observe the amount and characteristics of the returns from a continuous bladder irrigation for a patient after a transuretheral resection. (4) Observe a patient newly diagnosed with diabetes mellitus practice injection techniques using an orange.

Step 1. Reword the question. "Which task will you assign to a nursing assistant?" The fact that a nursing assistant is "experienced" is a distracter. Do not fall for this trap! Just answer the question.

Step 2. Eliminate answer choices using the Rules of Management.

(1) Obtain a 24-hour diet recall from a patient recently admitted with anorexia nervosa. Some students may consider this answer choice because eating is certainly a recurring daily activity, but this answer isn't about feeding a patient. Eating has special significance for a patient with anorexia nervosa. An important assessment that the nurse must make is the quantity of food consumed by this patient. The nurse cannot delegate assessment. Eliminate this answer choice.

(2) Obtain a clean catch urine specimen from a patient suspected of having an urinary tract infection. Rule # 4 states, "Delegate activities that involve standard, unchanging procedures." There is no indication that the patient has a catheter so this is a routine procedure. Keep it in for consideration.

Keep Your Focus!

The NCLEX is all about caring for patients.

(3) Observe the amount and characteristics of the returns from a continuous bladder irrigation for a patient after a transuretheral resection. The color of the fluid needs to be assessed to determine if hemorrhage is occurring. This is an assessment. Eliminate this answer choice.

(4) Observe a patient newly diagnosed with diabetes mellitus practice injection techniques using an orange. This answer choice involves the evaluation of patient teaching. According to Rule #1, the nurse cannot delegate evaluation of patient care. This choice should be eliminated.

That leaves only answer choice (2), the correct answer.

Let's try one more question.

Which of the following patients should the nurse on a pediatric unit assign to a LPN/LVN?	1) A 3-year-old girl admitted yesterday with larnygotracheogronchitis who has a tracheostomy. 2) A 5-year-old girl admitted after gastric lavage for Tylenol ingestion. 3) A 6-year-old boy admitted for a fracture of the femur in balanced suspension traction. 4) A 10-year-old boy admitted for observation after an acute asthmatic attack.

What Should You Do First?

Establish priorities.

Step 1. Reword the question in your own words. The question is asking for the appropriate assignment for a LPN/LVN.

Step 2. Eliminate answer choices using the Rules of Management. Remember, "Delegate activities for stable patients with predictable outcomes."

(1) A 3-year-old girl admitted yesterday with larnygotracheobronchitis who has a tracheostomy. Ask yourself, is this a stable patient with a predictable outcome? A 3 year-old with a new tracheostomy is not stable or predictable. Eliminate this answer choice.

(2) A 5-year-old girl admitted after gastric lavage for Tylenol ingestion. This child may be unstable and the outcome is of a poisoning is unpredictable. Eliminate this answer choice.

(3) A 6-year-old boy admitted for a fracture of the femur in balanced suspension traction. This child has a problem that has a predictable outcome. No information is provided in the choice to lead you to believe that this child is unstable at this time. Keep this answer choice in consideration.

(4) A 10-year-old boy admitted for observation after an acute asthmatic attack. Because of the narrow airway of a child, this child may be unstable and the outcome is unpredictable. Eliminate this answer choice.

Answer choice (3) is the correct answer.

Establishing Priority

Is this getting easier for you? Let's try a couple of more questions with a slightly different focus: priority. Many students are uncomfortable with these types of questions because more than one answer looks right.

A home care nurse is planning her visits for the day. Which of the following patients should the nurse visit first?	(1) A 62-year-old man two days after an inguinal hernia repair. (2) A 40-year-old woman with type 1 diabetes mellitus (IDDM) with a foot ulcer. (3) A 76-year-old man with chronic obstructive pulmonary disease (COPD). (4) A 50-year-old woman three days after a right mastectomy.

Step 1. Reword the question in your own words. This question is a priority question: Which patient takes highest priority? As with all priority questions, more than one answer will seem correct.

Step 2. Eliminate answers using the Rules of Management.

(1) A 62-year-old man two days after an inguinal hernia repair. There is nothing stated that leads you to believe that this patient is unstable. Usually, recovery from hernia repairs are uneventful. Eliminate this answer.

(2) A 40-year-old woman with type 1 diabetes mellitus (IDDM) with a foot ulcer. Impaired circulation is a complication of diabetes, and this client's situation is potentially unstable. Leave this in for consideration.

(3) A 76-year-old man with chronic obstructive pulmonary disease (COPD). While this client has a chronic condition that requires close monitoring by the nurse, there is no indication of an acute situation. Eliminate this answer.

(4) A 50-year-old woman three days after a right mastectomy. This is a relatively new postop client that has the potential for major complications. This patient should be assessment by the nurse. Leave this in for consideration.

You are now choosing from answers (2) and (4). Which client do you consider the least stable? The correct answer is (4). Remember, the *only* way to answer priority questions correctly is to eliminate answer choices. It is too difficult to just pick the correct answer from four answer choices.

Let's look at one more question.

After receiving a report from the night nurse, which of the following patients should the nurse see first?	(1) A 31-year-old woman refusing Carafate before breakfast. (2) A 40-year-old man with left-sided weakness asking for assistance to the bedside commode. (3) A 52-year-old woman complaining of chills who is scheduled for a cholecystectomy. (4) A 65-year-old man with a nasogastric tube who had a bowel resection yesterday.

Step 1. Reword the question in your own words. This question asks, "Who is the highest priority for the nurse?"

Step 2. Eliminate answers using the Rules of Management.

(1) A 31-year-old woman refusing Carafate before breakfast. You're not told what's wrong with this patient or why she's receiving Carafate, but this patient is probably not the priority. Let's look at the other answers.

(2) A 40-year-old man with left-sided weakness asking for assistance to the bedside commode. This can certainly be a messy situation if not attended to in a timely manner, but assisting a patient to the bedside commode does not require a registered professional nurse. Eliminate this answer.

(3) A 52-year-old woman complaining of chills who is scheduled for a cholecystectomy. This is an unstable situation since chills are indicative of an infectious process and the patient is scheduled for surgery. Leave this answer in for consideration.

(4) A 65-year-old man with a nasogastric tube who had a bowel resection yesterday. A patient who is one day into postop certainly has the potential for complications even though none are indicated. Leave this in for consideration.

You can now choose between answers (3) and (4). Which patient is the highest priority? The woman is complaining of chills and is scheduled for surgery. This patient has a problem that requires the immediate attention of the RN.

Although you may still feel slightly uncomfortable when answering management questions, continue to practice answering questions using the Rules of Management. You will choose more correct answers!

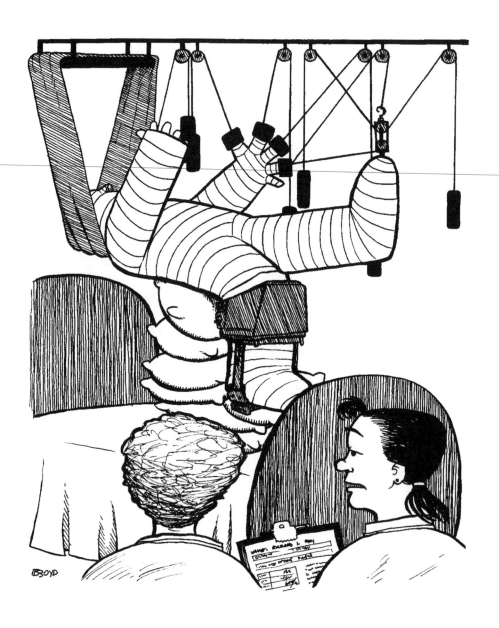

"I hope I don't see this on the NCLEX!"

CHAPTER NINE

"It Sounds Great, but . . ."

Now that you've read about the Kaplan Critical Thinking Strategies, you are probably thinking, "Wow! This is great!" Most of you have started identifying why you are having difficulty answering application/analysis-level test questions. Some of you have already formulated a plan to master your NCLEX questions using the strategies outlined in this book, and are confident that you *will* pass the NCLEX. Others are thinking, "This sounds great, but can I really answer questions using these strategies?" Let's talk about some of the questions that you may be asking yourself.

Question: "I'm terrible at standardized tests. Is this really going to help me?"

Answer: Yes, these strategies will help you choose more correct responses when you take the NCLEX. Read this book—more than once if necessary—to learn the strategies. Then practice, practice, practice. Use the strategies to answer many, many test questions, and you will find yourself answering more and more questions correctly. Tear out the chart in Appendix A that contains the critical thinking strategies chart and consult it while you are answering practice test questions. This will help get you comfortable with putting the strategies into practice. As you answer more and more questions, put the diagram aside and rely on your memory to identify and implement a critical thinking strategy.

Practice Makes Perfect

Practice answering test questions using the chart in Appendix A.

Question: "Am I going to have enough time when I take the NCLEX to figure out which strategy to use?"

Answer: Timing is a concern on the NCLEX. You need to maximize your efforts on each test question. Practice answering test questions using the critical thinking strategies. As you get more proficient, you will discover that it takes you less time to identify the strategy or path that will lead you to the correct answer.

Question: "I don't have to use these strategies on every question, do I? I think I'll only use them when I can't figure our the correct answer on my own."

Answer: Wrong! You should use critical thinking to answer *every* question on the NCLEX exam to make sure that you pass. Go through the steps that we have outlined for *every* practice question that you answer as you prepare for the NCLEX. If you practice these steps, you will not need to "throw a dart" to select the correct answer on the NCLEX.

Stick to the Plan

Don't "throw a dart" to select correct answers on the NCLEX.

Question: "So all I have to do is memorize the strategies, right?"

Answer: Just memorizing the critical thinking strategies will not ensure your success on NCLEX. Remember, NCLEX does *not* test your ability to memorize either critical thinking strategies or nursing content. NCLEX tests your ability to think critically and use the nursing knowledge that you have. It's relatively easy to just memorize nursing content. The hard part is to figure out how to use this knowledge to make nursing judgments. It's relatively easy to memorize the critical thinking strategies. The hard part is to figure out which strategy to use on each and every question. That takes practice.

Question: "What if I use the strategies, but still can't figure out the correct answer?"

Answer: It's not unusual that students will read a question, read the answers, and think "Huh? Something is missing!" If you feel like something is missing, reread the question to determine if you have correctly identified what the question is asking. If you have identified the question correctly, then read the answer choices to make sure that you haven't missed the nursing concept contained in the answer choices.

Question: "Will these strategies work on every practice question that I answer?"

Answer: The critical thinking strategies discussed in this book will enable you to answer all kinds of multiple-choice test questions. The critical thinking strategies apply to application/analysis-level test questions and do not work with knowledge-based test questions. If you feel that the strategies don't work with the practice questions you are answering, determine the level of difficulty of the questions you are working with. Are the practice questions knowledge based, or are they at the application/analysis level of difficulty? Remember, the majority of questions that are of a passing level of difficulty on the NCLEX are at the application/analysis level of difficulty.

Do you see a study plan developing? You need to answer questions, questions, and more questions using the Kaplan critical thinking strategies. Don't make the mistake of focusing only on content when preparing for the NCLEX exam. You are required to prove your competence on the NCLEX by answering application/analysis questions. That means that you should practice answering questions at the same level of difficulty. It's time for you to start your successful preparation for the NCLEX!

CHAPTER TEN

How to Study for the NCLEX

The authors of this book work for Kaplan, the oldest test prep company in the nation. We have been preparing graduate nurses and international nurses for the NCLEX for more than 15 years. We know what works to prepare for the NCLEX and what doesn't work. Here is some of the wisdom we've acquired.

Ineffective Ways to Prepare

Relying on False Hopes
Some students use what is knows as the "hope" method of study. "I hope that I don't have questions about chest tubes on the test." "I hope that I don't have questions about medication on my test." "I hope that I have questions about ABGs because I did great on that test in school." The "hope" method usually doesn't work very well. The test pool contains thousands of questions. How many topics do you "hope" won't be on your test?

Lacking Respect for the Exam
Many candidates for the NCLEX are good students in school. Because of their school success, they expect to pass the NCLEX with minimal preparation. After all, it's just a test of minimum competency. These students do some studying, but they really believe there is no chance they might fail this exam. You might think that you can't possibly fail, but if you do not respect this exam and prepare for it correctly, you run the risk of failure!

All students know why they take the NCLEX. But after interviewing hundreds of students, we have discovered that many graduate nurses have no idea what the exam content is. How can you effectively study for a test

Hope Springs Eternal . . . Not!

Hoping a certain topic won't be on the exam is not an effective way to prepare for the NCLEX.

R-E-S-P-E-C-T

Respect the NCLEX.

if you don't know what content the exam tests? Learn what is on the NCLEX and then you will realize that preparation with a review course or a planned method of study at home is essential.

Cramming

Some students completed nursing school with a minimal understanding of nursing content. These students studied long and hard on the night before a nursing school test, cramming as many facts into their heads as they could remember. Since the test questions primarily involved recognition and recall, cramming worked for tests in nursing school. But as we said earlier, the NCLEX is not an exam about facts. It tests your ability to apply the knowledge that you have learned and to think critically. Recognition and recall will not work!

Poor Planning

As with all standardized exams, you must work on your areas of weaknesses. This is hard to do because there's usually a reason you're weak in an area. Some graduate nurses, for example, profess a weakness in or dislike for obstetrical nursing. Some students didn't understand the theory, while other students had a poor clinical experience or didn't get to see many deliveries; still other students simply didn't like this rotation. Whatever the reason, it causes you to have a weakness in a particular area. In order to pass a standardized test, you must work on your areas of weakness.

Some students don't establish a plan of study. Other students establish a plan of study, but don't follow it. You can enroll in a review course or buy review books, but if you don't apply yourself, they will do you no good.

To pass the NCLEX you need to:

(1) Know nursing content.
(2) Be able to apply critical thinking skills.
(3) Cope with the CAT testing experience.

"All-Nighters" Won't Work

Don't cram for the NCLEX. It is not a test about recognition and recall.

You Hold the Keys

The keys to passing the NCLEX:

Nursing content
Critical thinking skills
Coping with the CAT

Effective Methods of Study

Become Knowledgeable About the NCLEX.

Find out:

- The content of the exam
- What topics are usually included on the NCLEX
- What kind of questions are asked
- How the content is organized

Identify Your Strengths and Weaknesses.

- Take as many diagnostic exams as you can.
- Identify your weaknesses in nursing content.
- Identify your weaknesses in test taking skills.

Decide If You Need to Take a Review Course.

If you decide that this is the best way for you to prepare, ask yourself these questions:

- Is the content integrated? The material should be organized according to the "Meeting the Client Needs" concept. Some review programs are still organized according to the "old" medical model of medical, surgical, psychiatric, obstetric, and pediatric nursing. This type of review won't help you put it all together for Test Day.
- Are testing strategies included? You can know everything about congestive heart failure (CHF), but if you don't know how to use this information to answer a question about CHF correctly on the NCLEX, you will have difficulty on the exam. Are the strategies useful for taking a computer adaptive test? Are the strategies specific for the NCLEX?
- Are there plenty of opportunities for practice testing? You need to prove your competence by answering NCLEX-style test questions, so you should practice answering these questions. If the exam were about opening a sterile pack, what you spend your time doing to prepare for the exam? Reading about opening a sterile pack or practicing opening a sterile pack? Are there NCLEX-style questions included in the course? Do the questions require recall and recognition of facts or application of nursing care principles? Remember, your NCLEX exam will consist mainly of application-level questions.
- What do students who have taken the course have to say about how it helped them prepare for the exam? If a review

You Can Procrastinate Later

Establish a study plan that includes working on your areas of weakness.

course boasts of a particularly high pass rate, ask to see their statistics. Be an informed consumer.

- Is there a guarantee? There are guarantees and there are empty promises. Make sure the course you are considering puts the guarantee in writing. Study the small print. Is your total tuition refunded? Do you have to fail the exam more than once?
- How much does it cost? This sounds easy, but "extras" can add up. Are there additional charges for books? Software? Registration fees?
- Is this course right for me?

Establish a Study Plan.

- Create a realistic study schedule that works for you.
- Make a vow to stick to that plan and reward yourself when you do.
- Prepare for at least three weeks before your exam date. Don't cram!
- Your content focus should be in understanding the principles of nursing care, not memorizing facts.
- Answer as many NCLEX-style test questions as possible.

Seek Help if Necessary.

If you are having difficulty, don't continue studying alone. Seek out help: a review course, a faculty advisor, or someone that is knowledgeable about the exam. They can help you identify your weaknesses, and establish a study plan to eliminate those weaknesses.

Prepare Mentally.

Stay away from people who are "prophets of doom." You know the type. With the proper preparation you can and will pass the NCLEX. Keep a positive attitude.

You may need to consider some techniques for battling stress and managing the test-day experience. Do any of these statements apply to you?

"I always freeze up on tests."
"I need to pass to get my new job, promotion, commission, etcetera."
"My best friend/girlfriend/sister/brother did really well, but I won't."
"My hospital/family/parents paid for my test prep course. They won't like it if I fail."
"I'm afraid of losing concentration."
"I'm afraid I'm not spending enough time preparing."

Know What You're Getting Into

Be prepared.

If these sound familiar, you may want to mentally prepare yourself by understanding ways to manage test stress. Forcing yourself to identify and face fears may make you edgy at first, but will significantly alleviate test stress in the long run by adding another dimension to your preparation.

Mental Preparation*

1. Visualize

You have probably learned how to do this with patients; now it's your turn. Close your eyes, sit back, and let your shoulders and arms relax. Imagine yourself escaping from the stressful world using the following steps:

Close your eyes and imagine yourself in a relaxing situation—it can be fictional, but a real-life memory is best. Make it as detailed as possible. Think about the sights, the sounds, the smells, even the tastes that you associate with the relaxing situation. Keep your eyes shut; keep sinking back into your chair. Now that you're in that situation, start bringing your test in—think about the experience of taking the test while *in* that relaxing situation. Imagine how much easier it would be if you could take your test in that situation. Notice how much easier your test seems in that situation.

Here's another variation. Close your eyes and start remembering a situation in which you did well on a test. If you can't come up with one, pick a situation in which you did some good academic work that you were really proud of, or some other kind of genuine accomplishment. Not a fiction, mind you: it has to be from real life. Make it as detailed as possible. Think about the sights, the sounds, the smells, even the tastes, that you associate with this experience of academic success. Now start thinking about your test in line with that experience. Don't make comparisons between them. Just start imagining taking your test with that same feeling of relaxed control.

2. Exercise

Whether it be jogging, walking, mild aerobics, pushups, or a pickup basketball game, physical exercise is a great way to stimulate the mind and body and improve one's ability to think and concentrate. A surprising number of those who prepare for standardized tests don't exercise regularly because they spend so much time preparing. Sedentary people—this is a medical fact—get less oxygen in the blood, and therefore to the brain, than active people.

3. Do the Following on Exam Day:

- *Keep moving forward.* By test day, do enough preparation with a review course or practice questions so that it becomes an instinct to keep moving forward instead of getting bogged down in a difficult question. You don't need to get everything right to pass, so don't linger on a question that is going nowhere. The best test takers don't get bothered by difficult questions because they accept that everyone encounters them on the NCLEX.

- *Don't listen to negative words or behavior.* Don't be distracted by the ignorant babble or the behavior of other, less prepared, less skilled candidates around you. Negative thoughts lead to negative feelings and may interfere with you performing your best on test day.

- *Don't be anxious if other test takers seem to be working harder or answering questions more quickly.* Continue to spend your time patiently but doggedly thinking through your answers; it's going to lead to higher-quality test taking and better results. Set your own pace and stick to it.

- *Keep breathing!* Weak standardized test takers tend to share one major trait—forgetting to breathe steadily as the test proceeds. They do not to know the value of proper breathing. They start holding their breath without realizing it, or begin breathing erratically or arrhythmically. This can hurt confidence and accuracy. Do what you can to instill an awareness of proper breathing before and during each study or testing section.

- *Do some quick isometrics during the test.* This is helpful especially if your concentration is wandering or energy is waning. For example, put your palms together and press intensely for a few seconds.

Attitude is Everything

Think positively!

*Some of these methods were originally conceptualized by Dr. Emile Coué, who in the 1920s told everyone that the key to a happy life was to constantly repeat the phrase, "Every day in every way I am getting better and better." As advice to test takers, that isn't bad at all!

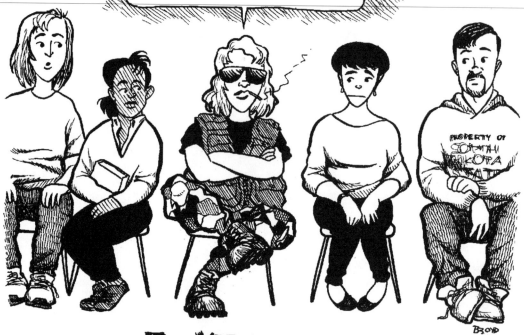

THE VETERAN

CHAPTER ELEVEN

The Licensure Process

The process of obtaining an American nursing license requires a definite sequence of actions by the candidate. Since this may be your first experience with the RN licensure process, and since there are no established test dates, you may have difficulty knowing exactly how to complete the paperwork and go through the licensure process. This chapter will give you a checklist to follow when planning to take the NCLEX. This is a general list, so you must individualize it according to the requirements for the state in which you wish to become licensed; see Appendix D for information on individual state licensing requirements. We will outline the questions that you need to ask, and the steps you need to take to complete the licensure process.

How to Apply for the NCLEX

During your last semester of nursing school, you will be given the following applications:

(1) Application for licensure that goes to your state board of nursing
(2) Application for the NCLEX that goes to The Chauncey Group,* a subsidiary of Educational Testing Services (ETS)

You will turn in the completed forms and the required licensure fees on a predetermined date to your nursing school.

Application Fees

- The NCLEX fee is $200. Additional licensure fees are determined by each state nursing board; see the state licensing requirements in Appendix D to determine your state's fee.

---

* Effective October 1, 2002, The Chauncey Group and Thomson Prometric will no longer be associated with the development or delivery of the NCLEX exam. At that time, VUE, a NCS-Pearson business, will assume both of these roles. This administrative change will **not** affect the format or content of the NCLEX exam. For more information, visit the NCSBN website at www.ncsbn.org.

The Registration Process

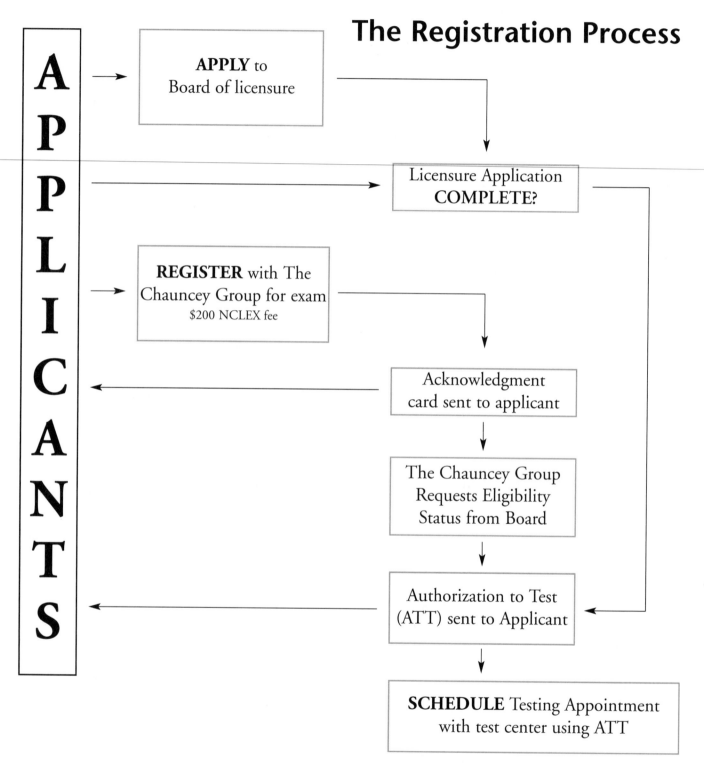

APPLICANTS

APPLY to
Board of licensure

Licensure Application
COMPLETE?

REGISTER with The
Chauncey Group for exam
$200 NCLEX fee

Acknowledgment
card sent to applicant

The Chauncey Group
Requests Eligibility
Status from Board

Authorization to Test
(ATT) sent to Applicant

SCHEDULE Testing Appointment
with test center using ATT

Applicant must **APPLY**, **REGISTER**, and **SCHEDULE**

- You are responsible for mailing the completed test application and the $200 fee to The Chauncey Group.
- Your application to The Chauncey Group can be completed by phone by dialing 800-551-1912. To do this you must use a credit card. A $12.00 fee will be added to the cost of the test.
- Some states require that the testing application form and fee be sent along with licensure application and fee.

How Do You Know Your Application Has Been Received?

You will receive a card from your state board stating that all of your information has been received.

Potential Problems with Licensure Application

Some states require that your permanent transcript be mailed with your application.

Here is a checklist to follow to avoid problems with your application:

- Have you met all requirements for graduation? Any electives still outstanding?
- Has your nursing school received a permanent transcript for any credits that you transferred from another institution?
- Do you owe any fines or have any unpaid parking tickets? (This can delay the release of your permanent transcript. Check at your nursing school office, just to be sure.)
- Some states require that a statement be sent from your nursing school stating that you have met all requirements for graduation.
- Did you change your mind about which state you want to apply in for licensure? If so, you must apply to a new state—and forfeit the original application fee.

What if You Want to Apply for Licensure in a Different State?

If you plan to apply for licensure in a different state from the one in which you are attending nursing school, contact the state board of nursing in the state in which you wish to become licensed (refer to the list in Appendix D).

Here's a checklist for obtaining a license in another state:

- Call or write the state board of nursing of that state and find out what their requirements are for licensure.
- What are their fees?
- Request a new candidate application for licensure.

Say When

You are responsible for scheduling your NCLEX.

One State at a Time

You can have licensure pending in only one state at a time.

Sample Copy of an Authorization to Test (ATT)

NCLEX®/The Chauncey Group
664 Rosedale Road
Princeton, NJ 08540

> ADMISSION TICKET
> Must present this whole page at
> the test center for admission to
> the NCLEX test

NATIONAL COUNCIL LICENSURE EXAMINATION
AUTHORIZATION TO TEST (ATT)
THIS IS YOUR ADMISSION TICKET, BRING THIS WITH YOU TO TEST

AUTHORIZATION NUMBER   IDENTIFICATION NUMBER   TEST
RN

VALID FROM – TO   STATE BOARD OF NURSING

IF THE NAME ON THIS AUTHORIZATION TO TEST DOES NOT EXACTLY MATCH YOUR NAME ON THE SIGNED PHOTOGRAPHIC IDENTIFICATION THAT YOU WILL BE USING AT THE TEST CENTER, PLEASE CALL THE NCLEX DATA CENTER AT 1-800-551-1912.

YOU MUST TAKE THE EXAMINATION DURING THE VALID TIME PERIOD LISTED ABOVE. TO MAKE AN APPOINTMENT:

* CALL ANY TESTING CENTER ON THE LIST THAT ACCOMPANIES THIS ATT;
* PROVIDE YOUR AUTHORIZATION NUMBER PRINTED ON THIS FORM;
* WRITE YOUR APPOINTMENT CONFIRMATION NUMBER, THE DATE AND TIME OF YOUR APPOINTMENT, AND THE ADDRESS AND DIRECTIONS TO THE TEST CENTER ON THE BOTTOM OF THIS FORM.

ON THE DAY OF YOUR EXAMINATION YOU MUST ARRIVE AT THE TEST CENTER THIRTY MINUTES BEFORE YOUR SCHEDULED APPOINTMENT TO COMPLETE THE ADMISSION PROCEDURES REQUIRED BEFORE TESTING BEGINS. YOU MUST BRING THE FOLLOWING WITH YOU TO BE ADMITTED TO THE EXAMINATION:

* THIS AUTHORIZATION TO TEST
* TWO PIECES OF IDENTIFICATION (ONE MUST HAVE A RECENT PHOTOGRAPH AND YOUR SIGNATURE, THE SECOND MUST HAVE YOUR SIGNATURE).

IF YOU DO NOT SHOW UP OR FAIL TO RESCHEDULE YOUR NCLEX EXAMINATION APPOINTMENT WITHOUT GIVING AT LEAST THREE BUSINESS DAYS' NOTICE, YOU WILL BE REQUIRED TO REGISTER AGAIN AND PAY AN ADDITIONAL $200 EXAMINATION FEE.

CONFIRMATION NUMBER _____ DIRECTIONS TO TEST CENTER:

APPOINTMENT DATE _____

APPOINTMENT TIME _____

Reprinted by permission of the National Council of State Boards of Nursing, Inc., Chicago, IL.

After you pass the NCLEX, you will receive your nursing license from the state in which you applied for licensure regardless of where you took your NCLEX. For example, if you applied for licensure in Michigan, you can take the test in Florida, if you wish. You would then receive a license to practice as an RN in Michigan because that is where you applied for licensure.

When Can You Schedule Your NCLEX Exam?

The Chauncey Group will send you a document entitled "Authorization to Test" (ATT). You will be unable to schedule your test date until you receive this form.

On the ATT is your assigned candidate number; you will need to refer to this when scheduling your exam. Your ATT is valid for a time determined by the individual state board of nursing, and you must test before your ATT expires. If you don't, you will need to reapply to take the exam and pay the testing fees again. With your ATT you will also receive a booklet entitled *Scheduling and Taking Your NCLEX Examination* and a list of test centers. You can schedule your test at any of the locations listed by calling the toll-free number on the list or or by calling any of the locations directly. Those with special testing requests, such as persons with disabilities, must call the number of the national registration center provided on the ATT.

There is a space on the ATT for you to record the date and time of your scheduled exam. It is very important that you record this information here because you won't receive written confirmation of your scheduled date and time.

Potential Rescheduling Problems

- You must test prior to the expiration date of your ATT. If you miss your appointment, you forfeit your testing fees and must reapply to both the state board of nursing and The Chauncey Group.

- If you wish to change your appointment, you must notify them within three days prior to the test date or you forfeit your testing fees and must reapply to both the state board of nursing and The Chauncey Group.

When Will You Take the Exam?

The earliest date on which you can take the NCLEX varies depending on your state, but the majority of students test approximately 45 days after

Can't Put It in Writing

You will not be sent written confirmation of your scheduled test date and time.

By the Book

Be knowledgeable about the rules for graduate nurses in your state. See Appendix D for state licensing requirements.

Dress Like an Onion

Wear layered clothing.

the date of their graduation. Variables include: when you submit the applications and fees, the length of time the ATT is valid, personal factors (weddings, births, vacations), and job requirements. Each state determines the requirements for graduate nurses, licensure pending. If you are working as a graduate nurse, you must be knowledgeable about the rules in your state.

Taking the Exam

What Happens on the Day of My NCLEX Exam?
Arrive at the test center at least 1/2 hour before your scheduled test time. Wear layered clothing, since the rooms may be cool in the morning but can warm up as the day progresses.

Here's a checklist of things to bring on the day of the exam:

- Your Authorization to Test (ATT).
- Two (2) forms of signed identification. One must be a picture I.D. If you have changed your hair color, lost weight, or grown a beard, have a new picture I.D. made before Test Day.
- A snack and something to drink. Plan on being at the test site for five hours.

Check-in procedure:

- Present your Authorization to Test (ATT).
- Present your two (2) forms of I.D.
- Sign in.
- A computer picture will be taken of you.
- You will be thumbprinted.
- All of your belongings will be placed in a locker outside the testing room.
- You will be offered ear plugs. Take them, in case you find yourself distracted by background noise.

Where Will I Take My Test?
You will be in a room separate from the rest of the test center. Many testing sites consist of a room with 10–15 computers placed around the outside walls. Each computer sits on a full-size desk, with an adjustable chair for you to sit on. There are dividers between desks, but you will be able to see the person sitting next to you. There is a picture window from which the proctor will observe each person testing. There are also video cameras and sound sensors mounted on the walls to monitor each candidate.

Well, I Lost Some Weight . . .
Make sure you look like your ID picture.

Food for the Mind
Bring something to feed your brain.

What Will the Computer Screen Look Like?

The number of the question you are answering is located in the upper right hand of your computer screen. On the upper left corner is a digital clock that begins at 5:00—representing the five hours you have to complete the short tutorial that begins the exam, the exam itself, and all breaks. The question stem is located on the left half of the screen, and the four answer choices are located on the right half of the screen (Figure 1). If the question involves a picture, the picture will appear on the left half of the screen, and the questions and four answer choices will appear on the right half of the screen.

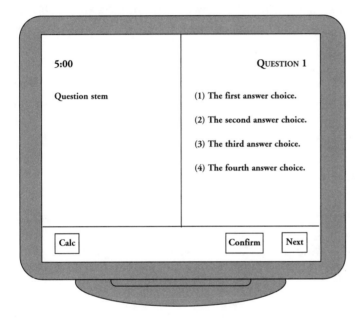

5:00   QUESTION 1

Question stem   (1) The first answer choice.

                        (2) The second answer choice.

                        (3) The third answer choice.

                        (4) The fourth answer choice.

Calc   Confirm   Next

Figure 1

You will notice that there are three icons at the bottom of the computer screen. The CALC icon is a drop-down calculator that can be used to perform drug calculations. The CONFIRM and NEXT icons are utilized to answer each question.

How Do I Use the Calculator?

Using the mouse, left click on the CALC icon, and a drop-down calculator will appear on the computer screen. Use the mouse to click on the calculator keys. The TRANSFER DISPLAY key will not function during the NCLEX exam. When you are through with your calculations, click on the CALC icon again, and the calculator will disappear.

How Do I Select an Answer Choice?

You will use the CONFIRM and NEXT icons to select an answer. Please note that when an icon is gray in color, it won't work. An icon will work only when it is dark in color.

Click on a Dark Icon

An icon will work only when it is dark in color. If an icon is gray, it won't work.

You will use a three-step process to answer each question. Read the question and select an answer by using the mouse to left click on the answer. Your answer is now highlighted. Next, left click on the NEXT icon. You will see the question with your chosen answer highlighted. Reread the question to make sure you agree with the highlighted answer. If the highlighted answer is your final answer, left click on the CONFIRM icon. Your answer is now locked in and a new question will appear on the screen.

After your answer is entered into the computer, the computer selects a new question for you based on the accuracy of your previous answer and the components of the NCLEX test plan. If you answer a question correctly, the next question selected by the computer is more difficult. If you answer a question incorrectly, the next question selected by the computer is easier.

What If I Don't Agree with the Answer that I Have Highlighted?

If you don't agree with the highlighted answer, click on a different answer choice. You will then click on the NEXT icon to get a second look at your answer. Your answer is not locked in until you click on the CONFIRM icon.

Even if you've never used a computer before, don't panic: You will be given instructions at the beginning of the test, and you will have to answer three tutorial questions before your test begins. These questions allow you to practice using the mouse to select an answer.

Time Out

Take a short break if you begin to experience trouble concentrating during the exam.

Do I Get Any Breaks?

You will receive a mandatory break at the end of two hours of testing. The computer will pause the test for ten minutes. Go out of the testing room, stretch your legs, eat your snack. Take some deep, cleansing breaths and get yourself ready to go back into the testing room. The computer will offer you an additional break after 3 1/2 hours of testing. This break is optional. We recommend that you take it unless you feel you're on a roll. You may take a break at any time during your test, but the time that you spend away from your computer is counted as a part of your five hours of total testing time. Kaplan recommends that you take a short (2–5 minute) break if you are having trouble concentrating. Take time to go to the restroom, eat your snack, or get a drink. This will enable you to maintain or regain your concentration for the test. Remember, every question counts!

How Will I Know When My Test Ends?

A screen will appear on your computer that states, "Your test is concluded." You will then be required to answer several exit questions. These are a few multiple-choice questions about your response to the examination experience. They do not count toward your results.

How Long Will It Take to Receive My Results?

Your results are sent to you by your state board of nursing. Each state board determines when the NCLEX results are released. For most states, you will receive your results approximately two to six weeks after your test date.

Next Generation NCLEX Testing

In the future, National Council of State Boards of Nursing, Inc., (NCSBN) may begin experimenting with new question types for the NCLEX exam. The new "innovative" question types are being developed under the direction of the NCSBN Examination Committee. These questions may involve formats such as *essay* (or *free-text entry*), *zone* (where portions of a graphic are selected), *order match* (which could be used to identify steps in a procedure), *numeric entry* (for calculations), and *shading* (for selecting an area of a graphic). Although the format of these questions is different from the text-based multiple-choice questions traditionally found on the NCLEX, the information tested by these questions is still minimum competency entry-level.

CHAPTER TWELVE

Taking the Test More Than Once

Some people may never have to read this chapter, but it's a certainty that others will. The most important advice we can give to repeat test takers is: Don't despair. There is hope. We can get you through the NCLEX.

You Are Not Alone

Think about that awful day when the big brown envelope arrived. You just couldn't believe it. You had to tell family, friends, your supervisor, and co-workers that you didn't pass the NCLEX. When this happens, each unsuccessful candidate feels like he or she is the only person that has failed the exam.

How to Interpret Unsuccessful Test Results

Most unsuccessful candidates on the NCLEX exam will usually say, "I almost passed." Some of you *did* almost pass, and some of you weren't very close. If you fail the exam, you will receive a diagnostic profile from National Council. In this profile, you will be told how many questions you answered on the exam. The more questions you answered, the closer you came to passing. The only way you will continue to get questions after you answer the first 75 is if you are answering questions close to the level of difficulty needed to pass the exam. If you are answering questions far above the level needed to pass or far below the level needed to pass, your exam will end at 75 questions.

Figure 1 on the next page shows a representation of what happens when a candidate fails in 75 questions. This student does not come close to passing. In 75 questions, this student demonstrates an inability to consistently answer questions correctly at or above the level of difficulty needed to pass the exam. This usually indicates a lack of nursing knowledge, considerable difficulties with taking a standardized test, or a deficiency in critical thinking skills.

Will It Ever End?

Your exam will end at 75 questions *only if* you are answering questions far above or far below the level of difficulty needed to pass.

KAPLAN 143

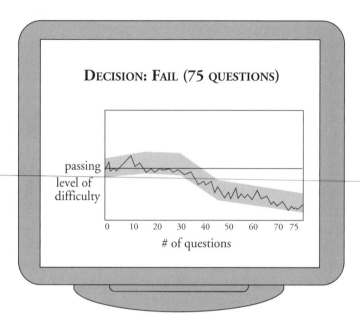

Figure 1

Figure 2 shows what happens when a candidate takes all 265 questions and fails. This candidate "almost passed." The candidate answers question 264 and the computer does not make a determination when it selects the last question. If the last question is below the level of difficulty needed to pass, the candidate fails.

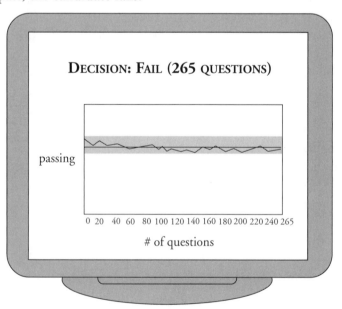

Figure 2

KAPLAN

If the last question is above the level of difficulty needed to pass, the candidate passes. If you took a test longer than 75 questions and failed, you were probably familiar with most of the content you saw on the exam but you may have difficulty using critical thinking skills or taking standardized tests.

The information contained on the diagnostic profile helps you identify your strengths and weaknesses on this particular NCLEX. This knowledge will help you identify where to concentrate your study when you prepare to retake the NCLEX.

Should You Test Again?

Absolutely! You completed your nursing education to become a RN. The initial response of many unsuccessful candidates is to declare, "I'm never going back! That was the worst experience of my life!" "What do I do now?"

When you first received your results, you went through a period of grieving—the same stages that you learned about in nursing school. Three to four weeks later, you find that you want to begin preparing to retake the NCLEX.

How Should You Begin?

You should prepare in a different way this time. Whatever you did to prepare last time didn't work well enough. The most common mistake that candidates who failed make is to assume that they did not study hard enough or learn enough content. For some of you, that's true. But for the majority of you, memorizing more content does not mean more right answers. It could simply means more frustration for you.

The first step in preparing for your next exam is to make a commitment that you will test again. Decide when you want to schedule your test and allow yourself enough time to prepare. Mark this test date on your calendar. You can do all of this before you send in your fees and receive your authorization to test. Remember, you cannot retake the NCLEX for a three-month period, so you may as well use this time wisely.

The next step is to figure out why you failed the NCLEX. Check off any reasons that pertain to you:

- ❑ I didn't know the nursing content.
- ❑ I memorized facts without understanding the principles of patient care.
- ❑ I had unrealistic expectations about the NCLEX test questions.

To Thine Own Self Be True

Be honest about your performance on the NCLEX. Figuring out why you failed is the key to passing your next attempt.

Are You Cramming Again?

Don't assume that you need to learn more facts. More facts doesn't always equal more right answers.

❏ I had difficulty correctly identifying THE REWORDED QUESTION.

❏ I had difficulty staying focused on THE REWORDED QUESTION.

❏ I found myself predicting answer choices.

❏ I did not carefully consider each answer choice.

❏ I am not good at choosing answers that require me to establish priorities of care.

❏ I answered question based on my "real world" experiences.

❏ I did not cope well with the computer adaptive experience.

❏ I thought I would complete the exam in 75 questions.

❏ When I got to question 200 I totally lost my concentration, and just answered questions to get through the rest of the exam.

After determining why you failed, the next step is to establish a plan of action for your next test. Remember, you should prepare differently this time. Consider the following when setting up your new plan of study:

You've seen the test.

You may wish that you didn't have to walk back into the testing center again, but if you want to be a registered professional nurse, you must go back. But this time you have an advantage over the first time test taker: you've seen the test! You know exactly what you are preparing for, and there are no unknowns. The computer will remember what questions you took before, and you will not be given any of the same questions. But the content of the question, the style of the question, and the kinds of answer choices will not change. You will not be surprised this time!

Study both content and test questions.

By the time you retest, you will be out of nursing school for 6 months or longer. Remember that old saying, "What you are not learning, you are forgetting"? Because this is a content-based test about safe and effective nursing care, you must remember all you can about nursing theory in order to select correct answers. You must study content that is integrated and organized like the NCLEX.

You must also master NCLEX-style test questions. It is essential that you be able to correctly identify what each question is asking. You will *not* pre-

Time For a Change of Plan

You must prepare differently for the second NCLEX!

No Reruns on This Channel

You will not see any of the questions you answered on your previous test

dict answers. You will *think* about each and every answer choice to decide if it answers the reworded question. In order to master test questions, you must practice answering them. We recommend that you answer hundreds of NCLEX-style test questions, especially at the application level of difficulty.

Know all of the words and their meanings.

Some students who have to learn a great deal of material in a short period of time have trouble learning the extensive vocabulary of the discipline. For example, difficulty with terminology is a problem for many good students who study history. They enjoy the concepts but find it hard to memorize all of the names and dates to allow them to do well on history tests. If you are one of those students who have trouble memorizing terms, you may find it useful to review a list of the terminology that you must know to pass the NCLEX. There is a list of those words at the end of this book.

Practice test-taking strategies.

There is no substitute for mastering the nursing content. This knowledge, combined with test-taking strategies, will help you to select a greater number of correct answers. For many students, the strategies mean the difference between a passing test and a failing test. Using strategies effectively can also determine whether you take a short test (75 questions) or a longer test (up to 265 questions).

Evaluate your CAT experience.

Some students attribute their failure to the CAT experience. Comments we have heard include:

> *"I didn't like answering questions on the computer."*
> *"I found the background noise distracting. I should have taken the earplugs!"*
> *"I looked up every time the door opened."*
> *"I should have taken a snack. I got so hungry!"*
> *"After 2 1/2 hours I didn't care what I answered. I just wanted the computer to shut off!"*
> *"I didn't expect to be there for four hours!"*
> *"I should have rescheduled my test, but I just wanted to get it over with!"*
> *"I wish I had taken aspirin with me. I had such a headache before it was over!"*

Do any of these comments sound familiar? It is important for you to take charge of your CAT experience. Here's how:

You're the Boss

Take charge of your CAT experience. If you felt uncomfortable taking the CAT the first time around, figure out how to remedy the situation before your second NCLEX.

- Choose a familiar testing site.
- Select the time of day that you test your best. (Are you a morning person or an afternoon person?)
- Accept the earplugs when offered.
- Take a snack and a drink for your break.
- Take a break if you become distracted or fatigued during the test.
- Contact the proctors at the test site if something bothers you during the test.
- Plan on testing for five hours. Then, if you get out early, it's a pleasant surprise.
- Say to yourself every day, "I will pass the NCLEX."

CHAPTER THIRTEEN

Notes for International Nurses

Many of you have years of nursing experience in your home country. Now you are preparing for the NCLEX so you can be licensed to practice your profession in the United States. Because of Kaplan's extensive experience preparing nurses educated in other countries, we are very aware of the special issues that you face when trying to pass the NCLEX. Your special concerns will be discussed in this chapter.

Many nurses educated outside of the United States have not had the experience of taking an objective multiple-choice test. Your testing experience may have been limited to oral exams or writing answers to essay and fill-in-the-blank questions. Multiple-choice tests are used in the United States because they measure knowledge more objectively and are easier to administer to large groups of people. In order to pass the NCLEX, you must demonstrate that you are a safe and effective nurse by correctly answering multiple-choice questions.

The CGFNS Certificate

In order to apply for licensure as a registered nurse, many U.S. state boards of nursing require internationally-educated nurses to obtain a certificate from the Commission on Graduates of Foreign Nursing Schools (CGFNS) before applying for initial licensure as a registered nurse. The process of obtaining a CGFNS certificate includes (1) a comparison of your nursing education credentials to what is required of U.S. nursing graduates, (2) passing the CGFNS exam that tests nursing knowledge, and (3) obtaining a score of 540 on the Test of English as a Foreign Language (TOEFL) that tests knowledge of English.

Know What's Required of You

Be sure to find out if your state board of nursing requires you to obtain a CGFNS certificate. Contact information for each state's nursing board can be found in Appendix D of this book.

The CGFNS exam is a two-part test of nursing knowledge. Nurses who pass this exam have been shown to have a higher degree of likelihood to pass the NCLEX on the first try than nurses who have not passed the CGFNS. This exam can be taken overseas at a number of international testing sites run by CGFNS or at selected sites in the United States.

Applications for the CGFNS exam are free and can be obtained by calling CGFNS at (215) 349-8767. To find out about a particular state's requirements for international nurses, call that state's board of nursing and request an application packet for initial licensure as an internationally educated nurse. The phone numbers and addresses for each of the state boards of nursing in the United States are listed in Appendix D of this book.

Work Visas

For the most current information on visa requirements, contact the nearest U.S. embassy or consulate in your home country or the nearest regional office of the Immigration and Naturalization Service if you already live in the United States. You can also contact the International Commission on Healthcare Professions by telephone at (215) 349-6735, or by mail at 3600 Market Street, Suite 400, Philadelphia, PA 19104-2651.

Nursing Practice in the United States

Some international nurses find nursing in the United States similar to nursing as they learned it in their country. For others, nursing in the United States is very different from what they learned or experienced in their country. NCLEX may ask you questions about procedures that are unfamiliar to you. You may be asked questions about diets and foods that are new to you. In order to be successful on the NCLEX, you must be able to correctly answer questions about nursing as it is practiced in the United States.

Here is an overview of services and skills that nurses are expected to perform:

- Nurses are involved with prevention, early detection, and treatment of illness for people of all ages.
- Nurses care for the whole person, not just an illness. Their focus is on patient needs, that is, how a patient will respond to an illness.

- Nurses are professionals who are responsible for their actions.
- Nurses must communicate with patients and all the members of the health care team: other nurses, unlicensed assistive personnel, physicians, dietitians, and social workers.
- Nurses serve as patients' advocates; that is, they counsel patients and make sure their rights are protected.
- Nurses help patients understand the health care system, and assist them to make decisions about their health care.
- Nurses are assertive and ask questions of health care professionals when necessary, including physicians. Their style of communication is polite but very direct.
- Nurses are responsible for meeting the needs of patients whose care involves high-tech equipment.
- Nurses are responsible for basing their actions on knowledge and acceptable nursing practice.
- Nurses, not families, are responsible for all the hands-on nursing care for patients in the hospital setting.
- Nurses are responsible for teaching patients and their families how to manage their health care needs.

American-Style Nursing Communication

An issue of special concern for international nurses is therapeutic communication. Correctly answering the questions about communication can be difficult for some nurses educated in the United States. These questions become a special challenge to test takers for whom English is a second language or for test-takers who do not yet fully understand American-style communication.

Key features of American-style communication in nursing:

- *Validate the client's experience and feelings by responding to the client verbally.* Ask questions that relate directly to what the client says.
- *Direct client's behavior to promote comfort and well-being.* Do not patronize or reject the client by imposing a value judgment.
- *Maintain eye contact with the client, especially during conversation.* Lean forward to face the client. Nod, smile, or frown to demonstrate agreement or disagreement while listening.

Responses used in American nursing are based on an assessment of the client's needs and are designed to foster growth and establish mutually formulated goals.

NCLEX questions concerning communication are best answered by:

- Conveying *respect* and *warmth,* making the client feel accepted and respected as an individual regardless of his or her words, actions, or behavior. This means that the nurse:
  * Assumes that all client behavior is purposeful and has meaning even though it may not make sense to others
  * Defines the social, physical, and emotional boundaries of the nurse-client relationship
  * Develops a contract with the client
  * Structures time to develop a nurse-client relationship
  * Creates a safe and secure environment
  * Accepts the dependency needs of the client while encouraging, assisting, and supporting movement toward health and independence
  * Intervenes when a client behaves inappropriately to directly reject the behavior but not the client
  * Intervenes directly to respond to the client, not to reinforce an inappropriate behavior

- Demonstrating *active listening* and *genuineness.* This means that the nurse:
  * Asks questions that relate directly to what the client says
  * Maintains good eye contact
  * Leans forward in the chair to face the client
  * Nods, smiles, or frowns to show agreement or disagreement
  * Understands that the personal feelings and past experiences of the nurse can negatively or positively affect relationships with clients

- Communicating *interest* and *empathy* by allowing the client to comfortably communicate concerns and behave in new ways. This means that the nurse:
  * Focuses conversation on the client's feelings
  * Understands that clients respond to the behavioral expectations of the nursing staff
  * Validates the client's feelings
  * Analyzes both verbal and nonverbal behavioral clues
  * Anticipates that there might be some difficulty as the client learns new behaviors

Nurses create barriers in the communication process when they demonstrate a poor understanding of the basics in therapeutic communication. They must convey *respect, warmth,* and *genuineness* through *active listening* and communicating *interest* and *empathy* about the concerns of clients, families, or staff.

Examples of barriers to communication:

- Minimizing concerns
- Giving false reassurance
- Giving approval
- Rejecting the person, not the behavior
- Choosing sides with the client, family member, or staff member in a conflict
- Blaming the external environment for the situation
- Disagreeing or arguing with the client or family member
- Offering advice about a situation
- Pressuring the client or family member for an explanation
- Defending one's own actions or behavior
- Belittling client, family member or staff concerns
- Giving one-word responses to questions
- Using denial
- Interpreting or analyzing both verbal and nonverbal behavioral clues in the situation to the client
- Shifting the focus of the conversation away from the client, family member, or staff concerns
- Using jargon or medical terminology without explanation in conversation with the client and/or family
- Invalidating the client's, family member's or staff's feelings
- Offering unrealistic hope for the future
- Ignoring client clues to help the client set appropriate limits on his or her behavior

The following are some questions that will allow you to practice the right approach to American-style questions.

Sample Questions

Directions: Carefully read the question and all answer choices. Examine each answer choice and determine whether it is an appropriate response. Indicate your decision in the column marked and give the reason for your choice.

QUESTION	CORRECT/ INCORRECT	REASON
1. A 35-year-old man has been hospitalized for two days for treatment of hepatitis A. When the nurse enters the client's room, he asks the nurse to leave him alone and stop bothering him. Which of the following responses by the nurse would be MOST appropriate? (1) "I understand and will leave you alone for now." (2) "Why are you angry with me?" (3) "Are you upset because you do not feel better?" (4) "You seem upset this morning."		
2. A 58-year-old woman states she is afraid to have her cast removed from her fractured arm. Which of the following is the MOST appropriate response by the nurse? (1) "I know it is unpleasant. Try not to be afraid. I will help you." (2) "You seem very anxious. I will stay with you while the cast is removed." (3) "I don't blame you. I'd be afraid also." (4) "My aunt just had a cast removed and she's just fine."		

QUESTION	CORRECT/ INCORRECT	REASON

3. A 28-year-old woman comes to the clinic because she thinks she is pregnant. She tells the nurse that she wants the pregnancy terminated because she and her husband do not want to have children, and then begins to cry. Which of the following statements by the nurse is the MOST appropriate?

    (1) "Are you upset because you forgot to use birth control?"

    (2) "Why are you so upset? You're married. There's no reason not to have the baby."

    (3) "If you're so upset, why don't you have the baby and put it up for adoption?"

    (4) "You seem upset. Let's talk about how you're feeling."

4. A 68-year-old man is in the terminal stages of carcinoma of the lung. A family member asks the nurse, "How much longer will it be?" Which of the following responses by the nurse would be MOST appropriate?

    (1) "I cannot say exactly. What are your concerns at this time?"

    (2) "I don't know. I'll call the doctor."

    (3) "This must be a terrible situation for you."

    (4) "Don't worry, it will be very soon."

QUESTION	CORRECT/ INCORRECT	REASON

5. A 51-year-old man is admitted to the hospital with a diagnosis of manic depressive disorder. The man approaches the nurse and says, "Hi, baby," and opens his robe, under which he is naked. Which of the following comments by the nurse would be MOST appropriate?

   (1) "This is inappropriate behavior. Please close your robe and return to your room."
   (2) "Please dress in your clothes and then join us for lunch in the dining room."
   (3) "I am offended by your behavior and will have to report you."
   (4) "Do you need some assistance dressing today?"

6. An 82-year-old woman is placed in Buck's traction. The nurse assigned to her prepares to assist her with a bath. The woman says, "You're too young to know how to do this. Get me somebody who knows what they're doing." Which of the following responses by the student nurse would be MOST appropriate?

   (1) "I am young, but I graduated from nursing school."
   (2) "If I don't bathe you now, you'll have to wait until I'm finished with my other clients."
   (3) "Can you be more specific about your concerns?"
   (4) "Your concerns are unnecessary. I know what I'm doing."

QUESTION	CORRECT/ INCORRECT	REASON

7. A 72-year-old woman is admitted to the hospital with an abdominal mass and is scheduled for an exploratory laparotomy. She asks the nurse admitting her, "Do you think I have cancer?" Which of the following responses by the nurse would be MOST appropriate?

   (1) "Would you like me to call your doctor so that you can discuss your specific concerns?"
   (2) "Your tests show a mass. It must be hard not knowing what is wrong."
   (3) "It sounds like you are afraid that you are going to die from cancer."
   (4) "Don't worry about it now; I'm sure you have many healthy years ahead of you."

8. A 23-year-old woman is admitted to the postpartum unit following a miscarriage. The next day the nurse finds the woman crying while looking at the babies in the newborn nursery. Which of the following approaches by the nurse would be MOST appropriate?

   (1) Assure the woman that the loss was "for the best."
   (2) Explain to her that she is young enough to have more children.
   (3) Ask her why she is looking at the babies.
   (4) Acknowledge the loss and be supportive.

QUESTION	CORRECT/ INCORRECT	REASON
9. An 84-year-old man is hospitalized with Alzheimer's disease. His daughter tells the nurse that caring for him is too hard, but that she feels guilty placing him in a nursing home. Which of the following statements by the nurse is MOST appropriate?		
(1) "It is hard to be caught between taking care of your needs and your father's needs." (2) "Would you like me to help you find a nursing home?" (3) "Don't feel guilty. The only solution is to place your father in a nursing home." (4) "I think I would feel guilty too if I had to place my father in a nursing home."		

Read the explanations to these questions and make sure that the American approach to these communications questions is understandable to you. It will help you to find the right answer on the NCLEX.

Answers

1. **(4) "You seem upset this morning,"** is the correct answer choice. This response is the best choice because the nurse seeks to verbally validate the client's behavior rather than simply respond to the behavior. This response promotes the nurse–client relationship by encouraging the client to share his feelings with the nurse.

   (1) *"I understand and will leave you alone for now,"* is not the best approach since it does not promote further communication between the nurse and the client about how the client is feeling. In order to interpret this client's behavior, the nurse must first validate it with the client.

   (2) *"Why are you angry with me?"* is incorrect. The nurse is drawing a conclusion about the client's behavior. This type of action is too confrontational. "Why" questions are considered nontherapeutic.

   (3) *"Are you upset because you do not feel better?"* is not the best choice. The nurse is drawing a conclusion about the client's behavior without validating it first. This type of response may also belittle the client's actual concerns.

2. **(2) "You seem very anxious. I will stay with you while the cast is removed,"** is the best response because the nurse responds to the client's feelings of fear. This is consistent with therapeutic communication used in American nursing. This response also provides an additional opportunity for the nurse to remain with the client in a supportive capacity enhancing the nurse–client relationship.

   (1) *"I know it is unpleasant. Try not to be afraid. I will help you,"* is not the best response. It is not clear what concerns the client has about this procedure. The nurse should establish this before responding. The nurse falsely reassures the client by saying, "I will help you." Since you do not know the nature of the client's concerns, you cannot honestly offer help.

(3) *"I don't blame you. I'd be afraid also,"* is not the correct response because the nurse shifts the focus of the conversation from the client to the nurse. This sets up a barrier to further communication. The nurse concedes the issue too quickly, leaving the source of the client's fear unknown.

(4) *"My aunt just had a cast removed and she's just fine,"* is not the best choice. The focus of the conversation is shifted from the client to the nurse's aunt, who is of no concern to the client. This response fails to explore the source of the client's anxiety and sets up a block to further communication.

3. **(4) "You seem upset. Let's talk about how you're feeling,"** is the best answer to this question. This promotes the nurse–client relationship and illustrates therapeutic communication used in American nursing. The nurse responds to the client's feelings in a nonjudgmental empathetic way.

(1) *"Are you upset because you forgot to use birth control?"* is inappropriate because it places blame on the client. The nurse should not assume that the client "forgot" to do something. This response also fails to respond to the client's feelings and does not encourage the client to discuss her concerns.

(2) *"Why are you so upset? You're married. There's no reason not to have the baby,"* is inappropriate in terms of American therapeutic communication. This response is harsh, presumptive, and assumes that the purpose of every marriage is to have children. This is not always the case in American culture. With this response, the nurse does not attempt to verify the reason for the client's tears, thereby discouraging further conversation about what the client is actually experiencing.

(3) *"If you're so upset, why don't you have the baby and put it up for adoption?"* is also inappropriate. This is a value-laden assumption placing positive value on adoption. Again, the nurse fails to explore with the client the reason for the client's tears, thereby discouraging further communication. The nurse is also offering advice.

4. **(1) "I cannot say exactly. What are your concerns at this time?"** is the most appropriate response since it is unclear why the family member has approached the nurse at this point. Perhaps the client is in pain and the family member wants to discuss it with the nurse. This response allows for that possibility. This response is also direct and factually correct.

(2) *"I don't know. I'll call the doctor,"* is not the most appropriate response. It shifts the focus of responsibility from the nurse to the physician, which prevents a nurse–family member relationship from developing.

(3) *"This must be a terrible situation for you,"* is not the most appropriate response. It is a value-laden statement that fails to explore the family member's reason for approaching the nurse.

(4) *"Don't worry, it will be very soon,"* is inappropriate because the nurse offers the family member false reassurance. It also offers advice by telling the family member not to worry. This statement is demeaning and may sound as if the nurse is too busy to discuss the family member's concerns.

5. **(1) "This is inappropriate behavior. Please close your robe and return to your room,"** is the correct answer choice. This statement by the nurse responds to the client's behavior, sets limits on the behavior, and directs the client towards more appropriate social behavior in the milieu. This statement rejects the client's behavior, not the client as a person.

(2) *"Please dress in your clothes and then join us for lunch in the dining room,"* is incorrect. It ignores the behavior of the client exposing himself. Instead it directs the client to dress and report to the dining room for lunch as though nothing has happened. This is inappropriate and nontherapeutic.

(3) *"I am offended by your behavior and will have to report you,"* is incorrect. It shifts the focus from the client to the nurse and the nurse's feelings. The nurse's personal feelings are irrelevant. Also, the nurse goes on to threaten the client by reporting him. This is nontherapeutic.

(4) *"Do you need some assistance dressing today?"* is incorrect. This question fails to respond to the client's behavior. It is also a yes/no question, which is nontherapeutic.

6. **(3) "Can you be more specific about your concerns?"** is the correct answer. This is the best answer choice because it seeks to validate the client's message. It is direct, not defensive, and allows the client to express her point of view.

(1) *"I am young, but I graduated from nursing school,"* is incorrect. It responds to only part of the message that the client sent to the student nurse. It assumes that the student nurse knows what the

client's concerns are and agrees that there is some problem associated with being too young. Further clarification is necessary in this situation.

(2) *"If I don't bathe you now, you'll have to wait until I'm finished with my other clients,"* is a nontherapeutic response. It fails to explore the client's concerns about the student nurse. It is an uncaring and punitive statement by the nurse that is inappropriate in a nurse–client relationship.

(4) *"Your concerns are unnecessary. I know what I'm doing,"* is incorrect. The nurse dismisses the client's concerns by telling her that she shouldn't be concerned. The nurse should not tell a client how he or she should be feeling. It may sound as if the nurse is trying to reassure the client by telling her that the nurse knows what he or she is doing; however, the nurse has yet to validate the concerns that underlie the client's statement.

7. **(2) "Your tests show a mass. It must be hard not knowing what is wrong,"** is the correct answer choice. This is the best answer choice because it responds to the patient's feelings. It allows the client to continue to identify and express her concerns regarding surgery, hospitalization, and the possibility of having a potentially life-threatening illness. The nurse validates that the client has appropriate concerns and invites her to elaborate on them.

(1) *"Would you like me to call your doctor so that you can discuss your specific concerns?"* This response is incorrect because it shifts the focus of responsibility from the nurse to the doctor thereby reducing the possibility of developing an ongoing nurse–client relationship.

(3) *"It sounds like you are afraid that you are going to die from cancer,"* is inappropriate. It fails to validate with the client that "dying from cancer" is in fact the issue. The nurse inappropriately concludes this on the basis of a brief statement made by the client without giving the client a chance to elaborate.

(4) *"Don't worry about it now; I'm sure that you have many healthy years ahead of you,"* is inappropriate. The nurse is telling the client how she should feel and then goes on to offer false reassurance. This response fails to address or explore the actual concerns of the client.

8. **(4) Acknowledge the loss and be supportive** is the best answer choice. It promotes the nurse–client relationship, and allows for the identification of feelings and the expression of sadness. The client is in an acute stage of grief. This type of response addresses this issue.

   (1) *Assure the woman that the loss was "for the best"* is incorrect. This statement is insensitive to the client, offers false reassurance, and belittles the client's most immediate concerns.

   (2) *Explain to her that she is young enough to have more children* is inappropriate because it is insensitive to the grief that the client is experiencing. The nurse offers false reassurance by telling the woman that she can have other children.

   (3) *Ask her why she is looking at the babies* is also incorrect. This is inappropriate because it is a "why" question and because the woman may become defensive when answering such a question. This response also fails to respond to the client's immediate grief.

9. **(1) "It is hard to be caught between taking care of your needs and your father's needs,"** is the correct response. This is the most therapeutic response as it allows for continued development of a relationship with the family member of the client. This response allows the nurse to explore and validate the daughter's feelings about the nursing home placement.

   (2) *"Would you like me to help you find a nursing home?"* is not the best answer choice. It is a yes/no question and doesn't encourage discussion of the daughter's feelings.

   (3) *"Don't feel guilty. The only solution is to place your father in a nursing home,"* is not the best therapeutic response. The daughter's concerns are minimized when the nurse tells the daughter not to worry. While it may be true that the daughter has done all that she can, this response cuts off an opportunity for further conversation with the nurse.

   (4) *"I think I would feel guilty too if I had to place my father in a nursing home,"* is also incorrect. This statement is value-laden and judgmental, and would immediately block any further communication between the nurse and the daughter. It is not important what the nurse thinks about the daughter's decision, nor is it the nurse's role to make the daughter feel more guilty about her decision.

Language

English is the predominant language spoken and written in the United States, and the NCLEX is administered only in English. With the exception of the medical terminology, the reading level of the NCLEX is that of a junior in an American high school. In order to be successful on the NCLEX, you must understand English—and the terminology—as it is used in the United States.

Vocabulary

Vocabulary can be a challenge for international nurses on the NCLEX. Not only must you know what each word means, but sometimes a word may have more than one meaning. You need to be able to correctly identify words as they are used in context. Refer to Appendix B for some of the commonly found words on the NCLEX. Some other ways to increase your vocabulary and learn how the words are used in every day English include:

- Talking with Americans
- Watching American movies and television
- Reading newspapers and magazines

Abbreviations

Many of you are unfamiliar with the abbreviations used in the United States. When studying, always look up unknown words in a medical dictionary. Consult Appendix C, a list of appreviations used by nurses in American health care settings.

As an internationally educated nurse, you face special challenges in preparing for the NCLEX. Following the tips and guidelines outlined in this chapter will increase your chances of passing the NCLEX and will allow you to reach your career goals.

Kaplan International Programs

Knowing something about American culture and how American nurses fit into the overall healthcare industry is important for nurses trained outside the United States. If you are not from the United States, but are interested in learning more about American nursing, wish to practice in the United States, or are exploring the possibilities of attending an American nursing school for graduate study, Kaplan is able to help you.

How Kaplan International Programs Can Help You

Kaplan's International Programs were designed to help students and professionals from outside the United States meet their educational and career goals. At locations throughout the United States, international students take advantage of Kaplan's programs to help them improve their academic and conversational English skills, raise their scores on the TOEFL and other standardized exams, and gain admission to the schools of their choice. Our staff and instructors give international students the individualized instruction they need to succeed. Here is a brief description of some of Kaplan's programs for international students and professionals:

General Intensive English

Kaplan's General Intensive English classes are designed to help you improve your skills in all areas of English and to increase your fluency in spoken and written English. Classes are available for beginning to advanced students.

English for TOEFL and Academic English

This course provides you with the skills you need to improve your TOEFL score and succeed in an American university or graduate program. It includes advanced reading, writing, listening, grammar, and conversational English. You will also receive training for the TOEFL using Kaplan's exclusive computer-based practice materials.

CGFNS (Commission on Graduates of Foreign Nursing Schools) Preparation for International Nurses

Many U.S. state boards of nursing require internationally educated nurses to obtain a CGFNS certificate before applying for initial licensure as a registered nurse. The certification process requires that a candidate pass a two-part test of nursing knowledge and to demonstrate English language proficiency on the TOEFL exam. Kaplan offers a comprehensive course of study to help you pass this exam.

NCLEX (National Council Licensure Examination) Preparation for International Nurses

An internationally educated nurse must pass the NCLEX in order to obtain a license to practice as a registered nurse in the United States. Kaplan has a comprehensive course and review products to help international nurses pass this exam.

Other Kaplan Programs

Since 1938, more than 3 million students have come to Kaplan to advance their studies, prepare for entry to American universities, and further their careers. In addition to the above programs, Kaplan offers courses to prepare for the SAT, ACT, GMAT, GRE, LSAT, MCAT, DAT, USMLE, and other standardized exams at locations throughout the United States.

Applying to Kaplan International Programs*

To get more information, or to apply for admission to any of Kaplan's programs for international students and professionals, contact us at:

Kaplan International Programs
700 South Flower, Suite 2900
Los Angeles, CA 90017 USA
Phone (if calling from within the United States): 800-818-9128
Phone (if calling from outside the United States): 213-452-5800
Fax: 213-892-1364
Website: www.kaplaninternational.com
Email: world@kaplan.com

*Kaplan is authorized under federal law to enroll nonimmigrant alien students.
Kaplan is authorized to issue Form IAP-66 needed for a J-1 (Exchange Visitor) visa.
Kaplan is accredited by ACCET (Accrediting Council for Continuing Education and Training).
Test names are registered trademarks of their respective owners.

PART TWO

THE NCLEX PRACTICE TEST

Practice Test

Directions: Each question or incomplete statement below is followed by four suggested answers or completions. In each case, HIGHLIGHT the statement that best answers the question or completes the statement.

1. The nurse is interviewing a client who is being treated for obsessive-compulsive disorder. What is the MOST important question the nurse should ask this patient?

   (1) "Do you find yourself forgetting simple things?"

   (2) "Do you find it hard to stay on a task?"

   (3) "Do you have trouble controlling upsetting thoughts?"

   (4) "Do you experience feelings of panic in a closed area?"

2. Which of the following actions, if performed by the nurse, would be considered negligence?

   (1) Obtaining a Guthrie blood test on a 4-day-old infant.

   (2) Massaging lotion on the abdomen of a 3-year-old diagnosed with Wilm's tumor.

   (3) Instructing a 5-year-old asthmatic to blow on a pinwheel.

   (4) Playing kickball with a 10-year-old with juvenile arthritis (JA).

3. The nurse on postpartum is preparing four clients for discharge. It would be MOST important for the nurse to refer which of the following patients for home care?

   (1) A 15-year-old primipara who delivered a 7-lb male two days ago.

   (2) An 18-year-old multipara who delivered a 9-lb female by cesarean section two days ago.

   (3) A 20-year-old multipara who delivered 1 day ago and is complaining of cramping.

   (4) A 22-year-old who delivered by cesarean section and is complaining of burning on urination.

4. A patient is telling the nurse about his perception of his thought patterns. Which of the following statements, if made by the patient, would validate the diagnosis of schizophrenia?

(1) "I can't get the same thoughts out of my head."

(2) "I know I sometimes feel on top of the world, then suddenly down."

(3) "Sometimes I look up and wonder where I am."

(4) "It's clear that this is an alien laboratory and I am in charge."

5. A nursing team consists of an RN, an LPN/LVN, and a nursing assistant. The nurse should assign which of the following patients to the LPN/LVN?

(1) A 72-year-old patient with diabetes who requires a dressing change for a stasis ulcer.

(2) A 42-year-old patient with cancer of the bone complaining of pain.

(3) A 55-year-old patient with terminal cancer being transferred to hospice home care.

(4) A 23-year-old patient with a fracture of the right leg who asks to use the urinal.

6. An 84-year-old man is admitted with a diagnosis of dementia. He attempts several times to pull out his nasogastric tube. An order for cloth wrist restraints is received by the nurse. Which of the following actions by the nurse is MOST appropriate?

(1) Attach the ties of the restraint to the bed frame.

(2) Perform circulation checks to the extremities, which are restrained once a shift.

(3) Remove the restraints when the patient is up in a wheelchair.

(4) Explain the need for restraints only to the family.

7. A 50-year-old man complains of pain in his right lower extremity. The physician orders codeine 60 mg and aspirin grains XPO every four hours, as needed for pain. Each codeine tablet contains 15 mg of codeine. Each aspirin tablet contains 325 mg of aspirin. Which of the following should the nurse administer?

(1) 2 codeine tablets and 4 aspirin tablets

(2) 4 codeine tablets and 3 aspirin tablets

(3) 4 codeine tablets and 2 aspirin tablets

(4) 3 codeine tablets and 3 aspirin tablets

8. The nurse is leading an inservice about management issues. The nurse would intervene if another nurse made which of the following statements?

(1) "It is my responsibility to ensure that the consent form has been signed and attached to the patient's chart prior to surgery."

(2) "It is my responsibility to witness the signature of the client before surgery is performed."

(3) "It is my responsibility to provide a detailed description of the surgery and ask the patient to sign the consent form."

(4) "It is my responsibility to answer questions that the patient may have prior to surgery."

9. A nurse in the outpatient clinic evaluates the Mantoux test of a 36-year-old woman whose history indicates that she has been treated during the past year for an AIDS-related infection. The nurse should document that there was a positive reaction if there was an area of induration measuring what?

(1) 3 mm

(2) 7 mm

(3) 11 mm

(4) 15 mm

10. The nurse in the newborn nursery has just received report. Which of the following infants should the nurse see first?

(1) A two-day-old infant is lying quietly alert with a heart rate of 185.

(2) A one-day-old infant is crying and the anterior fontanel is bulging.

(3) A 12-hour infant is being held; the respirations are 45 breaths per minute and irregular.

(4) A five-hour-old infant is sleeping and the hands and feet are blue bilaterally.

11. While inserting a nasogastric tube, the nurse should use which of the following protective measures?

(1) Gloves, gown, goggles, and surgical cap

(2) Sterile gloves, mask, plastic bags, and gown

(3) Gloves, gown, mask, and goggles

(4) Double gloves, goggles, mask, and surgical cap

12. The nurse is caring for patients in the outpatient clinic. Which of the following phone calls should the nurse return first?

(1) A client with hepatitis A who states, "My arms and legs are itching."

(2) A client with a cast on the right leg who states, "I have a funny feeling in my right leg."

(3) A client with osteomylitis of the spine who states, "I am so nauseous that I can't eat."

(4) A client with rheumatoid arthritis who states, "I am having trouble sleeping."

13. The nursing team consists of an RN, two LPNs/LVNs, and three nursing assistants. The RN should care for which of the following patients?

(1) A patient with a chest tube who is ambulating in the hall.

(2) A patient with a colostomy who requires assistance with a colostomy irrigation.

(3) A patient with a right-sided cerebral vascular accident (CVA) who requires assistance with bathing.

(4) A patient who is refusing medication to treat cancer of the colon.

14. The home care nurse is visiting a client during the icteric phase of hepatitis of unknown etiology. The nurse would be MOST concerned if the client made which of the following statements?

(1) "I must not share eating utensils with my family."

(2) "I must use my own bath towel."

(3) "I'm glad that my husband and I can continue to have intimate relations."

(4) "I must eat small, frequent feedings."

15. A nurse plans for care of a patient with anemia who is complaining of weakness. Which of the following tasks should the nurse assign to the nursing assistant?

(1) Listen to the patient's breath sounds.

(2) Set up the patient's lunch tray.

(3) Obtain a diet history.

(4) Instruct the client on how to balance rest and activity.

16. The nurse is caring for patients on the surgical floor and has just received report from the previous shift. Which of the following patients should the nurse see FIRST?

(1) A 35-year-old admitted three hours ago with a gunshot wound; 1.5 cm area of dark drainage noted on the dressing.

(2) A 43-year-old who had a mastectomy two days ago; 23 cc of serosanguinous fluid noted in the Jackson-Pratt drain.

(3) A 59-year-old with a collapsed lung due to an accident; no drainage noted in the previous eight hours.

(4) A 62-year-old who had an abdominal-perineal resection three days ago; patient complains of chills.

17. Which of the following actions, if performed by the nurse, would certainly be considered negligence?

(1) Inserting a 16 Fr NG tube and aspirating 15 cc of gastric contents.

(2) Administering Demerol IM to patient prior to using the incentive spirometer.

(3) Administering ferrous sulfate (Feosol) 325 mg with coffee.

(4) Initially administering blood at 5 cc per minute for 15 minutes.

18. A one-day-old newborn diagnosed with intrauterine growth retardation is observed by the nurse to be restless, irritable, fist-sucking, and having a high-pitched, shrill cry. Based on this data, the nurse should

(1) discourage stimulation of the baby by rocking.

(2) tightly swaddle the infant in a flexed position.

(3) schedule feeding times every three to four hours.

(4) encourage eye contact with the infant during feedings.

19. The nurse visits a neighbor who is 20 weeks gestation. The neighbor complains of nausea, headache, and blurred vision. The nurse notes that the neighbor appears nervous, is diaphoretic, and is experiencing tremors. It would be MOST important for the nurse to ask which of the following questions?

(1) "Are you having menstrual-like cramps?"

(2) "When did you last eat or drink?"

(3) "Have you been diagnosed with diabetes?"

(4) "Have you been lying on the couch?"

20. The school nurse notes that a first-grade child is scratching her head almost constantly. It would be MOST important for the nurse to take which of the following actions?

   (1) Discuss basic hygiene with the parents.

   (2) Instruct the child not to sleep with her dog.

   (3) Inform the parents that they must contact an exterminator.

   (4) Observe the scalp for small white specks.

21. A suicidal patient, who was admitted to the psychiatric unit for treatment and observation a week ago, suddenly appears cheerful and motivated. The nurse should be aware that

   (1) the patient is likely sleeping well because of the medication.

   (2) the patient has made new friends and has a support group.

   (3) the patient may have finalized a suicide plan.

   (4) the patient is responding to treatment and is no longer depressed.

22. The nurse is caring for patients in the GYN clinic. A client complains of an off-white vaginal discharge with a curd-like appearance. The nurse notes the discharge and vulvular erythema. It would be MOST important for the nurse to ask which of the following questions?

   (1) "Do you douche?"

   (2) "Are you sexually active?"

   (3) "What kind of birth control do you use?"

   (4) "Have you taken any cough medicine?"

23. The nurse is caring for a client in the prenatal clinic. He nurse notes that the patient's chart contains the following information: blood type AB, Rh negative; serology—negative; indirect Coombs test—negative; fetal paternity—unknown. The nurse should anticipate taking which of the following actions?

   (1) Administer Rho (D) immune globulin (RhoGAM).

   (2) Schedule an amniocentesis.

   (3) Obtain a direct Coombs test.

   (4) Assess maternal serum for alpha-fetal protein level.

24. The nurse is caring for a woman at 37 weeks gestation. The client was diagnosed with insulin-dependent diabetes mellitus (IDDM) at age 7. The client states, "I am so thrilled that I will be breastfeeding my baby." Which of the following responses by the nurse is BEST?

(1) "You will probably need less insulin while you are breastfeeding."

(2) "You will need to initially increase your insulin after the baby is born."

(3) "You will be able to take an oral hypoglycemic instead of insulin after the baby is born."

(4) "You will probably require the same dose of insulin that you are now taking."

25. The nurse is caring for clients in a pediatric clinic. The mother of a 14-year-old male privately tells you that she is worried about her son because she unexpectedly walked into his room and discovered him masturbating. Which of the following responses by the nurse is MOST appropriate?

(1) "Tell your son he could go blind doing that."

(2) "Masturbation is a normal part of sexual development."

(3) "He's really too young to be masturbating."

(4) "Why don't you give him more privacy?"

26. The nurse performs a home visit on a client who delivered two days ago. The client states that she is bottle-feeding her infant. The nurse notes white, curd-like patches on the newborn's oral mucous membranes. The nurse should take which of the following actions?

(1) Determine the newborn's blood glucose level.

(2) Suggest that the newborn's formula be changed.

(3) Remind the caretaker not to let the infant sleep with the bottle.

(4) Explain that the newborn will need to receive some medication.

27. The nurse at the birthing facility is caring for a primipara woman in labor, who is 4 cm dilated, 25 percent effaced, and whose fetal vertex is at +1. The physician informs the patient that an amniotomy is to be performed. The patient states, "My friend's baby died when the umbilical cord came out when her water broke. I don't want you to do that to me!" Which of the following responses by the nurse is BEST?

(1) "If you are that concerned, you should refuse the procedure."

(2) "The procedure will help your labor go faster."

(3) "That shouldn't happen to you since the baby's head is engaged."

(4) "We will monitor you carefully to prevent cord prolapse."

28. A primigravida woman comes to the clinic for her initial prenatal visit. She is 32 weeks gestation and says that she has just moved from out-of-state. The client says that she has had periodic headaches during her pregnancy, and that she is continually bumping into things. The nurse notes numerous bruises in various stages of healing around the client's breasts and abdomen. Vital signs are: B/P 120/80, pulse 72, resps 18, and FHT 142. Which of the following responses by the nurse is BEST?

(1) "Are you battered by your partner?"

(2) "How do you feel about being pregnant?"

(3) "Tell me about your headaches."

(4) "You may be more clumsy due to your size."

29. The nurse is teaching a class on natural family planning. Which of the following statements, if made by a client, indicates that teaching has been successful?

(1) "When I ovulate, my basal body temperature will be elevated for two days and then will decrease."

(2) "My cervical mucus will be thick, cloudy, and sticky when I ovulate."

(3) "Since I am regular, I will be fertile about 14 days after the beginning of my period."

(4) "When I ovulate, my cervix will feel firm."

30. The home care nurse plans care for a 10-year-old in a leg cast for treatment of a fractured right ankle. The nurse enters the following nursing diagnosis on the care plan: skin integrity, risk for impaired. Which of the following actions, if performed by the nurse, is BEST?

(1) Teaching the child how to perform isometric exercises of the right leg.

(2) Teaching the mother to gently massage the child's right foot with emollient cream.

(3) Instructing the mother to keep the leg cast clean and dry.

(4) Teaching the mother how to turn and position the child.

31. The nurse is caring for a 45-year-old patient who had a thyroidectomy 12 hours ago for treatment of Graves's disease. The nurse would be MOST concerned if which of the following was observed?

(1) Blood pressure 138/82, pulse 84, respirations 16, oral temp 99° F.

(2) The patient supports his head and neck when turning his head to the right.

(3) The client spontaneously flexes his wrist when the blood pressure is obtained.

(4) The client is drowsy and complains of a sore throat.

32. A 16-year-old boy is admitted with complaints of severe pain in the lower right quadrant of the abdomen. To assist with pain relief, the nurse should take which of the following actions?

(1) Encourage the patient to change positions frequently in bed.

(2) Administer Demerol 50 mg IM q 4 hours and PRN.

(3) Apply warmth to the abdomen with a heating pad.

(4) Use comfort measures and pillows to position the patient.

33. The nurse prepares a 50-year-old woman for peritoneal dialysis. Which of the following actions should the nurse take FIRST?

(1) Assess for a bruit and a thrill.

(2) Warm the dialysate solution.

(3) Position the client on the left side.

(4) Insert a Foley catheter.

34. The nurse teaches a 65-year-old man with right-sided weakness how to use a cane. Which of the following behaviors, if demonstrated by the client to the nurse, indicates that the teaching was effective?

(1) The man holds the cane with his right hand, moves the cane forward followed by the right leg, and then moves the left leg.

(2) The man holds the cane with his right hand, moves the cane forward followed by his left leg, and then moves the right leg.

(3) The man holds the cane with his left hand, moves the cane forward followed by the right leg, and then moves the left leg.

(4) The man holds the cane with his left hand, moves the cane forward followed by his left leg, and then moves the right leg.

35. While caring for a patient receiving TPN through a central line, the nurse notices a small trickle of opaque fluid leaking from around the central line dressing. It is MOST important for the nurse to take which of the following actions?

(1) Prepare to change the central line dressing.

(2) Verify that the patient is on antibiotics.

(3) Place the patient's head lower than his feet.

(4) Secure the Y-port where the lipids are infusing.

36. A 46-year-old man is admitted to the hospital with a fractured right femur. He is placed in balanced suspension traction with a Thomas splint and Pearson attachment. During the first 48 hours, the nurse should assess the patient for which of the following complications?

(1) Pulmonary embolism

(2) Fat embolism

(3) Avascular necrosis

(4) Malunion

37. The nurse is helping a nursing assistant provide a bed bath to a comatose patient who is incontinent. The nurse should intervene if which of the following actions is noted?

(1) The nursing assistant answers the phone while wearing gloves.

(2) The nursing assistant log rolls the patient to provide back care.

(3) The nursing assistant places an incontinent diaper under the patient.

(4) The nursing assistant positions the patient on the left side, head elevated.

38. A 70-year-old woman is brought to the emergency room for treatment after being found on the floor by her daughter. X-rays reveal a displaced subcapital fracture of the left hip and osteoarthritis. When comparing the legs, the nurse would most likely make which of the following observations?

(1) The patient's left leg is longer than the right leg and externally rotated.

(2) The patient's left leg is shorter than the right leg and internally rotated.

(3) The patient's left leg is shorter than the right leg and adducted.

(4) The patient's left leg is longer than the right leg and is abducted.

39. The nurse is caring for a patient with a cast on the left leg. The nurse would be MOST concerned if which of the following were observed?

(1) Capillary refill time was less than 3 seconds.

(2) Patient complained of discomfort and itching.

(3) Patient complained of tightness and pain.

(4) Patient's foot is elevated on a pillow.

40. The nurse is discharging a patient from an inpatient alcohol treatment unit. Which of the following statements, if made by the patient's wife, indicates to the nurse that the family is coping adaptively?

(1) "My husband will do well as long as I keep him engaged in activities that he likes."

(2) "My focus is learning how to live my life."

(3) "I am so glad that our problems are behind us."

(4) "I'll make sure that the children don't give my husband any problems."

41. A nurse is caring for clients in the mental health clinic. A woman comes to the clinic complaining of insomnia and anorexia. The patient tearfully tells the nurse that she was laid off from a job that she had held for 15 years. Which of the following responses, if made by the nurse, is MOST appropriate?

(1) "Did your company give you a severance package?"

(2) "Focus on the fact that you have a healthy, happy family."

(3) "Tell me what happened."

(4) "Losing a job is common nowadays."

42. A patient with a history of alcoholism is brought to the emergency room in an agitated state. He is vomiting and diaphoretic. He says he had his last drink five hours ago. The nurse would expect to administer which of the following medications?

(1) Chlordiazepoxide hydrochloride (Librium)

(2) Disulfiram (Antabuse)

(3) Methadone hydrochloride (Dolophine)

(4) Naloxone hydrochloride (Narcan)

43. A 72-year-old woman is admitted to the nursing home setting. The client is occasionally confused and her gait is often unsteady. Which of the following actions, if taken by the nurse, is MOST appropriate?

(1) Ask the woman's family to provide personal items such as photos or mementos.

(2) Select a room with a bed by the door so the woman can look down the hall.

(3) Suggest the woman eat her meals in the room with her roommate.

(4) Encourage the woman to ambulate in the halls twice a day.

44. The nurse teaches a 60-year-old man how to use a standard aluminum walker. Which of the following behaviors, if demonstrated by the client, indicates that the nurse's teaching was effective?

(1) The client slowly pushes the walker forward 12 inches, then takes small steps forward while leaning on the walker.

(2) The client lifts the walker, moves it forward two feet, and then takes several small steps forward.

(3) The client supports his weight on the walker while advancing it forward, then takes small steps while balancing on the walker.

(4) The client slides the walker 18 inches forward, then takes small steps while holding onto the walker for balance.

45. A nurse is supervising a group of elderly clients in a residential home setting. The nurse knows that the elderly are at greater risk of developing sensory deprivation for what reason?

(1) Increased sensitivity to the side effects of medications

(2) Decreased visual, auditory, and gustatory abilities

(3) Isolation from their families and familiar surroundings

(4) Decreased musculoskeletal function and mobility

46. After receiving report, which of the following patients should the nurse see FIRST?

(1) A 14-year-old patient in sickle-cell crisis with an infiltrated IV.

(2) A 59-year-old patient with leukemia who has received half of a packed red cell transfusion.

(3) A 68-year-old patient scheduled for a bronchoscopy.

(4) A 74-year-old patient complaining of a leaky colostomy bag.

47. The home care nurse is visiting a 32-year-old woman with a diagnosis of hepatitis of unknown etiology. The nurse knows that teaching has been successful if the patient makes which one of the following statements?

(1) "I am so sad that I am not able to hold my baby."

(2) "I will eat after my family eats."

(3) "I will make sure that my children don't eat or drink after me."

(4) "I'm glad that I don't have to get help taking care of my children."

48. The nurse calculates the IV flow rate for a postoperative patient. The patient is to receive 3,000 ml of Ringer's lactate solution IV to run over 24 hours. The IV infusion set has a drop factor of 10 drops per milliliter. The nurse should regulate the patient's IV to deliver how many drops per minute?

(1) 18

(2) 21

(3) 35

(4) 40

49. A 67-year-old patient with emphysema becomes restless and confused. What step should the nurse take next?

(1) Encourage the patient to perform pursed-lip breathing.

(2) Check the patient's temperature.

(3) Assess the patient's potassium level.

(4) Increase the patient's oxygen flow rate to 5 L/min.

50. The nurse is caring for a patient one day after an abdominal-perineal resection for cancer of the rectum. The nurse should question which of the following orders?

(1) Discontinue the nasogastric tube.

(2) Irrigate the colostomy.

(3) Place petrolatum gauze over the stoma.

(4) Administer Demerol 50 mg IM for pain.

51. The nurse is caring for a patient four hours after intracranial surgery. Which of the following actions should the nurse take immediately?

(1) Turn, cough, and deep-breathe the patient.

(2) Place the patient with the neck flexed and head turned to the side.

(3) Perform passive range of motion exercises.

(4) Move client to the head of the bed using a turning sheet.

52. A 6-year-old child with a congenital heart disorder is admitted with congestive heart failure. Digoxin (Lanoxin) 0.12 mg is ordered for the child. The bottle of Lanoxin contains .05 mg of Lanoxin in 1 cc of solution. The nurse should administer

(1) 1.2 cc

(2) 2.4 cc

(3) 3.5 cc

(4) 4.2 cc

53. The nurse is caring for a patient with an acute myocardial infarction. Which of the following laboratory findings would MOST concern the nurse?

(1) Erythrocyte sedimentation rate (ESR): 10 mm/h

(2) Hematocrit (Hct): 42 percent

(3) Creatine kinase (CK): 150 U/ml

(4) Serum glucose: 100 mg/dL

54. The nurse is caring for a patient with cervical cancer. The nurse notes that the radium implant has become dislodged. Which of the following actions should the nurse take FIRST?

(1) Stay with the patient and contact radiology.

(2) Wrap the implant in a blanket and place it behind a lead shield.

(3) Pick up the implant with long-handled forceps and place it in a lead container.

(4) Obtain a dosimeter reading on the patient and report it to the physician.

55. The nurse in a primary care clinic is caring for a 68-year-old man. History reveals that the client has smoked one pack of cigarettes per day for 45 years and drinks two beers per day. He is complaining of a non-productive cough, chest discomfort, and dyspnea. The nurse hears isolated wheezing in the right middle lobe. It would be MOST important for the nurse to complete which of the following orders?

(1) Pulmonary function tests

(2) Echocardiogram

(3) Chest X-ray

(4) Sputum culture

56. The nurse is caring for a patient with pernicious anemia. The nurse knows that her teaching has been successful if the patient makes which of the following statements?

    (1) "In order to get better, I will take iron pills."

    (2) "I am going to attend smoking cessation classes."

    (3) "I will learn how to perform IM injections."

    (4) "I will increase my intake of carbohydrates."

57. The nurse is caring for clients in the Emergency Department of an acute care facility. Four clients have been admitted in the last 20 minutes. Which of the admissions should the nurse see FIRST?

    (1) A patient complaining of chest pain that is unrelieved by nitroglycerine.

    (2) A patient with third-degree burns to the face.

    (3) A patient with a fractured left hip.

    (4) A patient complaining of epigastric pain.

58. The nurse is caring for a patient with a diagnosis of COPD, bronchitis-type, in the long-term care facility. The patient is wheezing, and his oxygen saturation is 85 percent. Four hours ago, the oxygen saturation was 88 percent. It is MOST important for the nurse to take which of the following actions?

    (1) Administer beclomethasone (Vanceril), two puffs per metered dose inhaler.

    (2) Listen to breath sounds.

    (3) Increase oxygen to 4 L per mask.

    (4) Administer albuterol (Proventil), two puffs per metered dose inhaler.

59. The nurse is caring for a patient hospitalized for observation following a fall. The patient states, "My friend fell last year, and no one thought anything was wrong. She died two days later!" Which of the following responses by the nurse is BEST?

    (1) "This happens to quite a few people."

    (2) 'We are monitoring you, so you'll be okay."

    (3) "Don't you think I'm taking good care of you?"

    (4) "You're concerned that it might happen to you?"

60. The nurse is caring for patients on the pediatric unit. An eight-year-old patient with second and third degree burns on the right thigh is being admitted. The nurse should assign the new patient to which one of the following roommates?

   (1) A two-year-old with chicken pox

   (2) A four-year-old with asthma

   (3) A nine-year-old with acute diarrhea

   (4) A ten-year-old with methicillin-resistant staph auerus (MRSA)

61. The nurse teaches a client about elastic stockings. Which of the following statements, if made by the client, indicates to the nurse that teaching was successful?

   (1) "I will wear the stockings until the physician tells me to remove them."

   (2) "I should wear the stockings even when I am asleep."

   (3) "Every four hours I should remove the stockings for a half hour."

   (4) "I should put on the stockings before getting out of bed in the morning."

62. The nurse is teaching a client who is scheduled for a paracentesis. Which of the following statements, if made by the client to the nurse, indicates that teaching has been successful?

   (1) "I will be in surgery for less than one hour."

   (2) "I must not void prior to the procedure."

   (3) "The physician will remove 2–3 L of fluid."

   (4) "I will lie on my back and breathe slowly."

63. The homecare nurse is performing chest physiotherapy on an elderly client with chronic airflow limitations (CAL). Which of the following actions should the nurse take FIRST?

   (1) Perform chest physiotherapy prior to meals.

   (2) Auscultate the chest prior to beginning the procedure.

   (3) Administer bronchiodilators after the procedure.

   (4) Percuss each lobe prior to asking the client to cough.

64. A 60-year-old man is admitted to the hospital with a diagnosis of chronic bronchitis. He has a 10-year history of emphysema. The nurse should place him in which of the following positions?

(1) Side-lying
(2) Supine
(3) High-Fowler's
(4) Semi-Fowler's

65. A patient is to receive 1,000 ml of 5% dextrose in 0.45 NaCl intravenous solution in an 8-hour period. The intravenous set delivers 15 drops per milliliter. The nurse should regulate the flow rate so it delivers how many drops of fluid per minute?

(1) 15
(2) 31
(3) 45
(4) 60

66. The nurse knows that the plan of care for a patient with severe liver disease would include which of the following actions?

(1) Administer Kayexelate enemas.
(2) Offer a low protein, high carbohydrate diet.
(3) Insert a Sengsteken-Blakemore tube.
(4) Administer salt-poor albumin IV.

67. A 59-year-old patient with a diagnosis of delirium is admitted to the hospital. To evaluate the cause of a patient's delirium, blood is sent to the laboratory for analysis. The results are as follows: Na^+ 156, Cl^- 100, K^+ 4.0, CO_2 21, BUN 86, glucose 100. Based on these laboratory results, the nurse should record which of the following nursing diagnoses on the patient's care plan?

(1) Alteration in patterns of urinary elimination
(2) Fluid volume deficit
(3) Nutritional deficit: less than body requirements
(4) Self-care deficit: feeding

68. A patient is to receive 3,000 ml of 0.9% NaCl IV in 24 hours. The intravenous set delivers 15 drops per milliliter. The nurse should regulate the flow rate so that the patient receives how many drops of fluid per minute?

    (1) 21
    (2) 28
    (3) 31
    (4) 42

69. The nurse is supervising care of a patient receiving total parenteral nutrition (TPN) through a single-lumen percutaneous central catheter. The nurse would be MOST concerned if which of the following was observed?

    (1) The patient receives insulin through the single-lumen.
    (2) A mask is worn when changing the patient's dressing.
    (3) The patient's dressing is changed daily using sterile technique.
    (4) The patient is weighed two to three times per week.

70. The nurse is caring for patients in the outpatient clinic. A client tells the nurse that he developed weakness and numbness in the legs the previous day and now his body feels the same way. The client's blood pressure is 120/80, P 86, R 20. The client denies any pain but appears anxious to the nurse. It would be MOST important for the nurse to ask which of the following questions?

    (1) "Have you recently fallen or had some other type of physical injury?"
    (2) "Have you recently had a viral infection such as a cold?"
    (3) "Have you recently taken any over-the-counter medication?"
    (4) "Have you recently experienced headaches?"

71. The nurse is admitting a patient who is jaundiced due to pancreatic cancer. The nurse should give the HIGHEST priority to which of the following needs?

    (1) Nutrition
    (2) Self-image
    (3) Skin integrity
    (4) Urinary elimination

72. Which of the following statements, if made by a client during a group therapy session, would the nurse identify as reflecting a client's narcissistic personality disorder?

    (1) "I'm sick of hearing about all your life tragedies."
    (2) "I know I'm interrupting others, so what?"
    (3) "I just can't stop wanting to slash myself."
    (4) "I just have no hope for the future."

73. A 15-year-old patient is admitted to the hospital with anorexia nervosa. Which of the following statements, if made by the patient, would require immediate follow-up by the nurse?

    (1) "My gums were bleeding this morning."
    (2) "I'm getting fatter every day."
    (3) "Nobody likes me because I'm so ugly."
    (4) "I'm feeling dizzy and weak today."

74. A client is admitted to the hospital for treatment of pneumocystis carinii pneumonia and Kaposi sarcoma. The client tells the nurse that he has been considering organ donation when he dies. Which of the following responses by the nurse is BEST?

    (1) "What does your family think about your decision?"
    (2) "You will help many people by donating your organs."
    (3) "Would you like to speak to the Organ Donor Representative?"
    (4) "That is not possible based on your illness."

75. The nurse is caring for a patient five hours after a pancreatectomy for cancer of the pancreas. On assessment, the nurse notes that there is minimal drainage from the nasogastric tube. It is MOST important for the nurse to take which of the following actions?

    (1) Notify the physician.
    (2) Monitor vital signs q 15 minutes.
    (3) Check the tubing for kinks.
    (4) Replace the NG tube.

76. When collecting a 24-hour urine specimen for creatinine clearance, it is MOST important for the nurse to do which of the following?

(1) Obtain an order from the physician for insertion of a Foley catheter.

(2) Obtain the client's weight prior to beginning the urine collection.

(3) Discard the last voided specimen prior to ending the collection.

(4) Ask if a preservative is present in the container.

77. The nurse is planning discharge teaching for a patient with Parkinson's disease. To maintain safety, the nurse should make which one of the following suggestions to the family?

(1) Install a raised toilet seat.

(2) Obtain a hospital bed.

(3) Instruct the patient to hold his arms in a dependent position when ambulating.

(4) Perform an exercise program during the late afternoon.

78. The nurse is performing discharge teaching for a patient with chronic pancreatitis. Which of the following statements, if made by the patient to the nurse, indicates that further teaching is necessary?

(1) "I do not have to restrict my physical activity."

(2) "I should take pancrelipase (Viokase) before meals."

(3) "I will eat three meals per day."

(4) "I am not allowed to drink any alcoholic beverages."

79. Following a laparoscopic cholecystectomy, the patient complains of abdominal pain and bloating. Which of the following responses by the nurse is BEST?

(1) "Increase your intake of fresh fruits and vegetables."

(2) "I'll give you the prescribed pain medication."

(3) "Why don't you take a walk in the hallway."

(4) "You may need an indwelling catheter."

80. The nurse in an outpatient clinic is supervising student nurses administering influenza vaccinations. The nurse should question the administration of the vaccine to which of the following clients?

(1) A 45-year-old male who is allergic to shellfish

(2) A 60-year-old female who says she has a sore throat

(3) A 66-year-old female who lives in a group home

(4) A 70-year-old female with congestive heart failure

81. An arterial blood gas is ordered for a man following a myocardial infarction. After obtaining the specimen, it would be MOST appropriate for the nurse to take which of the following actions?

(1) Obtain ice for the specimen.

(2) Apply direct pressure to the site.

(3) Apply a sterile dressing to the site.

(4) Observe the site for hematoma formation.

82. The nurse is caring for a man who was involved in an auto accident the previous day. The patient has a double-lumen tracheostomy tube with a cuff. The nurse should

(1) change the tracheostomy dressing every eight hours and PRN.

(2) change the tracheostomy ties every 48 hours.

(3) keep the inner cannula of the tracheostomy in place at all times.

(4) push the outer cannula back in if it accidentally "blows out."

83. The nurse performs discharge teaching with a patient with emphysema. Which statement, if made by the patient, indicates that teaching was successful?

(1) "Cold weather will help my breathing problems."

(2) "I should eat three balanced meals but limit my fluid intake."

(3) "My outside activity should be limited when pollution levels are high."

(4) "An intensive exercise program is important in regaining my strength."

84. The nurse assists the physician with the removal of a chest tube. Before the physician removes the chest tube, the nurse should instruct the patient to

(1) exhale and bear down.

(2) hold his breath for five seconds.

(3) inhale and exhale rapidly.

(4) cough as hard as he can.

85. A 45-year-old man comes into the emergency room with complaints of sudden onset of severe right flank pain. While tests are being performed, it is MOST important for the nurse to

(1) make sure that he does not eat or drink anything.

(2) strain all his urine through several layers of gauze.

(3) check his grip strength and pupil reactivity.

(4) send blood and urine specimens to the lab for analysis.

86. The nurse is preparing discharge teaching for a patient with a new colostomy. The nurse knows teaching was successful when the patient chooses which of the following menu options?

(1) Sausage, sauerkraut, baked potato, and fresh fruit

(2) Cheese omelet with bran muffin and fresh pineapple

(3) Pork chop, mashed potatoes, turnips, and salad

(4) Baked chicken, boiled potato, cooked carrots, and yogurt

87. A 59-year-old man is seen in the outpatient clinic to rule out acute renal failure. The nurse would be MOST concerned if the patient made which one of the following statements?

(1) "My urine is often pink-tinged."

(2) "It is hard for me to start the flow of urine."

(3) "It is quite painful for me to urinate."

(4) "I urinate in the morning and again before dinner."

88. The nurse is teaching a new mother how to breastfeed her newborn. The nurse knows that teaching has been successful if the client makes which of the following statements?

(1) "My baby's weight should equal her birthweight in five to seven days."

(2) "My baby should have at least six to eight wet diapers per day."

(3) "My baby will sleep at least six hours between feedings."

(4) "My baby will feed for about 10 minutes per feeding."

89. A man is admitted to the Telemetry Unit for evaluation of complaints of chest pain. Eight hours after admission, the patient goes into ventricular fibrillation. The physician defibrillates the patient. The nurse understands that the purpose of defibrillation is to

(1) increase cardiac contractility and cardiac output.

(2) cause asystole so the normal pacemaker can recapture.

(3) reduce cardiac ischemia and acidosis.

(4) provide energy for depleted myocardial cells.

90. A man is brought to the emergency room complaining of chest pain. The nurse performs an assessment of the patient. Which of the following symptoms would be MOST characteristic of an acute myocardial infarction?

(1) Colic-like epigastric pain

(2) Sharp, well-localized, unilateral chest pain

(3) Severe substernal pain radiating down the left arm

(4) Sharp, burning chest pain moving from place to place

91. The nurse is caring for patients on the medical unit. A patient is admitted with a diagnosis of deep vein thrombosis (DVT). Admission orders include heparin 2,000 units per hour in 5 percent dextrose in water. The nurse should have which of the following available?

(1) Propranolol (Inderal)

(2) Protamine zinc

(3) Protamine sulfate

(4) Vitamin K

92. A client returns to the clinic two weeks after discharge from the hospital. He is taking wafarin sodium (Coumadin) 2 mg po daily. Which of the following statements, if made by the client to the nurse, indicates that further teaching is necessary?

    (1) "I have been taking an antihistamine before bed."
    (2) "I take aspirin when I have a headache."
    (3) "I use sunscreen when I go outside."
    (4) "I take Mylanta if my stomach gets upset."

93. To enhance the percutaneous absorption of nitroglycerine ointment, it would be MOST important for the nurse to select a site that is

    (1) muscular.
    (2) near the heart.
    (3) non-hairy.
    (4) over a bony prominence.

94. A client with chronic alcohol abuse has been admitted to a rehabilitation unit. The nurse knows that the client is denying alcoholism when he makes which of the following statements?

    (1) "My brother did this to me."
    (2) "Drinking always calms my nerves."
    (3) "I can stop drinking anytime I feel like it."
    (4) "Let's all plan to play cards tonight."

95. During the acute phase of a cerebrovascular accident (CVA), the nurse should maintain the patient in which of the following positions?

    (1) Semi-prone with the head of the bed elevated 60–90 degrees
    (2) Lateral, with the head of the bed flat
    (3) Prone, with the head of the bed flat
    (4) Supine, with the head of the bed elevated 30–45 degrees

96. Which of the following statements, if made by a client during a group therapy session, would require immediate follow-up by the nurse?

(1) "I know I'm a chronically compulsive liar, but I can't help it."

(2) "I don't ever want to go home; I feel safer here."

(3) "I don't really care if I ever see my girlfriend again."

(4) "I'll make sure that doctor is sorry for what he said."

97. A patient newly diagnosed with Alzheimer's disease is admitted to the unit. Which action, if taken by the nurse, is BEST?

(1) Place the patient in a private room away from the nurses' station.

(2) Ask the family to wait in the waiting room while the nurse admits the patient.

(3) Assign a different nurse daily to care for the patient.

(4) Ask the patient to state today's date.

98. A 40-year-old woman visits the clinic with complaints of right calf tenderness and pain. It would be MOST important for the nurse to ask which of the following questions?

(1) 'Do you exercise excessively?"

(2) "Have you had any fractures in the last year?"

(3) "What type of birth control do you use?"

(4) "Are you under a lot of stress?"

99. A mother calls the well-baby clinic to report that her 4-month-old son has an upper respiratory infection (URI) with a temperature of 104° F (40° C). The infant is scheduled to receive his DPT and TOPV immunizations later that day. The mother asks the nurse if she should bring him in for his scheduled immunizations. Which of the following responses by the nurse would be MOST appropriate?

(1) "Keep him at home. We'll give him a double dose next time."

(2) "Bring him in. His illness will not interfere with his immunizations."

(3) "Keep him at home until his temperature and infection resolve."

(4) "Bring him in. We'll give some antibiotics with the immunizations."

100. The nurse in the postpartum unit cares for a 27-year-old woman who delivered her first child the previous day. During her assessment of the patient, the nurse notes multiple varicosities on the patient's lower extremities. The nurse should

(1) teach the patient to rest in bed when the baby sleeps.

(2) encourage early and frequent ambulation.

(3) apply warm soaks for 20 minutes every four hours.

(4) perform passive range of motion exercises three times daily.

101. A 26-year-old man fractures his left femur in a bicycle accident. A cast is applied. Which of the following exercises would be MOST beneficial for this patient?

(1) Passive exercise of the affected limb

(2) Quadriceps setting of the affected limb

(3) Active ROM exercises of the unaffected limb

(4) Passive exercise of the upper extremities

102. The nurse plans care for a patient receiving electroconvulsive treatments (ECT). Immediately following a treatment, the nurse should take which of the following actions?

(1) Orient the patient to time and place.

(2) Talk about events prior to the patient's hospitalization.

(3) Restrict fluid intake and encourage the patient to ambulate.

(4) Initiate comfort measures to relieve vertigo.

103. A patient is to receive 35 mg/hr of intravenous aminophylline. The nurse mixes 350 mg of aminophylline in 500 cc D_5W. At what rate should this solution be infused?

(1) 20 cc/hr

(2) 35 cc/hr

(3) 50 cc/hr

(4) 70 cc/hr

104. The nurse prepares an adult client for instillation of ear drops. The nurse should use which of the following methods to administer the ear drops?

    (1) Cool the solution for better adsorption. Drop the medication directly into the auditory canal.
    (2) Warm the solution. Flush the medication rapidly into the ear.
    (3) Warm the solution. Drop the medication along the side of the ear canal.
    (4) Warm the solution to 40° C. Drop the medication slowly into the ear canal.

105. A 52-year-old man is receiving intravenous cimetidine (Tagamet). After twenty minutes of the infusion, the patient complains of a headache and dizziness. Which of the following actions should the nurse take FIRST?

    (1) Stop the infusion.
    (2) Call the physician.
    (3) Take vital signs.
    (4) Call the pharmacist.

106. A 26-year-old man comes to the emergency room with complaints of nausea, vomiting, and abdominal pain. He is a type I diabetic (IDDM). Four days earlier, he reduced his insulin dose when flu symptoms prevented him from eating. The nurse performs an assessment of the patient which reveals poor skin turgor, dry mucous membranes, and fruity breath odor. The nurse should be alert for which of the following problems?

    (1) Hypoglycemia
    (2) Viral illness
    (3) Ketoacidosis
    (4) Hyperglycemic hyperosmolar nonketotic coma

107. A 45-year-old homeless man is hospitalized with tuberculosis. The physician's orders include isoniazid (INH) and pyridoxine (vitamin B_6). The patient asks why he is receiving pyridoxine. The nurse's response should be based on the knowledge that pyridoxine

    (1) increases INH absorption.
    (2) prevents the development of tolerance to INH.
    (3) decreases the severity of INH side effects.
    (4) prevents INH-associated neuritis.

108. An 11-year-old boy is admitted to the hospital for evaluation for a kidney transplant. During the initial assessment, the nurse learns that the patient received hemodialysis for three years due to renal failure. The nurse knows that his illness can interfere with this patient's achievement of

   (1) intimacy.
   (2) trust.
   (3) industry.
   (4) identity.

109. The nurse assesses a patient with a history of Addison's disease who has received steroid therapy for several years. The nurse could expect the patient to exhibit which of the following changes in appearance?

   (1) Buffalo hump, girdle-obesity, gaunt facial appearance.
   (2) Tanning of the skin, discoloration of the mucous membranes, alopecia, weight loss.
   (3) Emaciation, nervousness, breast engorgement, hirsutism.
   (4) Truncal obesity, purple striations on the skin, moon face.

110. Haloperidol (Haldol) 5 mg tid is ordered for a patient with schizophrenia. Two days later, the patient complains of "tight jaws and a stiff neck." The nurse should recognize that these complaints are

   (1) common side effects of antipsychotic medications that will diminish over time.
   (2) early symptoms of extrapyramidal reactions to the medication.
   (3) psychosomatic complaints resulting from a delusional system.
   (4) permanent side effects of Haldol.

111. The nurse is caring for a woman who states she was beaten and sexually assaulted by a male friend. What should the nurse do first?

   (1) Encourage the client to call her family lawyer.
   (2) Ask for a psychiatry consult.
   (3) Stay with the client during the physical exam.
   (4) Wash and dress the client's wounds before the physical exam.

112. The nurse cares for a 65-year-old woman following surgery for removal of a cataract in her right eye. The patient complaints of severe eye pain in her right eye. The nurse knows this symptom

(1) is expected and should administer analgesic to the patient.

(2) is expected and should maintain the patient on bed rest.

(3) is unexpected and may signify a detached retina.

(4) is unexpected and may signify hemorrhage.

113. A patient returns to his room following a lower GI series. When he is assessed by the nurse, he complains of weakness. Which of the following nursing diagnoses should receive priority in planning his care?

(1) Alteration in sensation-perception, gustatory

(2) Constipation, colonic

(3) High risk for fluid-volume deficit

(4) Nutrition, less than body requirements

114. A patient hospitalized with a gastric ulcer is scheduled for discharge. The nurse teaches the patient about an antiulcer diet. Which of the following statements, if made by the patient, would indicate to the nurse that dietary teaching was successful?

(1) "I must eat bland foods to help my stomach heal."

(2) "I can eat most foods, as long as they don't bother my stomach."

(3) "I cannot eat fruits and vegetables because they cause too much gas."

(4) "I should eat a low-fiber diet to delay gastric emptying."

115. A 6-year-old boy is returned to his room following a tonsillectomy. He remains sleepy from the anesthesia but is easily awakened. The nurse should place the child in which of the following positions?

(1) Sims'

(2) Side-lying

(3) Supine

(4) Prone

116. A 22-year-old woman is preparing to take her one-day-old infant home from the hospital. The nurse discusses the test for phenylketonuria (PKU) with the mother. The nurse's teaching should be based on an understanding that the test is MOST reliable

   (1) after a source of protein has been ingested.

   (2) after the meconium has been excreted.

   (3) after the danger of hyperbilirubinemia has passed.

   (4) after the effects of delivery have subsided.

117. A 54-year-old man is being treated for Addison's disease. The physician orders cortisone 25 mg PO daily. The nurse should explain to the patient that adjustment of the dosage may be required in which of the following situations?

   (1) Dosage is increased when the blood glucose level increases.

   (2) Dosage is decreased when dietary intake is increased.

   (3) Dosage is decreased when infection stimulates endogenous steroid secretion.

   (4) Dosage is increased relative to an increase in the level of stress.

118. A 48-year-old woman is hospitalized with a diagnosis of bipolar disorder. While she is in the patient activities room on the psychiatric unit, she flirts with male patients and disrupt unit activities. Which of the following approaches would be MOST appropriate for the nurse to take at this time?

   (1) Set limits on the patient's behavior and remind her of the rules.

   (2) Distract the patient and escort her back to her room.

   (3) Instruct the other patients to ignore this patient's behavior.

   (4) Tell the patient that she is behaving inappropriately and send her to her room.

119. A 33-year-old man is brought to the emergency room bleeding profusely from a stab wound in the left chest area. The nurse's assessment reveals a blood pressure of 80/50, pulse of 110, and respiratory rate of 28. The nurse should expect which of the following potential problems?

   (1) Hypovolemic shock

   (2) Cardiogenic shock

   (3) Neurogenic shock

   (4) Septic shock

120. A 42-year-old man is admitted to the hospital for surgical repair of a detached retina in the right eye. In planning care for this patient postoperatively, the nurse should

(1) encourage self-care activities.

(2) maintain patches over both eyes.

(3) limit movements of his eyes.

(4) caution him against excessive talking.

121. The nurse cares for a patient receiving full strength Ensure by tube feeding. The nurse knows that the MOST common complication of a tube feeding is

(1) edema.

(2) diarrhea.

(3) hypokalemia.

(4) vomiting.

122. A 6-week-old infant is brought to the hospital for treatment of pyloric stenosis. The nurse enters the following nursing diagnosis on the infant's care plan: "fluid volume deficit related to vomiting." Which of the following assessments supports this diagnosis?

(1) The infant eagerly accepts feedings.

(2) The infant vomited once since admission.

(3) The infant's skin is warm and moist.

(4) The infant's anterior fontanelle is depressed.

123. A 68-year-old woman is diagnosed with thrombocytopenia due to acute lymphocytic leukemia. She is admitted to the hospital for treatment. The nurse should assign the patient

(1) to a private room so she will not infect other patients and health care workers.

(2) to a private room so she will not be infected by other patients and health care workers.

(3) to a semiprivate room so she will have stimulation during her hospitalization.

(4) to a semiprivate room so she will have the opportunity to express her feelings about her illness.

124. A 28-year-old woman comes to the clinic because she thinks she is pregnant. Tests are performed and the pregnancy is confirmed. The patient's last menstrual period began on September 8 and lasted for 6 days. The nurse calculates that her expected date of confinement (EDC) is

(1) May 15.

(2) June 15.

(3) June 21.

(4) July 8.

125. A 2-month-old infant is brought to the pediatrician's office for a well-baby visit. During the examination, congenital subluxation of the left hip is suspected. The nurse knows that symptoms of congenital hip dislocation include

(1) lengthening of the limb on the affected side.

(2) deformities of the foot and ankle.

(3) asymmetry of the gluteal and thigh folds.

(4) plantar flexion of the foot.

126. After two weeks of receiving lithium therapy, a patient in the psychiatric unit becomes depressed. Which of the following evaluations of the patient's behavior by the nurse would be MOST accurate?

(1) The treatment plan is not effective; the patient requires a larger dose of lithium.

(2) This is a normal response to lithium therapy; the patient should continue with the current treatment plan.

(3) This is a normal response to lithium therapy; the patient should be monitored for suicidal behavior.

(4) The treatment plan is not effective; the patient requires an antidepressant.

127. A 67-year-old woman is admitted for treatment of pulmonary edema. During the admission interview, she states she has a six-year history of congestive heart failure (CHF). The nurse performs an initial assessment. When the nurse auscultates the breath sounds, the nurse should expect to hear

(1) crackling.

(2) wheezing.

(3) whistling.

(4) absent breath sounds.

128. A 63-year-old man is diagnosed with cancer of the larynx and comes to the hospital for a total laryngectomy. When admitting this patient, how should the nurse assess laryngeal nerve function?

(1) Assess the extent of neck edema.

(2) Check his ability to swallow.

(3) Observe for excessive drooling.

(4) Tap the side of his neck gently and observe for facial twitching.

129. The nurse supervises care at an adult day-care center. Four meal choices are available to the residents. The nurse should ensure that a resident on a low-cholesterol diet receives which of the following meals?

(1) Egg custard, boiled liver

(2) Fried chicken, potatoes

(3) Hamburger, french fries

(4) Grilled flounder, green beans

130. The nurse cares for a patient with a possible bowel obstruction. A nasogastric tube is to be inserted. Before inserting the tube, the nurse explains its purpose to the patient. Which of the following explanations, if made by the nurse, is MOST accurate?

(1) "It empties the stomach of fluids and gas."

(2) "It prevents spasms of the sphincter of Oddi."

(3) "It prevents air from forming in the small and large intestine."

(4) "It removes bile from the gall bladder."

131. A 25-year-old man is being treated in the burn unit for second- and third-degree burns over 45% of his body. The physician's orders include the application of silver sulfadiazine (Silvadene cream). The BEST way to apply this medication is to use a sterile

(1) 4 × 4 soaked in saline.

(2) tongue depressor.

(3) cotton-tipped applicator.

(4) gloved hand.

132. The nurse teaches a 20-year-old primigravida how to measure the frequency of uterine contractions. The nurse should explain to the patient that the frequency of uterine contractions is determined

    (1) from the beginning of one contraction to the end of the next contraction.

    (2) from the beginning of one contraction to the end of the same contraction.

    (3) by the number of contractions that occur within a given period of time.

    (4) by the strength of the contraction at its peak.

133. The nurse performs teaching with a 49-year-old woman receiving estrogen replacement therapy. Which of the following statements, if made by the nurse to the woman, indicates that the nurse is aware of the possible complications of estrogen therapy?

    (1) "Take an analgesic before you take estrogen, since estrogen may cause discomfort."

    (2) "Make sure you keep your clinic appointments, especially your gynecologic checkup."

    (3) "Limit your fluid intake since estrogen promotes the retention of fluids."

    (4) "Increase roughage in your diet to avoid constipation."

134. Several days after being admitted for depression, a man is observed sitting alone in the patient's dining room. The nurse notes that the patient has not finished his meal. Which of the following nursing measures would be MOST appropriate?

    (1) Allow the patient to eat in his room until he becomes more comfortable eating with other patients.

    (2) Ask the patient's family to bring foods that he likes to eat.

    (3) Order small frequent meals and sit with the patient while he eats in the dining room.

    (4) Do not focus on eating behaviors since his appetite will improve over time.

135. A 21-year-old woman is being treated for injuries sustained in an automobile accident. The patient has a central venous pressure (CVP) line in place. The nurse recognizes that CVP measurement reflects

    (1) cardiac output.

    (2) pressure in the left ventricle.

    (3) pressure in the right atrium.

    (4) pressure in the pulmonary artery.

136. A mother brings her 4-year-old daughter to the pediatrician for treatment of chronic otitis media. The mother asks the nurse how she can prevent her child from getting ear infections so often. The nurse's response should be based on an understanding that the recurrence of otitis media can be decreased by

   (1) covering the child's ears while bathing.

   (2) treating upper respiratory infections quickly.

   (3) administering nose drops at bedtime.

   (4) isolating her child from other children.

137. A patient receives 10 units of NPH insulin every morning at 8 A.M. At 4 P.M., the nurse observes that the patient is diaphoretic and slightly confused. The FIRST action the nurse should take is to

   (1) check vital signs.

   (2) check urine for glucose and ketones.

   (3) give 6 oz of skim milk.

   (4) call the physician.

138. Prior to the patient undergoing a scheduled intravenous pyelogram (IVP), the nurse reviews the patient's health history. It would be MOST important for the nurse to obtain the answer to which of the following questions?

   (1) Does the patient have difficulty voiding?

   (2) Does the patient have any allergies to shellfish or iodine?

   (3) Does the patient have a history of constipation?

   (4) Does the patient have frequent headaches?

139. A 6-year-old girl with chicken pox (varicella) is brought by her parents to the physician for evaluation. The nurse knows the rash characteristic of chicken pox can be described as

   (1) maculopapular.

   (2) small irregular red spots with minute bluish-white centers.

   (3) round or oval erythematous scaling patches.

   (4) petechiae.

140. A 37-year-old primigravida at 28 weeks gestation, takes a three-hour glucose tolerance test. The results indicate a fasting blood sugar of 100 mg/dL and a two-hour post-load blood sugar of 300 mg/dL. Which of the following nursing diagnoses should be considered the HIGHEST priority at this time?

(1) Potential impaired family coping related to diagnosis of gestational diabetes mellitus (GDM).

(2) Potential noncompliance related to lack of knowledge or lack of adequate support system.

(3) Potential for altered parenting related to disappointment.

(4) Ineffective family coping related to anticipatory grieving.

141. The nurse cares for a 45-year-old man admitted for a possible herniated intervertebral disk. Ibuprofen (Motrin), propoxyphene hydrochloride (Darvon), and cyclobenzaprine hydrochloride (Flexeril) are ordered PRN. Several hours after admission, the patient complains of pain. Which of the following actions should the nurse do FIRST?

(1) Administer ibuprofen (Motrin).

(2) Call the physician to determine which medication should be given.

(3) Gather more information from the patient about the complaint.

(4) Allow the patient some time to rest and see if the pain subsides.

142. When planning care for a 56-year-old man hospitalized with depression, the nurse includes measures to increase his self-esteem. Which of the following actions should the nurse take to meet this goal?

(1) Encourage him to accept leadership responsibilities in milieu activities.

(2) Set simple, realistic goals with him to help him experience success.

(3) Help him to accept his illness and the adjustments that are required.

(4) Assure him that when he is discharged, he will be able to resume his previous activities.

143. The nurse finds a visitor unconscious on the floor of a patient's room during visiting hours at the hospital. Which of the following nursing assessments is consistent with cardiopulmonary arrest?

(1) Absent pulse, fixed and dilated pupils

(2) Absent respirations, fixed and dilated pupils

(3) Absent pulse and respirations

(4) Thready pulse and pupillary changes

144. A 68-year-old man is transferred to an extended care facility following a cerebrovascular accident (CVA). The patient has right-sided paralysis and has been experiencing dysphagia. The nurse observes an aide prepare the patient to eat lunch. Which of the following situations would require an intervention by the nurse?

(1) The patient is in bed in high-Fowler's position.

(2) The patient's head and neck are positioned slightly forward.

(3) The aide puts the food in the back of his mouth on the unaffected side.

(4) The aide waters down the pudding to help the patient swallow.

145. The home care nurse plans care for a patient with pernicious anemia. A monthly intramuscular injection is ordered for the patient. The nurse knows that the best muscle to administer an intramuscular injection in an adult is the

(1) gluteus maximus.

(2) deltoid.

(3) vastus lateralis.

(4) dorsogluteal.

146. A 56-year-old man comes to the emergency room complaining of nausea, vomiting, and severe right upper quadrant pain. His temperature is 101.3° F (38.5° C) and an abdominal X-ray reveals an enlarged gall bladder. He is given a diagnosis of acute cholecystitis and is scheduled for surgery. After administering an analgesic to the patient, the nurse recognizes that which of the following actions is a priority?

(1) Assessing the patient's need for dietary teaching.

(2) Assessing the patient's fluid and electrolyte status.

(3) Examining the patient's health history for allergies to antibiotics.

(4) Determining whether the patient has signed consent for surgery.

147. A mother with four children calls the clinic for advice on how to care for her oldest child, who has developed chickenpox. Which of the following statements, if made by the mother, indicates a need for further teaching?

(1) "I should keep my child home from school until the vesicles are crusted."

(2) "I can use calamine lotion if needed."

(3) "I should remove the crusts so the skin can heal."

(4) "I can use mittens if scratching becomes a problem."

148. A 23-year-old woman comes the clinic at 32 weeks gestation. A diagnosis of pregnancy-induced hypertension (PIH) is made. The nurse performs teaching. Which of the following statements, if made by the patient, indicates to the nurse that further teaching is required?

(1) "Lying in bed on my left side is likely to increase my urinary output."

(2) "If the bed rest works, I may lose a pound or two in the next few days."

(3) "I should be sure to maintain a diet that has a good amount of protein."

(4) "I will have to keep my room darkened and not watch much television."

149. The nurse evaluates the care provided to a 42-year-old man hospitalized for treatment of adrenal crisis. Which of the following changes would indicate to the nurse that the patient is responding favorably to medical and nursing treatment?

(1) The patient's urinary output has increased.

(2) The patient's blood pressure has increased.

(3) The patient has lost weight.

(4) The patient's peripheral edema has decreased.

150. After completing an assessment, the nurse determines that a 45-year-old woman is exhibiting early symptoms of a dystonic reaction related to the use of an antipsychotic medication. Which of the following actions by the nurse would be MOST appropriate?

(1) Reality test with the patient and assure her that her physical symptoms are not real.

(2) Teach the patient about common side effects of antipsychotic medications.

(3) Explain to the patient that there is no treatment that will relieve these symptoms.

(4) Notify the physician and obtain an order for I.M. Benadryl.

151. The physician orders heparin for a 46-year-old woman. In order to evaluate the effectiveness of the patient's heparin therapy, the nurse should monitor which of the following laboratory values?

(1) Platelet count

(2) Clotting time

(3) Bleeding time

(4) Prothrombin time

152. A 50-year-old woman comes to the clinic for evaluation of acute onset of seizures. A thorough history and physical examination is performed. The nurse would expect which of the following diagnostic tests to be performed FIRST?

(1) Magnetic resonance imaging (MRI)

(2) Cerebral angiography

(3) Electroencephalogram (EEG)

(4) Electromyogram (EMG)

153. The nurse performs dietary teaching with a patient on a low-protein diet. The nurse would know that teaching had been successful if the patient identified which of the following meals as LOWEST in protein?

(1) Cranberries and broiled chicken

(2) Tomatoes and flounder

(3) Broccoli and veal

(4) Spinach and tofu

154. A patient has a vagotomy with antrectomy to treat a duodenal ulcer. Postoperatively, the patient develops dumping syndrome. Which of the following statements, if made by the patient, should indicate to the nurse that further dietary teaching is necessary?

(1) "I should eat bread with each meal."

(2) "I should eat smaller meals more frequently."

(3) "I should lie down after eating."

(4) "I should avoid drinking fluids with my meals."

155. A 25-year-old man is admitted to the hospital with a diagnosis of acquired immune deficiency syndrome (AIDS). He is being treated for *pneumocystis carinii* pneumonia. The nurse evaluates the care provided to this patient by other members of the health care team. The nurse should intervene in which of the following situations?

(1) A housekeeper cleans up spilled blood with a bleach solution.

(2) A nursing student takes his blood pressure wearing a mask and gloves.

(3) A technician wears gloves to perform a veinipuncture.

(4) A nurse attendant allows visitors to enter his room without masks.

156. An 18-year-old woman comes to the physician's office for a routine prenatal checkup at 34 weeks gestation. Abdominal palpation reveals the fetal position as right occipital anterior (ROA). At which of the following sites would the nurse expect to find the fetal heart tone?

(1) Below the umbilicus, on the mother's left side.

(2) Below the umbilicus, on the mother's right side.

(3) Above the umbilicus, on the mother's left side.

(4) Above the umbilicus, on the mother's right side.

157. A 20-year-old man is admitted to the hospital with complaints of seizures and a high fever. A brain scan is ordered. Before the scan, the patient asks the nurse what position he will be in while the procedure is being done. Which of the following statements, if made by the nurse, is MOST accurate?

(1) "You will be in a side-lying position, with the foot of the bed elevated."

(2) "You will be in a Fowler's position, with your knees flexed."

(3) "You will be lying supine with a small pillow under your head."

(4) "You will be in Trendelenburg's position, with your head elevated by two pillows."

158. A 28-year-old man is admitted to the psychiatric hospital with a diagnosis of obsessive-compulsive disorder. He is unable to stay employed because his ritualistic behavior causes him to be late for work. Which of the following interpretations of the patient's behavior, by the nurse, is MOST accurate?

(1) He is responding to auditory hallucinations and trying to gain control over his behavior.

(2) He is fulfilling an unconscious desire to punish himself.

(3) He is attempting to reduce anxiety by taking control of the environment.

(4) He is malingering in order to avoid responsibilities at work.

159. A 58-year-old man, diagnosed with chronic lympho-cytic leukemia, is admitted to the hospital for treatment of hemolytic anemia. Which of the following measures, if incorporated into the nursing care plan, would BEST address the patient's needs?

(1) Encourage activities with other patients in the day room.

(2) Isolate him from visitors and patients to avoid infection.

(3) Provide a diet high in vitamin C.

(4) Provide a quiet environment to promote adequate rest.

160. The nurse plans morning care for a 69-year-old man hospitalized after a cerebrovascular accident (CVA) resulting in left-sided paralysis and homonymous hemianopia. During morning care, the nurse should

(1) provide care from the patient's right side.

(2) speak loudly and distinctly when talking with the patient.

(3) reduce the level of lighting in the patient's room to prevent glare.

(4) provide all of the patient's care to reduce his energy expenditure.

161. The nurse prepares for the admission of a client with a perforated duodenal ulcer. Which of the following should the nurse expect to observe as the primary initial symptom?

(1) Fever

(2) Pain

(3) Dizziness

(4) Vomiting

162. A 3-week-old boy is admitted with a diagnosis of pyloric stenosis. The mother tells the nurse that this is her first child and asks if there is anything she can do to prevent this from happening to her next child. Which of the following statements, if made by the nurse, BEST addresses her concern?

(1) "This type of thing generally happens to first children."

(2) "When you have your second child at least you'll know what signs to look for."

(3) "This is a structural problem; it is not a reflection of your parenting skills."

(4) "This is an inherited condition; it is not your fault."

163. The nurse in a well-child clinic assesses a 4-year-old girl and observes multiple bruises on her back and buttocks. The parents state they don't know how the girl sustained the injury. The nurse should

(1) confront the parents about the suspected abuse.

(2) report the suspected child abuse to the appropriate authority.

(3) refer the family to social services for counseling.

(4) document the suspicions about child abuse in the child's medical record.

164. The nurse is caring for a Rh negative mother who has delivered an Rh positive child. The mother states, "The doctor told me about RhoGAM, but I'm still a little confused." Which of the following responses, if made by the nurse, is MOST appropriate?

(1) "RhoGAM is given to your child to prevent the development of antibodies."

(2) "RhoGAM is given to your child to supply the necessary antibodies."

(3) "RhoGAM is given to you to prevent the formation of antibodies."

(4) "RhoGAM is given to you to encourage the production of antibodies."

165. The nurse performs patient teaching with a 45-year-old woman with osteoarthritis. The patient asks what she can do to effectively decrease pain and stiffness in her joints before beginning her daily routine. The nurse should instruct the patient to

(1) perform isometric exercise for 10 minutes.

(2) do range-of-motion exercises, then apply ointment to her joints.

(3) take a warm bath and rest for a few minutes.

(4) stretch all muscles groups.

166. When caring for a patient with anorexia nervosa, which of the following observations indicate to the nurse that the patient's condition is improving?

(1) The patient eats all the food on her meal tray.

(2) The patient asks friends to bring her special foods.

(3) The patient weighs herself daily.

(4) The patient's weight has increased.

167. A 44-year-old man returns to his room following a cardiac catheterization. Which of the following assessments, if made by the nurse, would justify calling the physician?

(1) Pain at the site of the catheter insertion

(2) Absence of a pulse distal to the catheter insertion site

(3) Drainage on the dressing covering the catheter insertion site

(4) Redness at the catheter insertion site

168. An 8-year-old boy is seen in a clinic for treatment of Attention Deficit Disorder (ADD). Medication has been prescribed for the child along with family counseling. The nurse teaches the parents about the medication and discusses parenting strategies. Which of the following statements, if made by the parents, would indicate that further teaching is necessary?

(1) "We will give the medication at night so it doesn't decrease his appetite."

(2) "We will provide a regular routine for sleeping, eating, working, and playing."

(3) "We will establish firm, but reasonable limits on his behavior."

(4) "We will reduce distractions and external stimuli to help him concentrate."

169. A client has been taking Amphojel daily for three weeks. The nurse should be alert for which of the following side effects?

(1) Nausea

(2) Hypercalcemia

(3) Constipation

(4) Anorexia

170. The nurse cares for a 38-year-old man after an appendectomy. The patient continues to complain of discomfort to the nurse shortly after receiving an analgesic. Which of the following measures, if taken by the nurse, would be MOST appropriate?

(1) Notify the physician.

(2) Place him in Fowler's position.

(3) Massage his abdomen.

(4) Provide him with reading material.

171. A 68-year-old man returns to his room following a transurethral resection of the prostate (TURP) for benign prostatic hypertrophy (BPH). Which of the following would cause the nurse to suspect postoperative hemorrhage?

(1) Decreased blood pressure, increased pulse, increased respirations

(2) Fluctuating blood pressure, decreased pulse, rapid respirations

(3) Increased blood pressure, bounding pulse, irregular respirations

(4) Increased blood pressure, irregular pulse, shallow respirations

172. A 22-year-old woman is admitted to the hospital and delivers a healthy 7 lb, 2 oz girl. The mother decides to bottle-feed her infant. Which of the following statements, if made by the mother after a teaching session, indicates to the nurse that the patient needs further instruction?

(1) "I'll pump my breasts and use warm packs to relieve breast pain."

(2) "I'll use a tight bra and ice packs to relieve engorgement discomfort."

(3) "I'll take the medication prescribed by the doctor for pain."

(4) "I'll take the pills ordered by my doctor to help stop the production of milk."

173. The nurse performs teaching with a 52-year-old man undergoing a paracentesis for treatment of cirrhosis. The patient asks what position he will be in for the procedure. The nurse's reply should be based on an understanding that the MOST appropriate position for the patient is

(1) sitting with his lower extremities well supported.

(2) side-lying with a pillow between his knees.

(3) prone, with his head turned to the left side.

(4) dorsal-recumbent with a pillow at the back of his head.

174. A man calls the Suicide Prevention Hotline and states that he is going to kill himself. Which of the following questions should the nurse ask FIRST?

(1) "What has happened to cause you to want to end your life?"

(2) "How have you planned to kill yourself?"

(3) "When did you start to feel as though you wanted to die?"

(4) "Do you want me to prevent you from killing yourself?"

175. A 45-year-old man is admitted for treatment of congestive heart failure (CHF). The physician orders an IV of 125 cc of normal saline per hour and central venous pressure (CVP) readings every 4 hours. Sixteen hours after admission, the patient's CVP reading is 3 cm/H_2O. Which of the following evaluations of the patient's fluid status, if made by the nurse, would be MOST accurate?

(1) The patient has received enough fluid.

(2) The patient's fluid status remains unaltered.

(3) The patient has received too much fluid.

(4) The patient needs more fluid.

176. An agitated 20-year-old patient throws a chair across the dayroom on the psychiatry floor and threatens the other patients with physical harm. The nurse's initial action should be to

(1) tell the patient that his wife will be called to the hospital.

(2) ask the patient why he is so angry.

(3) remove the other patients from the dayroom.

(4) assemble staff and put the patient in preventive seclusion.

177. The nurse is caring for a depressed 40-year-old male patient who spends most of the day sitting at a window, and is about to implement a physical activity plan for him. The nurse knows that the purpose of this plan is to

(1) help the patient understand the problems creating the depression.

(2) reduce the patient's risk for obesity and diabetes.

(3) transform self-destructive impulses into positive behaviors.

(4) encourage socialization and improve self-esteem.

178. The nurse is caring for a patient with bipolar disorder. Which behavior, if demonstrated by the patient, would indicate to the nurse that a manic episode is subsiding?

(1) The patient tells several jokes at a group meeting.

(2) The patient sits and talks with other patients at mealtimes.

(3) The patient begins to write a book about his life.

(4) The patient initiates an effort to start a radio station on the unit.

179. A patient hospitalized for treatment of delusions tells the nurse that he is really the head of the hospital system and that his cover is being a patient to get information on patient abuse. The nurse's initial response should be:

(1) "Tell me what you mean about being head of the hospital system and getting patient abuse information."

(2) "I think you should share this story with the other patients at dinnertime and see what they say."

(3) "You are not the head of the hospital system, you are an accountant under treatment for a mental disorder."

(4) "It worries me when you say these things; it means you are not responding to the medication."

180. The nurse is caring for a patient in labor. The nurse palpates a firm, round form in the uterine fundus, small parts on the woman's right side, and a long, smooth, curved section on the left side. Based on these findings, the nurse should anticipate auscultating the fetal heart in which of the following locations?

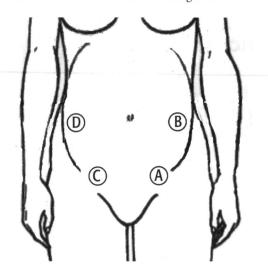

(1) A
(2) B
(3) C
(4) D

END OF TEST

ANSWER KEY

1. 3	37. 1	73. 4	109. 4	145. 3
2. 2	38. 3	74. 4	110. 2	146. 2
3. 4	39. 3	75. 3	111. 3	147. 3
4. 4	40. 2	76. 4	112. 4	148. 4
5. 1	41. 3	77. 1	113. 3	149. 2
6. 1	42. 1	78. 3	114. 2	150. 4
7. 3	43. 1	79. 3	115. 2	151. 2
8. 3	44. 2	80. 2	116. 1	152. 3
9. 2	45. 2	81. 2	117. 4	153. 1
10. 1	46. 1	82. 1	118. 2	154. 1
11. 3	47. 3	83. 3	119. 1	155. 2
12. 2	48. 2	84. 1	120. 3	156. 2
13. 4	49. 1	85. 2	121. 2	157. 3
14. 3	50. 2	86. 4	122. 4	158. 3
15. 2	51. 4	87. 4	123. 2	159. 4
16. 4	52. 2	88. 2	124. 2	160. 1
17. 3	53. 3	89. 2	125. 3	161. 2
18. 2	54. 3	90. 3	126. 3	162. 3
19. 2	55. 3	91. 3	127. 1	163. 2
20. 4	56. 3	92. 2	128. 2	164. 3
21. 3	57. 2	93. 3	129. 4	165. 3
22. 3	58. 4	94. 3	130. 1	166. 4
23. 1	59. 4	95. 4	131. 4	167. 2
24. 1	60. 2	96. 4	132. 3	168. 1
25. 2	61. 4	97. 4	133. 2	169. 3
26. 4	62. 3	98. 3	134. 3	170. 2
27. 3	63. 2	99. 3	135. 3	171. 1
28. 1	64. 3	100. 2	136. 2	172. 1
29. 3	65. 2	101. 2	137. 3	173. 1
30. 1	66. 2	102. 1	138. 2	174. 2
31. 3	67. 2	103. 3	139. 1	175. 4
32. 4	68. 3	104. 3	140. 2	176. 4
33. 2	69. 3	105. 1	141. 3	177. 4
34. 3	70. 2	106. 3	142. 2	178. 2
35. 3	71. 1	107. 4	143. 3	179. 1
36. 2	72. 1	108. 3	144. 4	180. 1

PRACTICE TEST EXPLANATIONS

1 The nurse is interviewing a client who is being treated for obsessive-compulsive disorder. What is the MOST important question the nurse should ask this patient?

REWORDED QUESTION: What are the signs and symptoms of obsessive-compulsive disorder?

STRATEGY: "MOST important" indicates there may be more than one correct response.

NEEDED INFO: Obsessive-compulsive disorder is characterized by a history of obsessions and compulsions. Obsessions are recurrent and persistent thoughts, ideas, impulses or images that are experienced as intrusive and senseless. The patient knows that the thoughts are ridiculous or morbid, but cannot stop, forget, or control them. Compulsions are repetitive behaviors performed in a certain way to prevent discomfort and neutralize anxiety.

CATEGORY: Assessment/Psychosocial Integrity

(1) "Do you find yourself forgetting simple things?"—*should be used to assess patient with suspected cognitive disorder*
(2) "Do you find it hard to stay on a task?"—*assesses for disorders that disrupt the ability to concentrate, such as depression*
(3) "Do you have trouble controlling upsetting thoughts?"—**CORRECT: one feature of obsessive-compulsive disorder is the patient's inability to control intrusive thoughts that repeat over and over**
(4) "Do you experience feelings of panic in a closed area?"—*appropriate for patient with suspected panic disorder related to closed spaces or claustrophobia*

2 Which of the following actions, if performed by the nurse, would be considered negligence?

REWORDED QUESTION: What is an incorrect behavior?

STRATEGY: Think about the consequence of each action.

NEEDED INFO: Negligence is the unintentional failure of nurse to perform an act that a reasonable person would or would not perform in similar circumstances; can be an act of commission or omission. Standards of care: the actions that other nurses would do in the same or similar circumstances that provide for quality client care. Nurse practice acts: state laws that determine the scope of the practice of nursing.

CATEGORY: Analysis/Safe and Effective Care

(1) Obtaining a Guthrie blood test on a 4-day-old infant—*obtain after ingestion of protein, no later than 7 days after delivery*
(2) Massaging lotion on the abdomen of a 3-year-old diagnosed with Wilm's tumor—**CORRECT: manipulation of mass may cause dissemination of cancer cells**
(3) Instructing a 5-year-old asthmatic to blow on a pinwheel—*exercise that will extend expiratory time and increase expiratory pressure*
(4) Playing kickball with a 10-year-old with juvenile arthritis (JA)—*excellent moving and stretching exercise*

3 The nurse on postpartum is preparing four clients for discharge. It would be MOST important for the nurse to refer which of the following patients for home care?

REWORDED QUESTION: Who is the most unstable patient?

STRATEGY: Think ABC's.

NEEDED INFO: Need to meet the client's needs. Physical stability is the nurse's first concern. Most unstable patient should be seen first.

CATEGORY: Implementation/Safe and Effective Care

(1) A 15-year-old primipara who delivered a 7-lb male two days ago—*stable situation, no indication of problems with mother or baby*
(2) An 18-year-old multipara who delivered a 9-lb female by cesarean section two days ago—*stable situation, no indication of problems with mother or baby*
(3) A 20-year-old multipara who delivered 1 day ago and is complaining of cramping—*stable patient, cramping due to uterine contraction*
(4) A 22-year-old who delivered by cesarean section and is complaining of burning on urination—**CORRECT: unstable patient, indicates urinary tract infection, requires follow-up**

4 A patient is telling the nurse about his perception of his thought patterns. Which of the following statements, if made by the patient, would validate the diagnosis of schizophrenia?

REWORDED QUESTION: What behaviors or thought patterns characterize schizophrenia?

NEEDED INFO: Schizophrenia is generally characterized by delusions (grandiose, religious, paranoid, nihilistic, or delusions of reference or influence), confusion, hallucinations, and illusions (misinterpretations of real external stimuli).

CATEGORY: Assessment/Psychosocial Integrity

(1) "I can't get the same thoughts out of my head."—*recurrent, intrusive thoughts are characteristic of obsessive-compulsive disorder*

(2) "I know I sometimes feel on top of the world, then suddenly down."—*rapid, changing moods are characteristic of manic phase of bipolar disorder*

(3) "Sometimes I look up and wonder where I am."—*confused, disoriented thoughts are characteristic of cognitive disorders*

(4) "It's clear that this is an alien laboratory and I am in charge."—**CORRECT: illogical, disorganized thoughts are typical of schizophrenia**

5 A nursing team consists of an RN, an LPN/LVN, and a nursing assistant. The nurse should assign which of the following patients to the LPN/LVN?

REWORDED QUESTION: Which patient is an appropriate assignment for the LPN/LVN?

STRATEGY: Think about the skill level involved in each patient's care.

NEEDED INFO: LPN/LVN: assists with implementation of care; performs procedures; differentiates normal from abnormal; cares for stable patients with predictable conditions; has knowledge of asepsis and dressing changes; administers medications (varies with educational background and state nurse practice act).

CATEGORY: Planning/Safe and Effective Care

(1) A 72-year-old patient with diabetes who requires a dressing change for a stasis ulcer—**CORRECT: stable patient with an expected outcome**

(2) A 42-year-old patient with cancer of the bone complaining of pain—*requires assessment; RN is the appropriate caregiver*

(3) A 55-year-old patient with terminal cancer being transferred to hospice home care—*requires nursing judgment; RN is the appropriate caregiver*

(4) A 23-year-old patient with a fracture of the right leg who asks to use the urinal—*standard unchanging procedure; assign to the nursing assistant*

6 An 84-year-old man is admitted with a diagnosis of dementia. He attempts several times to pull out his nasogastric tube. An order for cloth wrist restraints is received by the nurse. Which of the following actions by the nurse is MOST appropriate?

REWORDED QUESTION: What is appropriate care for a patient requiring restraints?

STRATEGY: "MOST appropriate" indicates there may be more than one correct response.

NEEDED INFO: Informed consent is needed to use restraints; if client is unable to consent, then consent of proxy must be obtained after full disclosure of risks and benefits; restraint of patient without informed consent or sufficient justification is false imprisonment. Assess and document need for restraints; consider use of alternative measures and document. Physician's order is required specifying duration and circumstances under which restraints should be used; cannot order restraints to be used PRN. Monitor patient closely and periodically reassess continued need for restraints, and document.

CATEGORY: Implementation/Safe and Effective Care

(1) Attach the ties of the restraint to the bed frame—**CORRECT: allows the raising and lowering of the side rail without causing injury to the patient**

(2) Perform circulation checks to the extremities, which are restrained once a shift—*circulation checks should be done every 1–2 hours; vascular injury may result from poor circulation from a restraint that's too tight*

(3) Remove the restraints when the patient is up in a wheelchair—*restraints should be secured when patient is at risk for harm to himself and is unattended; should be removed every 2 hours and skin assessed and area massaged; patient should not be left unattended when restraint is removed for care*

(4) Explain the need for restraints only to the family—*restraints can increase patient's confusion or combativeness; patient and family should receive explanation for the need for the restraint, the type of restraint, and the anticipated duration of use*

7 A 50-year-old man complains of pain in his right lower extremity. The physician orders codeine 60 mg and aspirin grains XPO every four hours, as needed for pain. Each codeine tablet contains 15 mg of codeine. Each aspirin tablet contains 325 mg of aspirin. Which of the following should the nurse administer?

REWORDED QUESTION: What amount of medication should you give?

STRATEGY: Remember how to calculate dosages.

NEEDED INFO: 60 mg = 1 grain.

CATEGORY: Implementation/Physiological Integrity

(1) 2 codeine tablets and 4 aspirin tablets—*inaccurate*
(2) 4 codeine tablets and 3 aspirin tablets—*inaccurate*
(3) 4 codeine tablets and 2 aspirin tablets—**CORRECT: $60/x = 15/1$, $x = 4$; 10 grains = 600 mg; $325/1 = 600/x$, $x = 2$**
(4) 3 codeine tablets and 3 aspirin tablets—*inaccurate*

8 The nurse is leading an inservice about management issues. The nurse would intervene if another nurse made which of the following statements?

REWORDED QUESTION: What are the nurse's responsibilities regarding obtaining consent?

STRATEGY: Think about each answer. Does it describe the nurse's responsibility for consent?

NEEDED INFO: Requirements: capacity-age (adult), competence, voluntary; info must be given in understandable form. Legal responsibility: physician's responsibility to get consent form signed; when nurse witnesses a signature it means there's reason to believe client is informed about upcoming treatment.

CATEGORY: Evaluation/Safe and Effective Care

(1) "It is my responsibility to ensure that the consent form has been signed and attached to the patient's chart prior to surgery."—*describes the nurse's responsibility*
(2) "It is my responsibility to witness the signature of the client before surgery is performed."—*signature indicates that the nurse saw the patient sign the form*
(3) "It is my responsibility to provide a detailed description of the surgery and ask the patient to sign the consent form."—**CORRECT: physician should provide explanation and obtain signature**
(4) "It is my responsibility to answer questions that the patient may have prior to surgery."—*describes the nurse's responsibility*

9 A nurse in the outpatient clinic evaluates the Mantoux test of a 36-year-old woman whose history indicates that she has been treated during the past year for an AIDS-related

infection. The nurse should document that there was a positive reaction if there was an area of induration measuring what?

REWORDED QUESTION: What is a positive reaction for a patient who is immunocompromised?

STRATEGY: Think about each answer choice.

NEEDED INFO: Given intradermally in the forearm; read in 48–72 hours. 10 mm induration (hard area under skin) = significant (positive) reaction. Greater than 5 mm for clients with AIDS = positive reaction. Does not mean active disease is present but indicates exposure to TB or the presence of inactive (dormant) disease. Multiple puncture test done for routine screening.

CATEGORY: Analysis/Safe and Effective Care

(1) 3 mm—*nonsignificant reaction*
(2) 7 mm—**CORRECT: greater than 5 mm area positive for patient with HIV-infection history**
(3) 11 mm—*area of 10 mm or more indicates positive reaction for patient without an HIV infection*
(4) 15 mm—*area of 10 mm or more indicates positive reaction for patient without an HIV infection*

10 The nurse in the newborn nursery has just received report. Which of the following infants should the nurse see first?

REWORDED QUESTION: Which infant is most unstable?

STRATEGY: Remember the ABC's.

NEEDED INFO: Need to meet client's needs. Physical stability of patient is nurse's first concern. Most unstable patient should be seen first.

CATEGORY: Evaluation/Safe and Effective Care

(1) A two-day-old infant is lying quietly alert with a heart rate of 185—**CORRECT: infant has tachycardia; normal resting rate is 120–160; requires further investigation**
(2) A one-day-old infant is crying and the anterior fontanel is bulging—*crying causes increased intracranial pressure, which causes fontanel to bulge*
(3) A 12-hour infant is being held; the respirations are 45 breaths per minute and irregular—*normal respiratory rate is 30–60 breaths per minute with apneic episodes*
(4) A five-hour-old infant is sleeping and the hands and feet are blue bilaterally—*acrocyanosis is normal for 2–6 hours postdelivery due to poor peripheral circulation*

11 While inserting a nasogastric tube, the nurse should use which of the following protective measures?

REWORDED QUESTION: What is the correct universal precaution?

STRATEGY: Think about each answer choice. How is each measure protecting the nurse?

NEEDED INFO: Mask, eye protection, face shield protect mucous membrane exposure; used if activities are likely to generate splash or sprays. Gowns used if activities are likely to generate splashes or sprays.

CATEGORY: Planning/Safe and Effective Care

(1) Gloves, gown, goggles, and surgical cap—*surgical caps offer protection to hair but aren't required*
(2) Sterile gloves, mask, plastic bags, and gown—*plastic bags provide no direct protection and aren't part of universal precautions*
(3) Gloves, gown, mask, and goggles—**CORRECT: must use universal precautions on ALL patients; prevent skin and mucous membrane exposure when contact with blood or other body fluids is anticipated**
(4) Double gloves, goggles, mask, and surgical cap—*surgical cap not required; unnecessary to double glove*

12 The nurse is caring for patients in the outpatient clinic. Which of the following phone calls should the nurse return first?

REWORDED QUESTION: Which client should the nurse call back first?

STRATEGY: Think ABC's.

NEEDED INFO: Need to meet client's needs. Physical stability is nurse's first concern. Most unstable patient should be contacted first.

CATEGORY: Analysis/Safe and Effective Care

(1) A client with hepatitis A who states, "My arms and legs are itching."—*caused by accumulation of bile salts under the skin; treat with calamine lotion and antihistamines*
(2) A client with a cast on the right leg who states, "I have a funny feeling in my right leg."—**CORRECT: may indicate neurovascular compromise; requires immediate assessment**
(3) A client with osteomylitis of the spine who states, "I am so nauseous that I can't eat."—*requires follow-up, but not highest priority*

(4) A client with rheumatoid arthritis who states, "I am having trouble sleeping."—*requires assessment, but not a priority*

13 The nursing team consists of an RN, two LPNs/LVNs, and three nursing assistants. The RN should care for which of the following patients?

REWORDED QUESTION: Which patient is an appropriate assignment for the RN?

STRATEGY: Think about the skill level involved in each patient's care.

NEEDED INFO: Determine nursing care required to meet clients' needs; take into account time required, complexity of activities, acuity of patient, infection control issues. Consider knowledge and abilities of staff members and decide which staff person is best able to provide care. Give assignments to staff members (assign responsibility for total patient care; avoid assigning only procedures). Provide additional help as needed.

CATEGORY: Planning/Safe and Effective Care

(1) A patient with a chest tube who is ambulating in the hall—*LPN/LVN can care for patient*
(2) A patient with a colostomy who requires assistance with a colostomy irrigation—*assign to the LPN/LVN*
(3) A patient with a right-sided cerebral vascular accident (CVA) who requires assistance with bathing—*assign to a nursing assistant*
(4) A patient who is refusing medication to treat cancer of the colon—**CORRECT: requires the assessment skills of the RN**

14 The home care nurse is visiting a client during the icteric phase of hepatitis of unknown etiology. The nurse would be MOST concerned if the client made which of the following statements?

REWORDED QUESTION: What is an incorrect statement about caring for a patient with hepatitis?

STRATEGY: "MOST concerned" indicates you are looking for an incorrect statement.

NEEDED INFO: Hepatitis A (HAV): high risk groups include young children, institutions for custodial care, international travelers; transmission by fecal/oral, poor sanitation; nursing considerations include prevention, improved sanitation, treat with gamma globulin early post-exposure, no preparation of food. Hepatitis B (HBV): high risk groups include drug addicts, fetuses from infected mothers, homosexually active men, transfusions, healthcare workers; transmission by parenteral, sexual contact, blood/body fluids; nursing considerations include vaccine (Heptavax-B, Recombivax HB), immune globulin (HBLg) postexposure, chronic carriers (potential for chronicity 5–10%). Hepatitis C (HVC): high risk groups include transfusions, international travelers; transmission by blood/body fluids; nursing considerations include great potential for chronicity. Delta hepatitis: high risk groups same as for HBV; transmission coinfects with HBV, close personal contact.

CATEGORY: Evaluation/Safe and Effective Care

(1) "I must not share eating utensils with my family."—*prevents transmission; handwashing before eating and after toileting very important*
(2) "I must use my own bath towel."—*prevents transmission; don't share bed linens*
(3) "I'm glad that my husband and I can continue to have intimate relations."—**CORRECT: avoid sexual contact until serologic indicators return to normal**
(4) "I must eat small, frequent feedings."—*easier to tolerate than three standard meals; diet should be high in carbohydrates and calories*

15 A nurse plans for care of a patient with anemia who is complaining of weakness. Which of the following tasks should the nurse assign to the nursing assistant?

REWORDED QUESTION: What is an appropriate assignment for the nursing assistant?

STRATEGY: Think about the skill level involved in each task.

NEEDED INFO: Unlicensed assistive personnel (UAPs): assist with direct patient care activities (bathing, transferring, ambulating, feeding, toileting, obtaining vital signs/height/weight/intake/output, housekeeping, transporting, stocking supplies); includes nurse aides, assistants, technicians, orderlies, nurse extenders; scope of nursing practice is limited.

CATEGORY: Planning/Safe and Effective Care

(1) Listen to the patient's breath sounds—*requires assessment; should be performed by RN*
(2) Set up the patient's lunch tray—**CORRECT: standard, unchanging procedure; decreases cardiac workload**
(3) Obtain a diet history—*involves assessment; should be performed by RN*

(4) Instruct the client on how to balance rest and activity—*assessment and teaching required; should be performed by RN*

16 The nurse is caring for patients on the surgical floor and has just received report from the previous shift. Which of the following patients should the nurse see FIRST?

REWORDED QUESTION: Which patient is the least stable?

STRATEGY: Think ABC's.

NEEDED INFO: Need to meet the client's needs. Physical stability is the nurse's first concern. Most unstable patient should be seen first.

CATEGORY: Analysis/Safe and Effective Care

(1) A 35-year-old admitted three hours ago with a gunshot wound; 1.5 cm area of dark drainage noted on the dressing—*does not indicate acute bleeding; small amount of blood*
(2) A 43-year-old who had a mastectomy two days ago; 23 cc of serosanguinous fluid noted in the Jackson-Pratt drain—*expected outcome*
(3) A 59-year-old with a collapsed lung due to an accident; no drainage noted in the previous eight hours—*indicates resolution*
(4) A 62-year-old who had an abdominal-perineal resection three days ago; patient complains of chills—**CORRECT: at risk for peritonitis; should be assessed for further symptoms of infection**

17 Which of the following actions, if performed by the nurse, would certainly be considered negligence?

REWORDED QUESTION: What is negligent behavior?

STRATEGY: Think about the consequences of each action.

NEEDED INFO: Negligence: unintentional failure of nurse to perform an act that a reasonable person would or would not perform in similar circumstances; can be an act of commission or omission. Standards of care: the actions that other nurses would do in same or similar circumstances that provide for quality client care. Nurse practice acts: state laws that determine the scope of the practice of nursing.

CATEGORY: Evaluation/Safe and Effective Care

(1) Inserting a 16 Fr NG tube and aspirating 15 cc of gastric contents—*correct procedure; verify placement by checking the pH*

(2) Administering Demerol IM to patient prior to using the incentive spirometer—*reducing the patient's pain enables the patient to take a deep breath*

(3) Administering ferrous sulfate (Feosol) 325 mg with coffee—**CORRECT: do not give together, may impair iron absorption; give with orange juice**

(4) Initially administering blood at 5 cc per minute for 15 minutes—*correct procedure; start blood with normal saline and 19-gauge needle*

18 A one-day-old newborn diagnosed with intrauterine growth retardation is observed by the nurse to be restless, irritable, fist-sucking, and having a high-pitched, shrill cry. Based on this data, the nurse should

REWORDED QUESTION: What do you do for a newborn experiencing withdrawal?

STRATEGY: Determine the outcome of each answer.

NEEDED INFO: Drug withdrawal may manifest from as early as 12–24 hrs after birth up to 7–10 days after delivery. Symptoms: high-pitched cry, hyperreflexia, decreased sleep, diaphoresis, tachypnea, excessive mucus, vomiting, uncoordinated sucking. Nursing care: assess muscle tone, irritability, vital signs; administer phenobarbital as ordered; report symptoms of respiratory distress; reduce stimulation; provide adequate nutrition/fluids; monitor mother/child interactions.

CATEGORY: Implementation/Health Promotion and Maintenance

(1) discourage stimulation of the baby by rocking—*rocking helps infant feel more comfortable*

(2) tightly swaddle the infant in a flexed position—**CORRECT: promotes infant's comfort and security**

(3) schedule feeding times every three to four hours—*small, frequent feedings are preferable*

(4) encourage eye contact with the infant during feedings—*may result in overstimulation of infant*

19 The nurse visits a neighbor who is 20 weeks gestation. The neighbor complains of nausea, headache, and blurred vision. The nurse notes that the neighbor appears nervous, is diaphoretic, and is experiencing tremors. It would be MOST important for the nurse to ask which of the following questions?

REWORDED QUESTION: What is the priority assessment question?

STRATEGY: "MOST important" indicates there may be more than one correct response.

NEEDED INFO: Assessment: Irritability, confusion, tremors, blurring of vision, coma, seizures, hypotension, tachycardia, skin cool and clammy, diaphoresis. Plan/Implementation: Liquids containing sugar if conscious, skim milk is ideal if tolerated; dextrose 50% IV if unconscious, glucagon; follow with additional carbohydrate in 15 minutes; determine and treat cause; patient education; exercise regimen.

CATEGORY: Assessment/Health Promotion and Maintenance

(1) "Are you having menstrual-like cramps?"—*symptoms of preterm labor*

(2) "When did you last eat or drink?"—**CORRECT: classic symptoms of hypoglycemia; offer carbohydrate**

(3) "Have you been diagnosed with diabetes?"—*need to determine if she is hypoglycemic*

(4) "Have you been lying on the couch?"—*not relevant to hypoglycemia*

20 The school nurse notes that a first-grade child is scratching her head almost constantly. It would be MOST important for the nurse to take which of the following actions?

REWORDED QUESTION: What is the best assessment?

STRATEGY: Determine if assessment or implementation is appropriate.

NEEDED INFO: Pediculosis (lice). Assessment: scalp—white eggs (nits) on hair shafts, itchy; body—macules and papules; pubis—red macules. Nursing consideration: OTC pyrethin (RID, A-200), permethrin 1% (Nix); kills both lice and nits with one application; may suggest repeating in 7 days if necessary.

CATEGORY: Assessment/Health Promotion and Maintenance

(1) Discuss basic hygiene with parents—*makes an assumption; must assess first*

(2) Instruct the child not to sleep with her dog—*must first assess to determine the problem*

(3) Inform the parents that they must contact an exterminator—*not enough information to make this determination*

(4) Observe the scalp for small white specks—**CORRECT: nits (eggs) appear as small, white, oval flakes attached to hair shaft**

21 A suicidal patient, who was admitted to the psychiatric unit for treatment and observation a week ago, suddenly appears cheerful and motivated. The nurse should be aware that

REWORDED QUESTION: What is the significance of sudden mood changes in a depressed patient?

STRATEGY: Know the signs of impending suicide.

NEEDED INFO: Assessment for suicidal ideation, suicidal gestures, suicidal threats, and actual suicidal attempt. Patients who have developed a suicide plan are more serious about following through, and are at grave risk. Patients emerging from severe depression have more energy with which to formulate and carry out a suicide plan (for which they had no energy before treatment). The nurse should determine risk for suicide; suspect suicidal ideation in depressed patient; ask the patient if he is thinking about suicide; ask the patient about the advantages and disadvantages of suicide to determine how patients sees his situation; evaluate patient's access to a method of suicide; develop a formal "no suicide" contract with patient; and support the patient's reason to live.

CATEGORY: Analysis/Psychosocial Integrity

(1) the patient is likely sleeping well because of the medication—*improved sleep patterns would not explain the patient's sudden mood change*
(2) the patient has made new friends and has a support group—*support on the nursing unit would not explain the mood change*
(3) the patient may have finalized a suicide plan—**CORRECT: as depressed patients improve, their risk for suicide is greater because they are able to mobilize more energy to plan and execute suicide**
(4) the patient is responding to treatment and is no longer depressed—*sudden cheerful and energetic mood does not indicate resolution of depression*

22 The nurse is caring for patients in the GYN clinic. A client complains of an off-white vaginal discharge with a curd-like appearance. The nurse notes the discharge and vulvular erythema. It would be MOST important for the nurse to ask which of the following questions?

REWORDED QUESTION: What is a predisposing factor to developing candidiasis?

STRATEGY: "MOST important" indicates there may be more than one correct response.

NEEDED INFO: Candida albican. Symptoms: odorless, cheesy white discharge; itching, inflames vagina and perineum. Treatment: topical clotrimazole (Gyne-Lotrimin), Hystatin (Mycostatin).

CATEGORY: Assessment/Health Promotion and Maintenance

(1) "Do you douche?"—*not a factor in the development of candidiasis*
(2) "Are you sexually active?"—*candidiasis not usually sexually transmitted; predisposing factors include glycosuria, pregnancy, and oral contraceptives*
(3) "What kind of birth control do you use?"—**CORRECT: oral contraceptives predispose individuals to candidiasis**
(4) "Have you taken any cough medicine?"—*no relationship between cough medicine and candidiasis*

23 The nurse is caring for a client in the prenatal clinic. He nurse notes that the patient's chart contains the following information: blood type AB, Rh negative; serology—negative; indirect Coombs test—negative; fetal paternity—unknown. The nurse should anticipate taking which of the following actions?

REWORDED QUESTION: What should the nurse do in this situation?

STRATEGY: Determine if it is appropriate to assess or implement.

NEEDED INFO: RhoGAM: given to unsensitized Rh-negative mother after delivery or abortion of an Rh-positive infant or fetus to prevent development of sensitization. Direct Coombs test done on cord blood after delivery; if both are negative and neonate is Rh-positive, mother is given RhoGAM. RhoGAM is ususally given to unsensitized mothers within 72 hours of delivery, but may be effective up to 3–4 weeks after delivery. Administration of RhoGAM at 26–28 weeks gestation also recommended. RhoGAM is ineffective against Rh-positive antibodies already present in the maternal circulation.

CATEGORY: Implementation/Health Promotion and Maintenance

(1) Administer Rho (D) immune globulin (RhoGAM)—**CORRECT: no indication of sensitization; RhoGAM will prevent possibility that she'll become sensitized; given at 28 weeks gestation if Coombs test is negative**
(2) Schedule an amniocentesis—*amniotic fluid aspirated by needle through abdominal and uterine walls to detect a genetic disorder*

(3) Obtain a direct Coombs test—*obtained from newborns, not from pregnant woman*

(4) Assess maternal serum for alpha-fetal protein level—*predicts neural tubal defects, done between 16 and 18 weeks*

24

The nurse is caring for a woman at 37 weeks gestation. The client was diagnosed with insulin-dependent diabetes mellitis (IDDM) at age 7. The client states, "I am so thrilled that I will be breastfeeding my baby." Which of the following responses by the nurse is BEST?

REWORDED QUESTION: What are the insulin requirements of the breastfeeding diabetic?

STRATEGY: Determine the outcome of each answer choice.

NEEDED INFO: Nursing care of diabetic during pregnancy: reinforce need for careful monitoring throughout pregnancy; evaluate understanding of modifications in diet/insulin coverage. Teach client and significant other: diet (eat prescribed amount of food daily at same times); home glucose monitoring; insulin (purpose, dosage, administration, action, side effects, potential change in amount needed during pregnancy as fetus grows and immediately after delivery; no oral hypoglycemics (teratogenic). Assist with stress reduction; fetal surveillance.

CATEGORY: Planning/Health Promotion and Maintenance

(1) "You will probably need less insulin while you are breastfeeding."—**CORRECT: breastfeeding has an antidiabetogenic effect; less insulin is needed**

(2) "You will need to initially increase your insulin after the baby is born."—*insulin needs will decrease due to antidiabetogenic effect of breastfeeding and physiological changes during immediate postpartum period*

(3) "You will be able to take an oral hypoglycemic instead of insulin after the baby is born."—*client has IDDM: insulin required*

(4) "You will probably require the same dose of insulin that you are now taking."—*during third trimester insulin requirements increase due to increased insulin resistance*

25

The nurse is caring for clients in a pediatric clinic. The mother of a 14-year-old male privately tells you that she is worried about her son because she unexpectedly walked into his room and discovered him masturbating. Which of the following responses by the nurse is MOST appropriate?

REWORDED QUESTION: What is the most therapeutic response?

STRATEGY: Remember therapeutic communication.

NEEDED INFO: Male changes in puberty: increase in genital size; breast swelling; pubic, facial, axillary, and chest hair; deepening voice; production of functional sperm; nocturnal emissions. Psychosexual development: masturbation as expression of sexual tension; sexual fantasies; experimental sexual intercourse.

CATEGORY: Implementation/Health Promotion and Maintenance

(1) "Tell your son he could go blind doing that."—*false information*

(2) "Masturbation is a normal part of sexual development."—**CORRECT: true statement provides opportunity for sexual self-exploration**

(3) "He's really too young to be masturbating."—*boys typically begin masturbating in early adolescence*

(4) "Why don't you give him more privacy?"—*judgmental; doesn't take advantage of opportunity to teach*

26

The nurse performs a home visit on a client who delivered two days ago. The client states that she is bottle-feeding her infant. The nurse notes white, curd-like patches on the newborn's oral mucous membranes. The nurse should take which of the following actions?

REWORDED QUESTION: What is the treatment for thrush?

STRATEGY: Determine the outcome of each answer choice.

NEEDED INFO: Thrush (oral candidiasis): white plaque on oral mucous membranes, gums, or tongue; treatment includes good handwashing, nystatin (Mycostatin).

CATEGORY: Implementation/Health Promotion and Maintenance

(1) Determine the newborn's blood glucose level—*thrush in newborns is caused by poor handwashing or exposure to an infected vagina during birth*

(2) Suggest that the newborn's formula be changed—*not related to thrush*

(3) Remind the caretaker not to let the infant sleep with the bottle—*not related to thrush*

(4) Explain that the newborn will need to receive some medication—**CORRECT: thrush most often treated with nystatin (Mycostatin)**

27 The nurse at the birthing facility is caring for a primipara woman in labor, who is 4 cm dilated, 25 percent effaced, and whose fetal vertex is at +1. The physician informs the patient that an amniotomy is to be performed. The patient states, "My friend's baby died when the umbilical cord came out when her water broke. I don't want you to do that to me!" Which of the following responses by the nurse is BEST?

REWORDED QUESTION: What is the most therapeutic response?

STRATEGY: "BEST" indicates that there may be more than one correct response.

NEEDED INFO: Amniotomy: artificial rupture of membranes. Presenting part should be engaged to prevent cord prolapse. Obtain FHR before and after procedure. Assess color, odor, consistency of amniotic fluid. Check maternal temperature q 2 hr; notify head care provider if temp is 38 degrees C or higher.

CATEGORY: Implementation/Health Promotion and Maintenance

(1) "If you are that concerned, you should refuse the procedure."—*giving advice, nontherapeutic*
(2) "The procedure will help your labor go faster."—*doesn't respond to patient's concerns*
(3) "That shouldn't happen to you since the baby's head is engaged."—**CORRECT: umbilical prolapse usually occurs when the presenting part isn't engaged**
(4) "We will monitor you carefully to prevent cord prolapse."—*monitoring will not prevent prolapsed cord*

28 A primigravida woman comes to the clinic for her initial prenatal visit. She is 32 weeks gestation and says that she has just moved from out-of-state. The client says that she has had periodic headaches during her pregnancy, and that she is continually bumping into things. The nurse notes numerous bruises in various stages of healing around the client's breasts and abdomen. Vital signs are: B/P 120/80, pulse 72, resps 18, and FHT 142. Which of the following responses by the nurse is BEST?

REWORDED QUESTION: What is the best assessment?

STRATEGY: Determine if it is appropriate to assess or implement.

NEEDED INFO: Symptoms of domestic abuse: frequent visits to physician's office or emergency room for unexplained trauma; client being cued, silenced, or threatened by an accompanying family member; evidence of multiple old injuries, scars, healed fractures seen on X-ray; fearful, evasive, or inconsistent replies, or nonverbal behaviors such as flinching when approached or touched. Nursing care: provide privacy during initial interview to ensure perpetrator of violence does not remain with client; carefully document all injuries (with consent); determine safety of client by asking specific questions about weapons, substance abuse, extreme jealousy; develop with client a safety or escape plan; refer client to community resources.

CATEGORY: Assessment/Health Promotion and Maintenance

(1) "Are you battered by your partner?"—**CORRECT: evidence of injury should be investigated; assess head, neck, chest, abdomen, breasts, upper extremities**
(2) "How do you feel about being pregnant?"—*injuries take priority*
(3) "Tell me about your headaches."—*headaches not related to hypertension; injuries take priority*
(4) "You may be more clumsy due to your size."—*assumption; need to assess*

29 The nurse is teaching a class on natural family planning. Which of the following statements, if made by a client, indicates that teaching has been successful?

REWORDED QUESTION: What is a true statement about natural family planning?

STRATEGY: Think about each statement. Is it true about natural family planning?

NEEDED INFO: Natural family planning—Action: periodic abstinence from intercourse during fertile period; based on regularity of ovulation; variable effectiveness. Teaching: fertile period may be determined by a drop in basal body temp before and a slight rise after ovulation, and/or a change in cervical mucus from thick, cloudy, and sticky during nonfertile period to more abundant, clear, thin, stretchy, and slippery during ovulation

CATEGORY: Evaluation/Health Promotion and Maintenance

(1) "When I ovulate, my basal body temperature will be elevated for two days and then will decrease."—*basal body temp decreased prior to ovulation; after ovulation, temp increases*
(2) "My cervical mucus will be thick, cloudy, and sticky when I ovulate."—*fertile mucus appears clear, thin, watery, and stretchy*

(3) "Since I am regular, I will be fertile about 14 days after the beginning of my period."—**CORRECT: ovulation occurs approx. 14 days after start of menstrual period**

(4) "When I ovulate, my cervix will feel firm."—*cervix softens slightly during ovulation*

30 The home care nurse plans care for a 10-year-old in a leg cast for treatment of a fractured right ankle. The nurse enters the following nursing diagnosis on the care plan: skin integrity, risk for impaired. Which of the following actions, if performed by the nurse, is BEST?

REWORDED QUESTION: What is the priority action to prevent skin breakdown?

STRATEGY: Determine the outcome of each answer choice.

NEEDED INFO: Immediate nursing care for plaster cast: Don't cover cast until dry (48 hours), handle with palms not fingertips; don't rest on hard surfaces; elevate affected limb above heart on soft surface until dry; don't use head lamp; check for blueness or paleness, pain, numbness, tingling (if present, elevate area; if it persists, contact physician); child should remain inactive while cast is drying. Intermediate nursing care: Mobilize patient, isometric exercises; check for break in cast or foul odor; tell patient not to scratch skin under cast and not to put anything underneath cast; if fiberglass cast gets wet, dry with hair dryer on cool setting. After-cast nursing care: Wash skin gently, apply baby powder/cornstarch/baby oil; have patient gradually adjust to movement without support of cast; swelling is common, elevate limb and apply elastic bandage.

CATEGORY: Implementation/Physiological Integrity

(1) Teaching the child how to perform isometric exercises of the right leg—**CORRECT: contraction of muscle without moving joint; promotes venous return and circulation, prevents thrombi; quadriceps setting (push back knees into bed) and gluteal setting (push heels into bed)**

(2) Teaching the mother to gently massage the child's right foot with emollient cream—*will help prevent dryness of foot but does not address skin under cast*

(3) Instructing the mother to keep the leg cast clean and dry—*since child is age 10, should be included in teaching of cast care; improving circulation is best way to prevent impaired skin integrity under cast*

(4) Teaching the mother how to turn and position the child—*no info provided about mobility of child; will prevent hazards of immobility*

31 The nurse is caring for a 45-year-old patient who had a thyroidectomy 12 hours ago for treatment of Graves' disease. The nurse would be MOST concerned if which of the following was observed?

REWORDED QUESTION: What is a complication after a thyroidectomy?

STRATEGY: "MOST concerned" indicates a complication.

NEEDED INFO: Nursing care for Graves' disease/hyperthyroidism: limit activities to quiet and provide frequent rest periods; advise light, cool clothing; avoid stimulants; use calm, unhurried approach; administer antithyroid medication, irradiation with I131 PO. Post-thyroidectomy care: low or semi-Fowler's position; support head, neck, shoulders to prevent flexion or hyperextension of suture line; tracheostomy set at bedside; observe for complications—laryngeal nerve injury, thyroid storm, hemorrhage, respiratory obstruction, tetany (decreased calcium from parathyroid involvement), check Chvostek's and Trousseau's signs.

CATEGORY: Assessment/Physiological Integrity

(1) Blood pressure 138/82, pulse 84, respirations 16, oral temp 99 degrees F—*vital signs within normal limits*

(2) The patient supports his head and neck when turning his head to the right—*prevents stress on the incision*

(3) The client spontaneously flexes his wrist when the blood pressure is obtained—**CORRECT: carpal spasms indicate hypocalcemia**

(4) The client is drowsy and complains of a sore throat—*expected outcome after surgery*

32 A 16-year-old boy is admitted with complaints of severe pain in the lower right quadrant of the abdomen. To assist with pain relief, the nurse should take which of the following actions?

REWORDED QUESTION: What is an appropriate non-pharmacological method for pain relief?

STRATEGY: Determine the outcome of each answer choice.

NEEDED INFO: Establish a 24-hour pain profile. Teach patient about pain and its relief: explain quality and location of impending pain; slow, rhythmic breathing to promote relaxation; effects of analgesics and benefits of preventative approach; splinting techniques to reduce pain. Reduce anxiety and fears. Provide comfort measures: proper positioning; cool, well ventilated, quiet room; back rub; allow for rest.

CATEGORY: Implementation/Physiological Integrity

(1) Encourage the patient to change positions frequently in bed—*unnecessary movement will increase pain, should be avoided*

(2) Administer Demerol 50 mg IM q 4 hours and PRN—*pain medications usually withheld until a definite diagnosis is made; may be appendicitis*

(3) Apply warmth to the abdomen with a heating pad—*if pain is caused by appendicitis, increased circulation from heat may cause appendix to rupture*

(4) Use comfort measures and pillows to position the patient—**CORRECT: non-pharmacological methods of pain relief**

33 The nurse prepares a 50-year-old woman for peritoneal dialysis. Which of the following actions should the nurse take FIRST?

REWORDED QUESTION: What is the priority action for a patient undergoing peritoneal dialysis?

STRATEGY: Determine if it is appropriate to assess or implement.

NEEDED INFO: Peritoneal dialysis: takes place within peritoneal cavity to remove excess fluids and waste products usually removed by the kidneys. Procedure: rubber catheter surgically inserted into abdominal cavity; 1–2 L of fluid infused into peritoneal space by gravity; fluid stays in cavity for approx. 20 minutes; fluid drained by gravity. Complications: peritonitis, abdominal pain, insufficient return of fluid. Nursing care before procedure: obtain baseline vitals, breath sounds, weight, glucose and electrolyte levels. During procedure: take vital signs, ongoing assessment for respiratory distress, pain, discomfort; use aseptic technique; check abdominal dressing around catheter for wetness.

CATEGORY: Implementation/Physiological Integrity

(1) Assess for a bruit and a thrill—*used with hemodialysis through an AV fistula, graft, or shunt*

(2) Warm the dialysate solution—**CORRECT: solution should be warmed to body temp in warmer or with heating pad; don't use microwave oven; cold dialysate increases discomfort**

(3) Position the client on the left side—*client should be in supine or low-Fowler's position wearing a mask*

(4) Insert a Foley catheter—*unnecessary, client can void without a catheter*

34 The nurse teaches a 65-year-old man with right-sided weakness how to use a cane. Which of the following behaviors, if demonstrated by the client to the nurse, indicates that the teaching was effective?

REWORDED QUESTION: What is the appropriate technique used to ambulate with a cane?

STRATEGY: Determine the outcome of each answer choice.

NEEDED INFO: Tip should have concentric rings (shock absorber for stability). Flex elbow 30 degrees and hold handle up; tip of cane should be 15 cm lateral to base of the fifth toe. Hold cane in hand opposite affected extremity; advance cane and affected leg; lean on cane when moving good leg. To manage stairs, step up on good leg, the place cane and affected leg on step; reverse when going down ("up with the good, down with the bad"); same sequence used with crutches.

CATEGORY: Evaluation/Physiological Integrity

(1) The man holds the cane with his right hand, moves the cane forward followed by the right leg, and then moves the left leg—*should hold cane with the stronger (left) hand*

(2) The man holds the cane with his right hand, moves the cane forward followed by his left leg, and then moves the right leg—*should hold cane with the stronger (left) hand*

(3) The man holds the cane with his left hand, moves the cane forward followed by the right leg, and then moves the left leg—**CORRECT: the cane acts as a support and aids in weight bearing for the weaker right leg**

(4) The man holds the cane with his left hand, moves the cane forward followed by his left leg, and then moves the right leg—*cane needs to be a support and aid in weight bearing for the weaker right leg*

35 While caring for a patient receiving TPN through a central line, the nurse notices a small trickle of opaque fluid leaking from around the central line dressing. It is MOST important for the nurse to take which of the following actions?

REWORDED QUESTION: What is the best action if the nurse suspects a break in the central line?

STRATEGY: "MOST important" indicates there may be more than one correct response.

NEEDED INFO: TPN: method of supplying nutrients to the body by the IV route. Nursing care: site of catheter changed every 4 weeks, change IV tubing and filters every 24 hours, dressing changed 2–3 times a week and PRN; initial rate of infusion 50 ml/h and gradually increased (100–125 ml/h) as patient's fluid and electrolyte tolerance permits; increased rate of infusion causes hyperosmolar state (headache, nausea, fever, chills, malaise); slowed rate of infusion results in "rebound" hypoglycemia caused by delayed pancreatic reaction to change in insulin requirements.

CATEGORY: Implementation/Physiological Integrity

(1) Prepare to change the central line dressing—*dressing might be removed later to further assess the situation, but this is not the most important action*

(2) Verify that the patient is on antibiotics—*no evidence of line infection*

(3) Place the patient's head lower than his feet—**CORRECT: indicates a break in the line, which places patient at risk for air embolism; turn patient on left side and place head lower than his feet; notify physician**

(4) Secure the Y-port where the lipids are infusing—*leakage is occurring at the IV site, not the Y site*

36 A 46-year-old man is admitted to the hospital with a fractured right femur. He is placed in balanced suspension traction with a Thomas splint and Pearson attachment. During the first 48 hours, the nurse should assess the patient for which of the following complications?

REWORDED QUESTION: What complication of a fracture is seen in the first 48 hours?

STRATEGY: Be careful! They are asking for the complication that occurs during the first 48 hours. Later complications may be included.

NEEDED INFO: Complications of fractures: 1) compartment syndrome (increased pressure externally [casts, dressings] or internally [bleeding, edema] resulting in compromised circulation); s/s: pallor, weak pulse, numbness, pain, 2) shock: bone is vascular, 3) fat embolism, 4) deep vein thrombosis, 5) infection, avascular necrosis, 6) delayed union, nonunion, malunion.

CATEGORY: Assessment/Physiological Integrity

(1) Pulmonary embolism—*obstruction of pulmonary system by thrombus from venous system or right side of heart; seen 2–3 days to several weeks after fracture*

(2) Fat embolism—**CORRECT: fat moves into blood stream from fracture; formed by alteration in lipids in blood; fat combines with platelets to form emboli; s/s: abnormal behavior due to cerebral anoxia (confusion, agitation, delirium, coma), abnormal ABGs (pO_2 below 60 mmHg), increased resp; chest pain, dyspnea, pallor, hypertension, petechiae on chest, upper arms, abdomen; treatment: high Fowler's, high conc O_2, ventilation with PEEP (positive end expiratory pressure) to decrease pulmonary edema, IVs, steroids, Dextran to prevent shock**

(3) Avascular necrosis—*(seen later than 48 hrs) bone looses blood supply and dies; seen with chronic renal disease or prolonged steroid use; treatment: bone graft, joint fusion, prosthetic replacement*

(4) Malunion—*bone fragments heal in deformed position as a result of inadequate reduction and immobilization; treatment: surgical or manual manipulation to realign*

37 The nurse is helping a nursing assistant provide a bed bath to a comatose patient who is incontinent. The nurse should intervene if which of the following actions is noted?

REWORDED QUESTION: What is an incorrect action?

STRATEGY: "Should intervene" indicates that you are looking for something wrong.

NEEDED INFO: Standard precautions (barrier) used with all patients: primary strategy for nosocomial infection control. Most important way to reduce transmission of pathogens. Gloves: use clean, nonsterile when touching blood, body fluids, secretions, excretions, contaminated articles; remove promptly after use, before touching items and environmental surfaces.

CATEGORY: Evaluation/Physiological Integrity

(1) The nursing assistant answers the phone while wearing gloves—**CORRECT: contaminated gloves should be removed before answering the phone**

(2) The nursing assistant log rolls the patient to provide back care—*correct way to roll a patient to maintain proper alignment*

(3) The nursing assistant places an incontinent diaper under the patient—*appropriate to use incontinent diapers for this patient*

(4) The nursing assistant positions the patient on the left side, head elevated—*appropriate position to prevent aspiration and protect the airway*

38 A 70-year-old woman is brought to the emergency room for treatment after being found on the floor by her daughter. X-rays reveal a displaced subcapital fracture of the left hip and osteoarthritis. When comparing the legs, the nurse would most likely make which of the following observations?

REWORDED QUESTION: What is a symptom of a hip fracture?

STRATEGY: Think about each answer choice.

NEEDED INFO: Symptoms of fracture: swelling, pallor, ecchymosis; loss of sensation to other body parts; deformity; pain/acute tenderness; muscle spasms; loss of function, abnormal mobility; crepitus (grating sound on movement); shortening of affected limb; decreased or absent pulses distal to injury; affected extremity colder than contralateral part. Emergency nursing care: immobilize joint above and below fracture by use of splints before patient is moved; in open fracture, cover the wound with sterile dressings or cleanest material available, control bleeding by direct pressure; check temp, color, sensation, capillary refill distal to fracture; in emergency room, give narcotic adequate to relieve pain (except in presence of head injury).

CATEGORY: Assessment/Physiological Integrity

(1) The patient's left leg is longer than the right leg and externally rotated—*leg is shorter due to contraction of muscles attached above and below fracture site*
(2) The patient's left leg is shorter than the right leg and internally rotated—*leg is usually externally rotated*
(3) The patient's left leg is shorter than the right leg and adducted—**CORRECT: extremity shortens due to contraction of muscles attached above and below fracture site, fragments overlap by 1–2 inches**
(4) The patient's left leg is longer than the right leg and is abducted—*extremity shortens and externally rotates*

39 The nurse is caring for a patient with a cast on the left leg. The nurse would be MOST concerned if which of the following were observed?

REWORDED QUESTION: What is a complication of a cast?

STRATEGY: "MOST concerned" indicates a complication.

NEEDED INFO: Immediate nursing care for plaster cast: Don't cover cast until dry (48 hours), handle with palms not fingertips; don't rest on hard surfaces; elevate affected limb above heart on soft surface until dry; don't use head lamp; check for blueness or paleness, pain, numbness, tingling (if present, ele-

vate area; if it persists, contact physician); patient should remain inactive while cast is drying. Intermediate nursing care: Mobilize patient, isometric exercises; check for break in cast or foul odor; tell patient not to scratch skin under cast and not to put anything underneath cast; if fiberglass cast gets wet, dry with hair dryer on cool setting. After-cast nursing care: Wash skin gently, apply baby powder/cornstarch/baby oil; have patient gradually adjust to movement without support of cast; swelling is common, elevate limb and apply elastic bandage.

CATEGORY: Analysis/Physiological Integrity

(1) Capillary refill time was less than 3 seconds—*capillary refill time is within normal limits*
(2) Patient complained of discomfort and itching—*a casted extremity may itch or feel uncomfortable due to prolonged immobility*
(3) Patient complained of tightness and pain—**CORRECT: patient with a pressure ulcer usually reports pain and tightness in the area; infection or necrosis will result in feeling of warmth and a foul odor**
(4) Patient's foot is elevated on a pillow—*newly casted extremity may be slightly elevated to help relieve edema; should remain in correct anatomical position and below heart level to allow sufficient arterial perfusion*

40 The nurse is discharging a patient from an inpatient alcohol treatment unit. Which of the following statements, if made by the patient's wife, indicates to the nurse that the family is coping adaptively?

REWORDED QUESTION: What indicates that the patient's family is coping with the patient's alcoholism?

STRATEGY: Think about what each statement means.

NEEDED INFO: Nursing care for chronic alcohol dependence: safety; monitor for withdrawal; reality orientation; increase self-esteem and coping skills; balanced diet; abstinence from alcohol; identify problems related to drinking in family relationships, work, etcetera; help patient to see/admit problem; confront denial with slow persistence; maintain relationship with patient; establish control of problem drinking; provide support; Alcoholics Anonymous; Disulfiram (Antabuse): drug used to maintain sobriety, based on behavioral therapy.

CATEGORY: Analysis/Psychosocial Integrity

(1) "My husband will do well as long as I keep him engaged in activities that he likes."—*wife is accepting responsibility, codependent behavior*

(2) "My focus is learning how to live my life."—**CORRECT: wife is working to change codependent patterns**

(3) "I am so glad that our problems are behind us."—*unrealistic; discharge is not the final step of treatment*

(4) "I'll make sure that the children don't give my husband any problems."—*wife is accepting responsibility, codependent behavior*

41 A nurse is caring for clients in the mental health clinic. A woman comes to the clinic complaining of insomnia and anorexia. The patient tearfully tells the nurse that she was laid off from a job that she had held for 15 years. Which of the following responses, if made by the nurse, is MOST appropriate?

REWORDED QUESTION: What is the most therapeutic response?

STRATEGY: Remember therapeutic communication.

NEEDED INFO: Nursing considerations, explore client's understanding of the problem: focus on the present; emphasize client's strengths; avoid blaming; determine how client handled similar situations; provide support; mobilize client's coping strategies.

CATEGORY: Implementation/Psychosocial Integrity

(1) "Did your company give you a severance package?"—*yes/no question, nontherapeutic*

(2) "Focus on the fact that you have a healthy, happy family."—*gives advice, false assurance*

(3) "Tell me what happened."—**CORRECT: explores situation; allows patient to verbalize**

(4) "Losing a job is common nowadays."—*dismisses the patient's concern*

42 A patient with a history of alcoholism is brought to the emergency room in an agitated state. He is vomiting and diaphoretic. He says he had his last drink five hours ago. The nurse would expect to administer which of the following medications?

REWORDED QUESTION: What is the best medication to treat acute alcohol withdrawal?

STRATEGY: Think about the action of each drug.

NEEDED INFO: Alcohol sedates the CNS; rebound during withdrawal. Early symptoms occur 4–6 hours after last drink. Symptoms: tremors; easily startled; insomnia; anxiety; anorexia; alcoholic hallucinosis (48 hours after last drink). Nursing

care: administer sedation as needed, usually benzodiazepines; monitor vital signs, particularly pulse; take seizure precautions; provide quiet, well-lit environment; orient patient frequently; don't leave hallucinating, confused patient alone; administer anticonvulsants as needed, thiamine IV or IM, and IV glucose.

CATEGORY: Planning/Psychosocial Integrity

(1) Chlordiazepoxide hydrochloride (Librium)—**CORRECT: antianxiety; used to treat symptoms of acute alcohol withdrawal; S/E: lethargy, hangover, agranulocytosis**

(2) Disulfiram (Antabuse)—*used as a deterrent to compulsive drinking; contraindicated if patient drank alcohol in previous 12 hours*

(3) Methadone hydrochloride (Dolophine)—*opioid analgesic; used to treat narcotic withdrawal; syndrome, S/E: seizures, respiratory depression*

(4) Naloxone hydrochloride (Narcan)—*narcotic antagonist used to reverse narcotic-induced respiratory depression; S/E: ventricular fibrillation, seizures, pulmonary edema*

43 A 72-year-old woman is admitted to the nursing home setting. The client is occasionally confused and her gait is often unsteady. Which of the following actions, if taken by the nurse, is MOST appropriate?

REWORDED QUESTION: What are visual cues for a client who is confused?

STRATEGY: Determine the outcome of each answer choice.

NEEDED INFO: Nursing care for Alzheimer's disease: provide calm, predictable environment with regular routine; give clear and simple explanations; display clock and calendar; color-code objects and areas; monitor medications and food intake; secure doors leading from house/unit; gently distract and redirect during wandering behavior; avoid restraints (increases combativeness); organize daily activities into short, achievable steps; discourage long naps during the day. If client experiences catastrophic reaction, remain calm and stay with client; provide distraction such as music, rocking, stroking.

CATEGORY: Implementation/Psychosocial Integrity

(1) Ask the woman's family to provide personal items such as photos or mementos—**CORRECT: provides visual stimulation to reduce sensory deprivation**

(2) Select a room with a bed by the door so the woman can look down the hall—*provides only occasional stimulation*

(3) Suggest the woman eat her meals in the room with her roommate—*needs to eat in the dining hall with others for stimulation*

(4) Encourage the woman to ambulate in the halls twice a day—*unsafe due to unsteady gait and confusion*

44 The nurse teaches a 60-year-old man how to use a standard aluminum walker. Which of the following behaviors, if demonstrated by the client, indicates that the nurse's teaching was effective?

REWORDED QUESTION: What is the correct technique when ambulating with a walker?

STRATEGY: Determine the outcome of each answer choice.

NEEDED INFO: Elbows flexed at 20–30 degree angle when standing with hands on grips. Lift and move walker forward 8–10 inches. With partial or non-weight-bearing, put weight on wrists and arms and step forward with affected leg, supporting self on arms, and follow with good leg. Nurse should stand behind patient, hold onto gait belt at waist as needed for balance. Sit down by grasping armrest on affected side, shift weight to good leg and hand, lower self into chair. Patient should wear sturdy shoes.

CATEGORY: Evaluation/Physiological Integrity

(1) The client slowly pushes the walker forward 12 inches, then takes small steps forward while leaning on the walker—*should not push the walker*
(2) The client lifts the walker, moves it forward 10 inches, and then takes several small steps forward—**CORRECT: walker needs to be picked up, placed down on all legs**
(3) The client supports his weight on the walker while advancing it forward, then takes small steps while balancing on the walker—*should not support weight on walker while trying to move it*
(4) The client slides the walker 18 inches forward, then takes small steps while holding onto the walker for balance—*walker should be picked up, not slid forward*

45 A nurse is supervising a group of elderly clients in a residential home setting. The nurse knows that the elderly are at greater risk of developing sensory deprivation for what reason?

REWORDED QUESTION: Why do the elderly have sensory deprivation?

STRATEGY: Think about each answer choice.

NEEDED INFO: Plan/Implementation: assist clients with adjusting to lifestyle changes; allow client to verbalize concerns; prevent isolation; provide assistance as required.

CATEGORY: Analysis/Psychosocial Integrity

(1) Increased sensitivity to the side effects of medications—*many medications alter GI functioning but do not cause decreased vision, hearing, or taste*
(2) Decreased visual, auditory, and gustatory abilities—**CORRECT: gradual loss of sight, hearing, and taste interferes with normal functioning**
(3) Isolation from their families and familiar surroundings—*clients are in contact with other residents and staff who provide stimulation*
(4) Decreased musculoskeletal function and mobility—*they can be placed in wheelchairs and moved*

46 After receiving report, which of the following patients should the nurse see FIRST?

REWORDED QUESTION: Who is the priority patient?

STRATEGY: Think ABC's.

NEEDED INFO: Consider the following factors: chief complaint; age of client; medical history; potential for life-threatening event

CATEGORY: Analysis/Physiological Integrity

(1) A 14-year-old patient in sickle-cell crisis with an infiltrated IV—**CORRECT: IV fluids are critical to reduce clotting and pain**
(2) A 59-year-old patient with leukemia who has received half of a packed red cell transfusion—*no indication that patient is unstable*
(3) A 68-year-old patient scheduled for a bronchoscopy—*stable patient*
(4) A 74-year-old patient complaining of a leaky colostomy bag—*stable patient*

47 The home care nurse is visiting a 32-year-old woman with a diagnosis of hepatitis of unknown etiology. The nurse knows that teaching has been successful if the patient makes which one of the following statements?

REWORDED QUESTION: What is a correct statement about hepatitis?

STRATEGY: Determine the outcome of each statement.

NEEDED INFO: Hepatitis A (HAV): high risk groups include young children, institutions for custodial care, international travelers; transmission by fecal/oral, poor sanitation; nursing considerations include prevention, improved sanitation, treat with gamma globulin early post-exposure, no preparation of food. Hepatitis B (HBV): high risk groups include drug addicts, fetuses from infected mothers, homosexually active men, transfusions, healthcare workers; transmission by parenteral, sexual contact, blood/body fluids; nursing considerations include vaccine (Heptavax-B, Recombivax HB), immune globulin (HBLg) postexposure, chronic carriers (potential for chronicity 5–10%). Hepatitis C (HVC): high risk groups include transfusions, international travelers; transmission by blood/body fluids; nursing considerations include great potential for chronicity. Delta hepatitis: high risk groups same as for HBV; transmission coinfects with HBV, close personal contact.

CATEGORY: Evaluation/Physiological Integrity

(1) "I am so sad that I am not able to hold my baby."—*hepatitis not spread by casual contact*

(2) "I will eat after my family eats."—*can eat with family; cannot share eating utensils*

(3) "I will make sure that my children don't eat or drink after me."—CORRECT: **to prevent transmission, families should not share eating utensils or drinking glasses; wash hands before eating and after using toilet**

(4) "I'm glad that I don't have to get help taking care of my children."—*need to alternate rest and activity to promote hepatic healing; mothers of young children will need help*

48 The nurse calculates the IV flow rate for a postoperative patient. The patient is to receive 3,000 ml of Ringer's lactate solution IV to run over 24 hours. The IV infusion set has a drop factor of 10 drops per milliliter. The nurse should regulate the patient's IV to deliver how many drops per minute?

REWORDED QUESTION: What is the IV flow rate?

STRATEGY: Remember the formula to calculate IV flow rate: Total volume × drop factor divided by the time in minutes.

NEEDED INFO: Ringer's lactate: electrolyte solution used to expand extracellular fluid vol, and reduce blood viscosity.

CATEGORY: Implementation/Physiological Integrity

(1) 18—*incorrect*
(2) 21—CORRECT: **3000 × 10 divided by 24 × 60**
(3) 35—*incorrect*
(4) 40—*incorrect*

49 A 67-year-old patient with emphysema becomes restless and confused. What step should the nurse take next?

REWORDED QUESTION: What should the nurse do to raise the oxygen levels of a patient with emphysema?

STRATEGY: Determine the outcome of each answer choice.

NEEDED INFO: Emphysema: overinflation of alveoli resulting in destruction of alveoli walls; predisposing factors include smoking, chronic infections, environmental pollution. Teaching includes breathing exercises; stop smoking; avoid hot/cold air or allergens; instructions regarding medications; avoid crowds or close contact with persons who have colds or flu; adequate rest and nutrition; oral hygiene; prophylactic flu vaccines; observe sputum for indications of infection.

CATEGORY: Implementation/Physiological Integrity

(1) Encourage the patient to perform pursed-lip breathing—CORRECT: **prevents collapse of lung unit and helps patient control rate and depth of breathing**

(2) Check the patient's temperature—*confusion is probably due to decreased oxygenation*

(3) Assess the patient's potassium level—*confusion is probably due to decreased oxygenation, not electrolyte imbalance*

(4) Increase the patient's oxygen flow rate to 5 L/min—*should receive low flow oxygen to prevent carbon dioxide narcosis*

50 The nurse is caring for a patient one day after an abdominal-perineal resection for cancer of the rectum. The nurse should question which of the following orders?

REWORDED QUESTION: What is an incorrect behavior?

STRATEGY: Determine the outcome of each answer choice.

NEEDED INFO: Skin care for stoma: effect on skin depends on composition, quality, consistency of drainage, medication, location of stoma, frequency of removal of appliance adhesive. Principles of skin protection: use skin sealant under all tapes; use skin barrier to protect skin around stoma; cleanse skin gently and pat dry, not rub; change appliance immediately when seal breaks.

CATEGORY: Analysis/Physiological Integrity

(1) Discontinue the nasogastric tube—*discontinued when peristalsis occurs*

(2) Irrigate the colostomy—CORRECT: **colostomy begins to function 3–6 days after surgery**

(3) Place petrolatum gauze over the stoma—*done if no pouch in place; keeps stoma moist; cover with dry, sterile dressing*

(4) Administer Demerol 50 mg IM for pain—*prevents post-op pain*

51

The nurse is caring for a patient four hours after intracranial surgery. Which of the following actions should the nurse take immediately?

REWORDED QUESTION: What is a priority after intracranial surgery?

STRATEGY: Determine the outcome of each answer choice.

NEEDED INFO: Monitor vital signs hourly. Elevate head 15 to 30 degrees to promote venous drainage from brain. Avoid neck flexion and head rotation (support in cervical collar or neck rolls). Reduce environmental stimuli. Prevent the Valsalva maneuver; teach client to exhale while turning or moving in bed. Administer stool softeners. Restrict fluids to 1,200–1,500 ml/day. Administer medications: osmotic diuretics, corticosteroid therapy, anticonvulsant meds.

CATEGORY: Implementation/Physiological Integrity

(1) Turn, cough, and deep-breathe the patient—*coughing is discouraged, can increase intracranial pressure*

(2) Place the patient with the neck flexed and head turned to the side—*will increase ICP; keep head in a neutral position*

(3) Perform passive range of motion exercises—*changes in patient's position can increase intracranial pressure*

(4) Move client to the head of the bed using a turning sheet—**CORRECT: patient's body should be moved as a unit to prevent increased ICP; prevent disruption of the ICP monitoring system**

52

A 6-year-old child with a congenital heart disorder is admitted with congestive heart failure. Digoxin (Lanoxin) 0.12 mg is ordered for the child. The bottle of Lanoxin contains .05 mg of Lanoxin in 1 cc of solution. The nurse should administer:

REWORDED QUESTION: How much of the med should you give?

STRATEGY: Remember how to calculate dosages. Be careful and don't make math errors.

NEEDED INFO: Formula: dose on hand over 1 cc = dose desired.

CATEGORY: Implementation/Physiological Integrity

(1) 1.2 cc—*inaccurate*

(2) 2.4 cc—**CORRECT: .05mg/1 cc = .12mg/x cc, .05x = .12, x = 2.4 cc**

(3) 3.5 cc—*inaccurate*

(4) 4.2 cc—*inaccurate*

53

The nurse is caring for a patient with an acute myocardial infarction. Which of the following laboratory findings would MOST concern the nurse?

REWORDED QUESTION: What is the most significant lab value for an MI?

STRATEGY: "MOST concerned" indicates that you are looking for a problem.

NEEDED INFO: Physical activity gradually increased after an MI; pulse rate not to exceed 100 to 125 bpm; stop activity if shortness of breath or chest pain occurs. Cardiac rehabilitation is essential; little or no exercise will not promote cardiac strength and healing. Lifestyle behavior change is often difficult; mild depression is not uncommon; positive behaviors should be encouraged and rewarded.

CATEGORY: Analysis/Physiological Integrity

(1) Erythrocyte sedimentation rate (ESR): 10 mm/h—*rate at which RBC's settle out of unclotted blood in one hour; indicates inflammation/neurosis; normal: men 1–15 mm/h, women 1–20 mm/h*

(2) Hematocrit (Hct): 42 percent—*relative volume of plasma to RBC; increased with dehydration; decreased with fluid volume excess; normal: men 40–45 percent, women 37–45 percent*

(3) Creatine kinase (CK): 150 U/ml—**CORRECT: enzyme specific to brain, myocardium, and skeletal muscles; indicates tissue necrosis or injury; normal: men 12–70 U/mL, women 10–55 U/mL**

(4) Serum glucose: 100 mg/dL—*indicates insulin production; normal: 60–110 mg/dL*

54

The nurse is caring for a patient with cervical cancer. The nurse notes that the radium implant has become dislodged. Which of the following actions should the nurse take FIRST?

REWORDED QUESTION: What is the best action when a radium implant becomes dislodged?

STRATEGY: Think about the outcome of each answer choice.

NEEDED INFO: Limit radioactive exposure: assign patient to private room; place "Caution: Radioactive Material" sign on door; wear dosimeter film badge at all times when interacting with patient (measures amount of exposure); do not assign pregnant nurse to patient; rotate staff caring for patient; organize tasks so limited time is spent in patient's room; limit visitors; encourage patient to do own care; provide shield in room. Patient care: use antiemetics for nausea; consider body image; provide comfort measures; provide good nutrition.

CATEGORY: Implementation/Physiological Integrity

(1) Stay with the patient and contact radiology—*need to secure the implant in a lead container kept in the patient's room*

(2) Wrap the implant in a blanket and place it behind a lead shield—*pick up implant with long-handled forceps*

(3) Pick up the implant with long-handled forceps and place it in a lead container—**CORRECT: never touch implant with bare hands; forceps and container should be placed in patient's room**

(4) Obtain a dosimeter reading on the patient and report it to the physician—*need to place implant in lead container*

55 The nurse in a primary care clinic is caring for a 68-year-old man. History reveals that the client has smoked one pack of cigarettes per day for 45 years and drinks two beers per day. He is complaining of a non-productive cough, chest discomfort, and dyspnea. The nurse hears isolated wheezing in the right middle lobe. It would be MOST important for the nurse to complete which of the following orders?

REWORDED QUESTION: Which order should the nurse complete first?

STRATEGY: "MOST important" indicates the possibility of more than one good answer.

NEEDED INFO: Symptoms to look for: cough; change in a chronic cough; wheezing; recurring fever.

CATEGORY: Analysis/Physiological Integrity

(1) Pulmonary function tests—*evaluates lung capacity; done for constrictive disease such as asthma*

(2) Echocardiogram—*determines cardiac structure*

(3) Chest X-ray—**CORRECT: patient's symptoms, smoking history, and age are suspicious of lung cancer; wheezing caused by constrictive airways**

(4) Sputum culture—*determines if infection is present; crackles present with infections*

56 The nurse is caring for a patient with pernicious anemia. The nurse knows that her teaching has been successful if the patient makes which of the following statements?

REWORDED QUESTION: What is true about pernicious anemia?

STRATEGY: Determine the outcome of each answer choice.

NEEDED INFO: Pernicious anemia is caused by failure to absorb vitamin B_{12} because of a deficiency of intrinsic factor from the gastric mucosa. Symptoms: pallor, slight jaundice, glossitis, fatigue, weight loss, paresthesias of hands and feet, disturbances of balance and gait. Treatment: vitamin B_{12} IM monthly.

CATEGORY: Evaluation/Physiological Integrity

(1) "In order to get better, I will take iron pills."—*pernicious anemia due to vitamin B deficiency*

(2) "I am going to attend smoking cessation classes."—*no direct link to smoking*

(3) "I will learn how to perform IM injections."—**CORRECT: many patients instructed how to give monthly IM B_{12} injection**

(4) "I will increase my intake of carbohydrates."—*pernicious anemia caused by faulty absorption of vitamin B_{12}*

57 The nurse is caring for clients in the Emergency Department of an acute care facility. Four clients have been admitted in the last 20 minutes. Which of the admissions should the nurse see FIRST?

REWORDED QUESTION: Who is the priority patient?

STRATEGY: Think ABC's.

NEEDED INFO: Factors to consider: chief complaint; age of client; medical history; potential for life-threatening event.

CATEGORY: Analysis/Physiological Integrity

(1) A patient complaining of chest pain that is unrelieved by nitroglycerine—*airway issue takes priority*

(2) A patient with third-degree burns to the face—**CORRECT: face, neck, chest, or abdominal burns result in severe edema, causing airway restriction**

(3) A patient with a fractured left hip—*airway issue takes priority*

(4) A patient complaining of epigastric pain—*airway issue takes priority*

58 The nurse is caring for a patient with a diagnosis of COPD, bronchitis-type, in the long-term care facility. The patient is wheezing, and his oxygen saturation is 85 percent. Four hours ago, the oxygen saturation was 88 percent. It is MOST important for the nurse to take which of the following actions?

REWORDED QUESTION: What is the best action for a patient with COPD?

STRATEGY: Determine the outcome of each answer choice.

NEEDED INFO: Emphysema: overinflation of alveoli resulting in destruction of alveoli walls; predisposing factors include smoking, chronic infections, environmental pollution. Teaching includes breathing exercises; stop smoking; avoid hot/cold air or allergens; instructions regarding medications; avoid crowds or close contact with persons who have colds or flu; adequate rest and nutrition; oral hygiene; prophylactic flu vaccines; observe sputum for indications of infection.

CATEGORY: Implementation/Physiological Integrity

(1) Administer beclomethasone (Vanceril), two puffs per metered dose inhaler—*administer brochodilator first to open passageways*

(2) Listen to breath sounds—*situation does not require further assessment*

(3) Increase oxygen to 4 L per mask—*increased oxygen levels in patient's blood may lead to respiratory depression*

(4) Administer albuterol (Proventil), two puffs per metered dose inhaler—**CORRECT: brochodilator, relaxes bronchial smooth muscles**

59 The nurse is caring for a patient hospitalized for observation following a fall. The patient states, "My friend fell last year, and no one thought anything was wrong. She died two days later!" Which of the following responses by the nurse is BEST?

REWORDED QUESTION: What is the most therapeutic response?

STRATEGY: Remember therapeutic communication.

NEEDED INFO: Therapeutic communication: using silence (allows patient time to think and reflect; conveys acceptance; allows patient to take lead in conversation); using general leads or broad openings (encourages patient to talk, indicates interest in patient); clarification (encourages description of feelings and details of particular experience; makes sure nurse understands patient); reflecting (paraphrases what patient says; reflects what patient says, especially feelings conveyed).

CATEGORY: Implementation/Psychosocial Integrity

(1) "This happens to quite a few people."—*nontherapeutic; doesn't address patient's concerns*

(2) 'We are monitoring you, so you'll be okay."—*nontherapeutic; "don't worry" response*

(3) "Don't you think I'm taking good care of you?"—*nontherapeutic; focus is on the nurse*

(4) "You're concerned that it might happen to you?"—**CORRECT: reflects patient's feelings**

60 The nurse is caring for patients on the pediatric unit. An eight-year-old patient with second and third degree burns on the right thigh is being admitted. The nurse should assign the new patient to which one of the following roommates?

REWORDED QUESTION: Who is the appropriate roommate for a patient with burns?

STRATEGY: Think about the transmission of diseases.

NEEDED INFO: Droplet precautions: used with pathogens transmitted by infectious droplets; involves contact of conjunctivae or mucous membranes of nose or mouth, or during coughing, sneezing, talking, or procedures such as suctioning or bronchoscopy; private room or with patient with same infection; spatial separation of three feet between infected patient and visitors or other patients; door may remain open; place mask on patient during transportation.

CATEGORY: Implementation/Physiological Integrity

(1) A two-year-old with chicken pox—*infectious disease*

(2) A four-year-old with asthma—**CORRECT: patient not infectious; lowest risk of cross-contamination**

(3) A nine-year-old with acute diarrhea—*requires contact precautions*

(4) A ten-year-old with methicillin-resistant staph auerus (MRSA)—*requires contact isolation*

61 The nurse teaches a client about elastic stockings. Which of the following statements, if made by the client, indicates to the nurse that teaching was successful?

REWORDED QUESTION: What is a correct statement about elastic stockings?

STRATEGY: Determine the outcome of each answer choice.

NEEDED INFO: Maintain pressure on muscles of the lower extremities. Don't use if there are any skin lesions or gangrenous areas. Remove and reapply at least two times per day. Stockings should be clean and dry.

CATEGORY: Evaluation/Physiological Integrity

(1) "I will wear the stockings until the physician tells me to remove them."—*remove daily for bathing and inspection of the extremities*

(2) "I should wear the stockings even when I am asleep."—*elastic stockings promote venous return; not necessary during prolonged periods of sleep*

(3) "Every four hours I should remove the stockings for a half hour."—*stockings should be worn when client is up to promote venous return*

(4) "I should put on the stockings before getting out of bed in the morning."—**CORRECT: promote venous return by applying external pressure on veins**

62 The nurse is teaching a client who is scheduled for a paracentesis. Which of the following statements, if made by the client to the nurse, indicates that teaching has been successful?

REWORDED QUESTION: What is a correct statement about paracentesis?

STRATEGY: Determine the outcome of each answer choice.

NEEDED INFO: Paracentesis: removal of fluid from the peritoneal cavity; 2–3 L may be removed. Prep: informed consent; void, take vital signs; measure abdominal girth; weigh patient. During procedure: take vital signs q 15 minutes. After procedure: document amount, color, characteristics of drainage obtained; assess pressure dressing for drainage; position in bed until vital signs are stable.

CATEGORY: Evaluation/Physiological Integrity

(1) "I will be in surgery for less than one hour."—*not a surgical procedure*

(2) "I must not void prior to the procedure."—*bladder is emptied prior to the procedure to prevent puncture*

(3) "The physician will remove 2–3 L of fluid."—**CORRECT: fluid removed slowly to decrease ascites; can remove up to 4–6 L in severe cases**

(4) "I will lie on my back and breathe slowly."—*positioned in an upright position with feet supported*

63 The homecare nurse is performing chest physiotherapy on an elderly client with chronic airflow limitations (CAL). Which of the following actions should the nurse take FIRST?

REWORDED QUESTION: What should the nurse do prior to beginning chest physiotherapy?

STRATEGY: Determine whether to assess or implement.

NEEDED INFO: Postural drainage: uses gravity to facilitate removal of bronchial secretions; patient is placed in a variety of positions to facilitate drainage into larger airways; secretions may be removed by coughing or suctioning. Percussion and vibration: usually performed during postural drainage to augment the effect of gravity drainage; percussion: rhythmic striking of chest wall with cupped hands over areas where secretions are retained; vibration: hand and arm muscles of person doing vibration are tensed, and a vibrating pressure is applied to chest as patient exhales.

CATEGORY: Assessment/Physiological Integrity

(1) Perform chest physiotherapy prior to meals—*prevents nausea, vomiting, aspiration*

(2) Auscultate the chest prior to beginning the procedure—**CORRECT: identify areas of the lung that require drainage; auscultate chest at end of procedure to determine effectiveness**

(3) Administer bronchiodilators after the procedure—*given before chest physiotherapy to dilate the bronchioles and to liquify secretions*

(4) Percuss each lobe prior to asking the client to cough—*may cause fractures of the ribs; percussion helps loosen thick secretions*

64 A 60-year-old man is admitted to the hospital with a diagnosis of chronic bronchitis. He has a 10-year history of emphysema. The nurse should place him in which of the following positions?

REWORDED QUESTION: What is the BEST position for a patient with a respiratory problem?

STRATEGY: Picture the patient as described.

NEEDED INFO: Fowler's position: 45–60°. High Fowler's position: 60–90°. Used to promote cardiac and respiratory function. Chronic bronchitis s/s: productive cough, wheezing, SOB, exercise intolerance. Treatment: bronchodilators, antihistamines, steroids, antibiotics, expectorants. Theophylline: bronchodilator. Side effects: restlessness, dizziness, palpitations, tachycardia, anorexia. Emphysema s/s: marked dyspnea on exertion that proceed to dyspnea at rest, use of accessory muscles for breathing, barrel chest, "pink puffer" (normal O_2 level and dyspnea). Treatment: low-flow O_2 (1–3 L/min), CO_2 resp stimulus obliterated.

CATEGORY: Implementation/Physiological Integrity

(1) Side-lying—*diaphragm against abdominal organs*
(2) Supine—*can't breath*
(3) High-Fowler's—**CORRECT: head of bed elevated 60–90°; gravity displaces abdominal organs**
(4) Semi-Fowler's—*head of bed elevated 15–30°*

65 A patient is to receive 1,000 ml of 5% dextrose in 0.45 NaCl intravenous solution in an 8-hour period. The intravenous set delivers 15 drops per milliliter. The nurse should regulate the flow rate so it delivers how many drops of fluid per minute?

REWORDED QUESTION: What is the correct IV flow rate?

STRATEGY: Use the correct formula and be careful not to make math errors.

NEEDED INFO: Formula: total volume × drip factor divided by the total time in minutes.

CATEGORY: Planning/Physiological Integrity

(1) 15—*incorrect*
(2) 31—**CORRECT: 1000 × 15 divided by 8 × 60**
(3) 45—*incorrect*
(4) 60—*incorrect*

66 The nurse knows the plan of care for a patient with severe liver disease would include which of the following actions?

REWORDED QUESTION: What is included in the plan of care?

STRATEGY: Determine the outcome of each answer choice.

NEEDED INFO: Nutrition—Early stages: high protein, high carb diet; advanced stages: fiber, protein, fat, and sodium restrictions; small, frequent feedings; fluid restriction; avoid alcohol. Administer blood products; observe vital signs for shock; monitor abdominal girth; maintain skin integrity; assess degree of jaundice; promote rest; promote adequate respiratory function; reduce exposure to infection; reduce ascites (sodium and fluid restrictions, diuretics).

CATEGORY: Implementation/Physiological Integrity

(1) Administer Kayexelate enemas—*decreases serum potassium levels*
(2) Offer a low protein, high carbohydrate diet—**CORRECT: hepatic coma caused by increased levels of ammonia from breakdown of protein**
(3) Insert a Sengsteken-Blakemore tube—*applies pressure against bleeding esophageal varices*
(4) Administer salt-poor albumin IV—*balances osmotic pressure*

67 A 59-year-old patient with a diagnosis of delirium is admitted to the hospital. To evaluate the cause of a patient's delirium, blood is sent to the laboratory for analysis. The results are as follows: NA^+ 156, CL^- 100, K^+ 4.0, HCO_3 21, BUN 86, glucose 100. Based on these laboratory results, the nurse should record which of the following nursing diagnoses on the patient's care plan?

REWORDED QUESTION: What nursing diagnosis is appropriate?

STRATEGY: Determine if each lab value is normal or abnormal. Decide what the abnormal lab values indicate about the patient and how it would influence your development of appropriate nursing diagnoses for that patient.

NEEDED INFO: Normal Na^+: 135–145 mEq/L. Hypernatremia: dehydration and insufficient water intake. Normal Cl: 95–105 mEq/L. Normal K: 3.5–5.0 mEq/L. Normal HCO_3: 22–26 mEq/L. Decreased levels seen with starvation, renal failure, diarrhea. Normal BUN (blood, urea, nitrogen): 6–20 mg/100 ml. Elevated levels indicate rapid protein catabolism, kidney dysfunction, dehydration. Normal glucose: 70–100 mg/dL.

CATEGORY: Analysis/Physiological Integrity

(1) Alteration in patterns of urinary elimination—*would have altered K^+*
(2) Fluid volume deficit—**CORRECT: elevated Na^+, decreased CO_2, elevated BUN, other values are normal; elevated Na^+ and BUN seen with dehydration**

(3) Nutritional deficit: less than body requirements—*seen with decreased CO_2, but would have altered K^+*

(4) Self-care deficit: feeding—*no information to support this*

68 A patient is to receive 3,000 ml of 0.9% NaCl IV in 24 hours. The intravenous set delivers 15 drops per milliliter. The nurse should regulate the flow rate so that the patient receives how many drops of fluid per minute?

REWORDED QUESTION: How should you regulate the IV flow rate?

STRATEGY: Use the formula and avoid making math errors.

NEEDED INFO: total volume × the drop factor divided by the total time in minutes

CATEGORY: Planning/Physiological Integrity

(1) 21—*inaccurate*
(2) 28—*inaccurate*
(3) 31—**CORRECT: 3,000 × 15 divided by 24 × 60**
(4) 42—*inaccurate*

69 The nurse is supervising care of a patient receiving total parenteral nutrition (TPN) through a single-lumen percutaneous central catheter. The nurse would be MOST concerned if which of the following was observed?

REWORDED QUESTION: What is an incorrect action?

STRATEGY: "MOST concerned" indicates that you are looking for an incorrect intervention.

NEEDED INFO: TPN: method of supplying nutrients to the body by the IV route. Nursing care: site of catheter changed every 4 weeks, change IV tubing and filters every 24 hours, dressing changed 2–3 times a week and PRN; initial rate of infusion 50 ml/h and gradually increased (100–125 ml/h) as patient's fluid and electrolyte tolerance permits; increased rate of infusion causes hyperosmolar state (headache, nausea, fever, chills, malaise); slowed rate of infusion results in "rebound" hypoglycemia caused by delayed pancreatic reaction to change in insulin requirements.

CATEGORY: Evaluation/Physiological Integrity

(1) The patient receives insulin through the single-lumen—*insulin compatible with TPN solution*
(2) A mask is placed on the patient when changing the patient's dressing—*decreases chance of airborne contamination; nurse also wears mask when changing dressing*
(3) The patient's dressing is changed daily using sterile technique—**CORRECT: dressing changed one to two times per week and PRN**
(4) The patient is weighed two to three times per week—*assess fluid balance*

70 The nurse is caring for patients in the outpatient clinic. A client tells the nurse that he developed weakness and numbness in the legs the previous day and now his body feels the same way. The client's blood pressure is 120/80, P 86, R 20. The client denies any pain but appears anxious to the nurse. It would be MOST important for the nurse to ask which of the following questions?

REWORDED QUESTION: What is a possible cause of Guillain-Barre syndrome?

STRATEGY: Determine the relationship between the answers and Guillain-Barre syndrome.

NEEDED INFO: GBS Plan/Implementation: intervention is symptomatic; steroids in acute phase; plasmapheresis; aggressive respiratory care; prevent hazards of immobility; maintain adequate nutrition; physical therapy; pain-reducing measures; eye care; prevention of complications (UTI, aspiration); psychosocial support.

CATEGORY: Assessment/Physiological Integrity

(1) "Have you recently fallen or had some other type of physical injury?"—*symptoms consistent with Guillain-Barre syndrome; not related to injury*
(2) "Have you recently had a viral infection such as a cold?"—**CORRECT: GBS often preceded by a viral infection as well as immunizations/vaccinations**
(3) "Have you recently taken any over-the-counter medication?"—*no association with symptoms; appropriate question for health history*
(4) "Have you recently experienced headaches?"—*GBS affects peripheral, not central nervous system*

71 The nurse is admitting a patient who is jaundiced due to pancreatic cancer. The nurse should give the HIGHEST priority to which of the following needs?

REWORDED QUESTION: What is the highest priority for a patient with pancreatic cancer?

STRATEGY: Remember Maslow.

NEEDED INFO: Medical treatment: high calorie, bland, low fat diet; small, frequent feedings; avoid alcohol; anticholinergics; antineoplastic chemotherapy

CATEGORY: Planning/Physiological Integrity

(1) Nutrition—**CORRECT: profound weight loss and anorexia occur with pancreatic cancer**

(2) Self-image—*jaundiced patients are concerned about how they look, but physiological needs take priority*

(3) Skin integrity—*jaundice causes dry skin and pruritis; scratching can lead to skin breakdown*

(4) Urinary elimination—*urine is dark due to obstructive process; kidney function is not affected*

72 Which of the following statements, if made by a client during a group therapy session, would the nurse identify as reflecting a client's narcissistic personality disorder?

REWORDED QUESTION: Which statement would a client with narcissistic personality disorder be most likely to make?

STRATEGY: Think about each answer choice.

NEEDED INFO: Clients with narcissistic personality disorder display grandiosity about their self-importance and achievements. These clients overvalue themselves and are indifferent to others' criticism; the feelings of others are not understood or considered. They have a sense of entitlement and expect special treatment, and also use rationalization to blame others, make excuses, and provide alibis for self-focused behaviors.

CATEGORY: Analysis/Psychosocial Integrity

(1) "I'm sick of hearing about all your life tragedies."— **CORRECT: lack of empathy is the main characteristic of a narcissistic personality disorder**

(2) "I know I'm interrupting others, so what?"—*prominent behavior in an antisocial personality disorder*

(3) "I just can't stop wanting to slash myself."—*characteristic of a borderline personality disorder*

(4) "I just have no hope for the future."—*characteristic of depression*

73 A 15-year-old patient is admitted to the hospital with anorexia nervosa. Which of the following statements, if made by the patient, would require immediate follow-up by the nurse?

REWORDED QUESTION: Which problem has the highest priority for this patient?

STRATEGY: Remember Maslow's hierarchy of needs.

NEEDED INFO: Anorexia nervosa: a disorder characterized by restrictive eating resulting in emaciation, disturbance in body image, and an intense fear of being obese. Physical needs must be met first in order to keep the patient in stable condition. A difficult area to maintain is that of appropriate hydration and fluid and electrolyte balance.

CATEGORY: Planning/Psychosocial Integrity

(1) "My gums were bleeding this morning."—*vitamin deficiencies occur in anorectic patients, but not the highest priority*

(2) "I'm getting fatter every day."—*body image disturbance is a perceptual problem with anorectics, but not the highest priority; this is a psychosocial need*

(3) "Nobody likes me because I'm so ugly."—*chronic low self-esteem is a psychodynamic factor, but not the highest priority; this is a psychosocial need*

(4) "I'm feeling dizzy and weak today."—**CORRECT: fluid volume deficit is client's highest priority; dehydration is common and could lead to irreversible renal damage and vital sign alterations**

74 A client is admitted to the hospital for treatment of pneumocystis carinii pneumonia and Kaposi sarcoma. The client tells the nurse that he has been considering organ donation when he dies. Which of the following responses by the nurse is BEST?

REWORDED QUESTION: Can this patient be an organ donor?

STRATEGY: Think about each answer choice.

NEEDED INFO: Criteria for organ/tissue donation: no history of significant disease process in organ/tissue to be donated; no untreated sepsis; brain death of donor; no history of extracranial malignancy; relative hemodynamic stability; blood group compatibility; newborn donors must be full-term (more than 200 g); only absolue restriction to organ donation is documented case of HIV infection. Family members can give consent. Nurse can discuss organ donation with other death-related topics (funeral home to be used, autopsy request).

CATEGORY: Implementation/Physiological Integrity

(1) "What does your family think about your decision?"— *client has the right to make the decision*

(2) "You will help many people by donating your organs."—*clients with documented HIV are prohibited from donating organs*

(3) "Would you like to speak to the Organ Donor Representative?"—*passing the buck*

(4) "That is not possible based on your illness."—**CORRECT: clients with documented HIV are prohibited from donating organs**

---

75 The nurse is caring for a patient five hours after a pancreatectomy for cancer of the pancreas. On assessment, the nurse notes that there is minimal drainage from the nasogastric tube. It is MOST important for the nurse to take which of the following actions?

REWORDED QUESTION: What is the best action when an NG tube is not draining?

STRATEGY: Determine whether it is appropriate to assess or implement.

NEEDED INFO: Insertion of Levin/Salem sump: Measure distance from tip of nose to earlobe, plus distance from earlobe to bottom of xyphoid process. Mark distance on tube with tape and lubricate end of tube. Insert tube through nose to stomach. Offer sips of water and advance tube gently; bend head forward. Observe for respiratory distress. Secure with hypoallergenic tape. Verify tube position initially and before feeding. Aspirate for gastric contents and check pH. Inject approx 15 cc of air into stomach while listening over epigastric area (not always accurate).

CATEGORY: Assessment/Physiological Integrity

(1) Notify the physician—*should assess first*

(2) Monitor vital signs q 15 minutes—*does not address lack of drainage*

(3) Check the tubing for kinks—**CORRECT: assess prior to implementing; maintain tubing in a dependent position**

(4) Replace the NG tube—*assess before implementing*

---

76 When collecting a 24-hour urine specimen for creatinine clearance, it is MOST important for the nurse to do which of the following?

REWORDED QUESTION: What is the correct procedure for a 24-hour urine analysis?

STRATEGY: "MOST important" indicates there may be more than one response that appears correct.

NEEDED INFO: Hydrate client before test. Encourage hourly intake of water during test. Have client void and discard urine; note the time; save all urine for specified time. Do not contaminate specimen with feces or toilet paper.

CATEGORY: Implementation/Physiological Integrity

(1) Obtain an order from the physician for insertion of a Foley catheter—*not necessary unless client is incontinent*

(2) Obtain the client's weight prior to beginning the urine collection—*not necessary*

(3) Discard the last voided specimen prior to ending the collection—*collect all urine voided during the time period*

(4) Ask if a preservative is present in the container—**CORRECT: save all urine in a container with no preservatives; refrigerate or keep on ice**

---

77 The nurse is planning discharge teaching for a patient with Parkinson's disease. To maintain safety, the nurse should make which one of the following suggestions to the family?

REWORDED QUESTION: What is a correct patient teaching for Parkinson's disease?

STATEGY: Determine the outcome of each answer choice.

NEEDED INFO: Symptoms: tremors, akinesia, rigidity, weakness, "motorized propulsive gait, slurred monotonous speech, dysphagia, drooling, mask-like expression. Nursing care: Encourage finger exercises. Administer Artane, Cogentin, L-Dopa, Parlodel, Sinemet, Symmetrel. Teach patient ambulation modification. Promote family understanding of the disease (intellect/sight/hearing not impaired, disease progressive but slow, doesn't lead to paralysis). Refer for speech therapy, potential stereotactic surgery.

CATEGORY: Implementation/Physiological Integrity

(1) Install a raised toilet seat—**CORRECT: helps client to be independent; slightly elevate the back leg of chairs**

(2) Obtain a hospital bed—*no indications that this is needed*

(3) Instruct the patient to hold his arms in a dependent position when ambulating—*should swing arms to assist in balance when walking*

(4) Perform an exercise program during the late afternoon—*activities should be scheduled for late morning when energy level is highest and patient won't be rushed*

78 The nurse is performing discharge teaching for a patient with chronic pancreatitis. Which of the following statements, if made by the patient to the nurse, indicates that further teaching is necessary?

REWORDED QUESTION: What is an incorrect statement about pancreatitis?

STRATEGY: This is a negative question; you are looking for incorrect information.

NEEDED INFO: Plan/Implementation: NPO, gastric decompression. Meds: antacids, analgesics, antibiotics, anticholinergics. Maintain fluid/electrolyte imbalance. Monitor for signs of infection. Cough and deep-breathe; semi-Fowler's position. Monitor for shock and hyperglycemia. TPN. Treatment of exocrine insufficiency: meds containing amylase, lipase, trypsin to aid digestion. Long-term: avoid alcohol; low-fat, bland diet; small, frequent meals. Monitor signs/symptoms of diabetes mellitus.

CATEGORY: Evaluation/Physiological Integrity

(1) "I do not have to restrict my physical activity."—*no specific restrictions on activity*
(2) "I should take pancrelipase (Viokase) before meals."—*pancreatic enzyme replacement; take before or with meals*
(3) "I will eat three meals per day."—**CORRECT: small, frequent feedings are most beneficial**
(4) "I am not allowed to drink any alcoholic beverages."—*complete absinence from alcohol required*

79 Following a laparoscopic cholecystectomy, the patient complains of abdominal pain and bloating. Which of the following responses by the nurse is BEST?

REWORDED QUESTION: What is the best intervention for a patient complaining of free air pain?

STRATEGY: "BEST" indicates there may be more than one response that appears correct.

NEEDED INFO: Cholecystectomy: removal of gall bladder. T-tube inserted to ensure drainage of bile from common bile duct until edema diminishes. Check amt of drainage (usually 500 to 1,000 ml/day, decreases as fluid begins to drain into duodenum). Protect skin around incision from bile drainage irritation (use zinc oxide or water soluble lubricant). Keep drainage bag at same level as gallbladder. Maintain patient in semi-Fowler position after T-tube is removed; observe dressing for bile; notify physician if there is significant drainage. Evaluate pain to check for other problems. Monitor for signs

of K^+ and Na^+ loss; flattened or inverted t-waves on EKG; muscle weakness; abdominal distension; headache; apathy; nausea or vomiting; jaundice.

CATEGORY: Implementation/Physiological Integrity

(1) "Increase your intake of fresh fruits and vegetables."—*no indication of constipation*
(2) "I'll give you the prescribed pain medication."—*less pain medication needed with laparoscopic procedure*
(3) "Why don't you take a walk in the hallway."—**CORRECT: "free air" pain caused by CO_2; ambulation will increase absorption**
(4) "You may need an indwelling catheter."—*pain due to retention of CO_2*

80 The nurse in an outpatient clinic is supervising student nurses administering influenza vaccinations. The nurse should question the administration of the vaccine to which of the following clients?

REWORDED QUESTION: What is a contraindication to receiving flu vaccine?

STRATEGY: Think about what each answer choice means.

NEEDED INFO: Influenza vaccine: given yearly, preferably Oct.–Nov.; recommended for people age 65 or older; people under 65 with heart disease, lung disease, diabetes, immuno-suppression, chronic care facility residents

CATEGORY: Assessment/Health Promotion and Maintenance

(1) A 45-year-old male who is allergic to shellfish—*allergy to eggs is a contraindication*
(2) A 60-year-old female who says she has a sore throat—**CORRECT: vaccine deferred in presence of acute respiratory disease**
(3) A 66-year-old female who lives in a group home—*vaccine deferred only if patient has an active immunization*
(4) A 70-year-old female with congestive heart failure—*no contraindication*

81 An arterial blood gas is ordered for a man following a myocardial infarction. After obtaining the specimen, it would be MOST appropriate for the nurse to take which of the following actions?

REWORDED QUESTION: What is the priority action after an ABG?

STRATEGY: Take care of the patient first.

NEEDED INFO: ABG: measurement of partial pressure of oxygen, CO_2, and pH of blood; assessment of acid-base status of body. Use a heparinized syringe. Needle inserted 45–60 degrees to skin surface and advanced into radial artery. Apply pressure after needle is removed. Put specimen on ice.

CATEGORY: Implementation/Physiological Integrity

(1) Obtain ice for the specimen—*should be done, but not the most important*

(2) Apply direct pressure to the site—**CORRECT: prevents bleeding, hematoma; maintain for 5 minutes, 15 minutes if on anticoagulant**

(3) Apply a sterile dressing to the site—*Band-Aid is applied*

(4) Observe the site for hematoma formation—*more important to prevent hematoma*

82 The nurse is caring for a man who was involved in an auto accident the previous day. The patient has a double-lumen tracheostomy tube with a cuff. The nurse should:

REWORDED QUESTION: What is a correct action when caring for a tracheostomy?

STRATEGY: Determine the outcme of each answer choice.

NEEDED INFO: Cuffed tracheostomy tube permits mechanical ventilation and seals off lower airways. Inject air with a syringe into one-way valve in pilot line. Nursing responsibilities: change patient's position frequently, provide humidification and hydration, suction as necessary.

CATEGORY: Implementation/Physiological Integrity

(1) change the tracheostomy dressing every eight hours and PRN—**CORRECT: prevents infection; use pre-cut gauze pads**

(2) change the tracheostomy ties every 48 hours—*change PRN; keep old ties on until new ties are in place; 1 finger space between tie and neck*

(3) keep the inner cannula of the tracheostomy in place at all times—*remove and clean q 8 hours and PRN using H_2O*

(4) push the outer cannula back in if it accidentally "blows out"—*maintain open airway and contact physician*

83 The nurse performs discharge teaching with a patient with emphysema. Which statement, if made by the patient, indicates that teaching was successful?

REWORDED QUESTION: What is true about emphysema?

STRATEGY: Determine the outcome of each answer choice.

NEEDED INFO: Emphysema: chronic progressive respiratory disease caused by destruction of alveolar walls. Complications: acute respiratory infections, cardiac failure or cor pulmonale, cardiac dysrhythmias. Symptoms: cough, dyspnea, wheezing, barrel chest, use of accessory muscles to breathe. Treatment: bronchodilators, corticosteroids, cromolyn sodium, oxygen, diaphragmatic and pursed-lip breathing maneuvers, energy conservation, diet therapy.

CATEGORY: Evaluation/Physiological Integrity

(1) "Cold weather will help my breathing problems."—*will exacerbate breathing problems by causing bronchiospasms*

(2) "I should eat three balanced meals but limit my fluid intake."—*need small, frequent feedings to increase caloric intake, limit SOB caused by eating; hydration will liquify secretions*

(3) "My outside activity should be limited when pollution levels are high."—**CORRECT: pollution will act as irritant by causing bronchiospasms**

(4) "An intensive exercise program is important in regaining my strength."—*unable to tolerate intensive exercise; conditioning program to conserve and increase pulmonary ventilation*

84 The nurse assists the physician with the removal of a chest tube. Before the physician removes the chest tube, the nurse should instruct the patient to

REWORDED QUESTION: What should the patient do when a chest tube is removed?

STRATEGY: Determine the outcome of each answer choice.

NEEDED INFO: Pneumothorax: air in pleural space causes collapse of lung. Chest tubes: used with Pleur-evac 3-chamber system to restore negative pressure in pleural space. Removal: chest tube is clamped, patient does Valsalva maneuver; apply petroleum gauze dressing sealed with tape.

CATEGORY: Implementation/Physiological Integrity

(1) exhale and bear down—**CORRECT: Valsalva maneuver; increased intrathoracic pressure; occlusive dressing applied**

(2) hold his breath for five seconds—*unnecessary*

(3) inhale and exhale rapidly—*unsafe*

(4) cough as hard as he can—*unnecessary*

85 A 45-year-old man comes into the emergency room with complaints of sudden onset of severe right flank pain. While tests are being performed, it is MOST important for the nurse to:

REWORDED QUESTION: What is the priority action for a patient with suspected renal calculi?

STRATEGY: "MOST important" indicates a priority question.

NEEDED INFO: Symptoms of renal calculi: pain (depends on location of stone), diaphoresis, nausea and vomiting, fever and chills, hematuria. Nursing care: monitor I/O and temp; force fluids; strain urine and check pH of urine; administer analgesics. Diet for prevention of stones (most stones contain calcium, phosphorus, and/or oxalate): consume foods low in calcium, sodium, and oxalates; avoid vitamin D-enriched foods; decrease purine sources; to make urine alkaline, restrict citrus fruits, milk, potatoes; to acidify urine, increase consumption of eggs, fish, cranberries.

CATEGORY: Implementation/Physiological Integrity

(1) make sure that he does not eat or drink anything—*not most important*

(2) strain all his urine through several layers of gauze— **CORRECT: symptoms suggestive of urinary calculi, should strain urine for passage of stone**

(3) check his grip strength and pupil reactivity—*symptoms suggestive of urinary calculi, not neurological*

(4) send blood and urine specimens to the lab for analysis— *not most important if urinary calculi is suspected*

86 The nurse is preparing discharge teaching for a patient with a new colostomy. The nurse knows teaching was successful when the patient chooses which of the following menu options?

REWORDED QUESTION: What is the appropriate diet for a patient with a colostomy?

STRATEGY: Recall the type of diet required and then select the menu that is appropriate.

NEEDED INFO: Skin care for stoma: effect on skin depends on composition, quality, consistency of drainage, medication, location of stoma, frequency of removal of appliance adhesive.

Principles of skin protection: use skin sealant under all tapes; use skin barrier to protect skin around stoma; cleanse skin gently and pat dry, not rub; change appliance immediately when seal breaks. Diet: a low-residue diet for 4–6 weeks post-op, avoiding gas-forming, odor-producing, or excessively laxative/constipating foods.

CATEGORY: Evaluation/Physiological Integrity

(1) Sausage, sauerkraut, baked potato, and fresh fruit— *sausage and sauerkraut are gas producing and should be avoided with a new colostomy*

(2) Cheese omelet with bran muffin and fresh pineapple— *bran muffin and fresh fruit are high fiber (residue)*

(3) Pork chop, mashed potatoes, turnips, and salad— *turnips are odor causing and salad is high residue*

(4) Baked chicken, boiled potato, cooked carrots, and yogurt—**CORRECT: provides balanced nutrition, high protein, low residue, low fat, and non-irritating foods**

87 A 59-year-old man is seen in the outpatient clinic to rule out acute renal failure. The nurse would be MOST concerned if the patient made which one of the following statements?

REWORDED QUESTION: What is a symptom of acute renal failure?

STRATEGY: "MOST concerned" indicates you are looking for a symptom of acute renal failure.

NEEDED INFO: Symptoms of oliguric phase of acute renal failure: urinary output less than 400 cc/day; irritability, drowsiness, confusion, coma; restlessness, twitching, seizures; increased serum K^+, BUN, creatinine, Ca^+, Na^+, pH; anemia; pulmonary edema, CHF, hypertension. Symptoms of diuretic or recovery phase: urinary output of 4–5 L/day; increased serum BUN; Na^+ and K^+ loss in urine; increased mental and physical activity.

CATEGORY: Assessment/Physiological Integrity

(1) "My urine is often pink-tinged."—*seen with urinary tract infections or trauma; hematuria not usually a symptom of acute renal failure*

(2) "It is hard for me to start the flow of urine."—*urinary hesitancy not usually seen with acute renal failure*

(3) "It is quite painful for me to urinate."—*dysuria seen with urinary tract infections, not with acute renal failure*

(4) "I urinate in the morning and again before dinner."— **CORRECT: symptoms of acute renal failure include**

decreased urinary output (anuria or ologuria), increased urinary output, hypotension, tachycardia, lethargy; normal output 1,200–1,500 cc/day or 50–63 cc/hr, normal voiding pattern 5–6 times/day and once at night

88 The nurse is teaching a new mother how to breast-feed her newborn. The nurse knows that teaching has been successful if the client makes which of the following statements?

REWORDED QUESTION: What indicates that a newborn is receiving adequate nutrition when breastfeeding?

STRATEGY: Think about each statement. Is it true?

NEEDED INFO: Breastfeeding is recommended for first 6–12 months of life; human milk is considered ideal food. Colostrum is secreted at first; clear and colorless; contains protective antibodies; high in protein and minerals. Milk is secreted after two to four days; milky white appearance; contains more fat and lactose than colostrum.

CATEGORY: Evaluation/Physiological Integrity

(1) "My baby's weight should equal her birthweight in five to seven days."—*breastfeeding infants should surpass birthweight in 10–14 days*
(2) "My baby should have at least six to eight wet diapers per day."—CORRECT: **indicates newborn is ingesting an adequate amount of nutrition; should have at least two bowel movements per day**
(3) "My baby will sleep at least six hours between feedings."—*newborns feed approximately every two to three hours during the day and every four hours at night*
(4) "My baby will feed for about 10 minutes per feeding."—*should feed for approx. 15–20 minutes per breast*

89 A man is admitted to the telemetry Unit for evaluation of complaints of chest pain. Eight hours after admission, the patient goes into ventricular fibrillation. The physician defibrillates the patient. The nurse understands that the purpose of defibrillation is to:

REWORDED QUESTION: Why is a patient defibrillated?

STRATEGY: Think about each answer choice.

NEEDED INFO: Defibrillation: produces asystole of heart to provide opportunity for natural pacemaker (SA node) to resume as pacer of heart activity

CATEGORY: Analysis/Physiological Integrity

(1) increase cardiac contractility and cardiac output—*inaccurate*
(2) cause asystole so the normal pacemaker can recapture—CORRECT: **allows SA node to resume as pacer of heart activity**
(3) reduce cardiac ischemia and acidosis—*inaccurate*
(4) provide energy for depleted myocardial cells—*inaccurate*

90 A man is brought to the emergency room complaining of chest pain. The nurse performs an assessment of the patient. Which of the following symptoms would be MOST characteristic of an acute myocardial infarction?

REWORDED QUESTION: What type of pain is characteristic in an MI?

STRATEGY: Think about the cause of each type of pain.

NEEDED INFO: MI signs and symptoms: chest pain radiating to neck, jaw, shoulder, back, or left arm; unrelieved by nitroglycerine. Also fever, apprehension, dizziness, diaphoresis, palpitations, shortness of breath.

CATEGORY: Assessment/Physiological Integrity

(1) Colic-like epigastric pain—*indicates GI disorder*
(2) Sharp, well-localized, unilateral chest pain—*symptoms of pneumothorax*
(3) Severe substernal pain radiating down the left arm—CORRECT: **crushing; may radiate; unrelated to emotion or exercise**
(4) Sharp, burning chest pain moving from place to place—*anxiety state*

91 The nurse is caring for patients on the medical unit. A patient is admitted with a diagnosis of deep vein thrombosis (DVT). Admission orders include heparin 2,000 units per hour in 5 percent dextrose in water. The nurse should have which of the following available?

REWORDED QUESTION: What is an antidote for heparin?

STRATEGY: Think about the action of each medication.

NEEDED INFO: Heparin: anticoagulant. Side effects: hemorrhage, thrombocytopenia. Antidote: protamine sulfate.

CATEGORY: Planning/Physiological Integrity

(1) Propranolol (Inderal)—*beta blocker; reduces myocardial oxygen consumption*

(2) Protamine zinc—*long-acting insulin*

(3) Protamine sulfate—**CORRECT: antidote, acts as base to neutralize heparin; give IV over three minutes**

(4) Vitamin K—*antidote to Coumadin*

92

A client returns to the clinic two weeks after discharge from the hospital. He is taking wafarin sodium (Coumadin) 2 mg PO daily. Which of the following statements, if made by the client to the nurse, indicates that further teaching is necessary?

REWORDED QUESTION: What is contraindicated for Coumadin?

STRATEGY: Think about what each statement means and how it relates to Coumadin.

NEEDED INFO: Coumadin: anticoagulant. Side effects: hemorrhage, fever, rash. Prrothrombin time (PT) used to monitor effectiveness; PT usually maintained at 1.5–2 times normal. Antidote: vitamin K (aquamephyton). Nursing responsibilities: check for bleeding gums, bruises, nosebleeds, petechiae, melena, tarry stools, hematuria. Use electric razor, soft toothbrush; green leafy vegetables (contain vitamin K).

CATEGORY: Evaluation/Physiological Integrity

(1) "I have been taking an antihistamine before bed."—*no contraindication*

(2) "I take aspirin when I have a headache."—**CORRECT: inhibits platelet aggregation; effect lasts 3–8 days**

(3) "I use sunscreen when I go outside."—*correct behavior*

(4) "I take Mylanta if my stomach gets upset."—*correct information*

93

To enhance the percutaneous absorption of nitroglycerine ointment, it would be MOST important for the nurse to select a site that is

REWORDED QUESTION: What is the best site for nitroglycerine ointment?

STRATEGY: Think about each site.

NEEDED INFO: Nitroglycerine: used in treatment of angina pectoris to reduce ischemia and relieve pain by decreasing myocardial oxygen consumption; dilates veins and arteries. Side effects: throbbing headache, flushing, hypotension, tachycardia. Nursing responsibilities: teach appropriate

administration, storage, expected pain relief, side effects. Ointment applied to skin; sites rotated to avoid skin irritation. Prolonged effect up to 24 hours.

CATEGORY: Implementation/Physiological Integrity

(1) muscular—*not most important*

(2) near the heart—*not most important*

(3) non-hairy—**CORRECT: skin site free of hair will increase absorption; avoid distal part of extremities due to less than maximal absorption**

(4) over a bony prominence—*most important is that the site be non-hairy*

94

A client with chronic alcohol abuse has been admitted to a rehabilitation unit. The nurse knows that the client is denying alcoholism when he makes which of the following statements?

REWORDED QUESTION: Which statement signifies denial?

STRATEGY: What are the defense mechanisms and how are they manifested?

NEEDED INFO: Defense mechanisms include: repression, denial, suppression, rationalization, intellectualization, identification, introjection, compensation, reaction formation, sublimation, displacement, projection, conversion, undoing, dissociation, regression.

CATEGORY: Analysis/Psychosocial Integrity

(1) "My brother did this to me."—*projection: blaming someone else for one's difficulties*

(2) "Drinking always calms my nerves."—*rationalization: the attempt to prove that one's feelings or behavior is justifiable*

(3) "I can stop drinking anytime I feel like it."—**CORRECT: denial is the unconscious refusal to admit an unacceptable idea or behavior**

(4) "Let's all plan to play cards tonight."—*suppression: the voluntary exclusion from awareness of feelings, ideas, or situations that produce anxiety*

95

During the acute phase of a cerebrovascular accident (CVA), the nurse should maintain the patient in which of the following positions?

REWORDED QUESTION: What is the best way to position a patient during the acute phase of a CVA?

STRATEGY: Remember the positioning strategy.

NEEDED INFO: Nursing responsibilities during acute phase: maintain patient airway; monitor vital signs; neurological assessment (Glasgow coma scale); passive ROM exercises; NPO for 24–48 hours; tube feedings.

CATEGORY: Implementation/Physiological Integrity

(1) Semi-prone with the head of the bed elevated 60–90 degrees—*on left side with legs flexed on abdomen, hip flexion increases intrathoracic pressure*

(2) Lateral, with the head of the bed flat—*helps with drainage of secretions, but not the best*

(3) Prone, with the head of the bed flat—*interferes with respiration*

(4) Supine, with the head of the bed elevated 30–45 degrees—**CORRECT: facilitates venous drainage from brain; reduces intracranial pressure; keeps head in midline**

96 Which of the following statements, if made by a client during a group therapy session, would require immediate follow-up by the nurse?

REWORDED QUESTION: Which statement indicates the possibility of impending danger?

STRATEGY: Think about which statement would make you question the client's intentions.

NEEDED INFO: In *Tarasoff v. The Regents of the University of California* (1976), the court established a duty to warn of threats of harm to others. Failure to warn, coupled with subsequent injury to the threatened person, exposes the mental health professional to civil damages for malpractice. Based on this and other rulings in many states, the mental health care giver must take responsibility to warn society of potential danger.

CATEGORY: Implementation/Psychosocial Integrity

(1) "I know I'm a chronically compulsive liar, but I can't help it."—*this statement is revealing, but does not indicate impending threat*

(2) "I don't ever want to go home; I feel safer here."—*this statement is a response to anxiety or fear, but does not indicate immediate danger*

(3) "I don't really care if I ever see my girlfriend again."—*this statement does not imply a threat or impending violence*

(4) "I'll make sure that doctor is sorry for what he said."—**CORRECT: under the Tarasoff Act, a threatened per-**son, including health professionals, must be warned about threats or potential threats to personal safety

97 A patient newly diagnosed with Alzheimer's disease is admitted to the unit. Which action, if taken by the nurse, is BEST?

REWORDED QUESTION: What is the best assessment?

STRATEGY: Determine whether to assess or implement.

NEEDED INFO: Alzheimer's disease (senile dementia): chronic, progressive, degenerative, resulting in cerebral atrophy. S/S: changes in memory, confusion, disorientation, change in personality; most common after age 65. Nursing responsibilities: reorient as needed; speak slowly; place clocks and calendars in room; place bed in low position with side rails up.

CATEGORY: Assessment/Psychosocial Integrity

(1) Place the patient in a private room away from the nurses' station—*should be in a semi-private room near nurses' station; needs frequent assessment*

(2) Ask the family to wait in the waiting room while the nurse admits the patient—*familiar people decrease confusion of unfamiliar environment*

(3) Assign a different nurse daily to care for the patient—*consistency is important*

(4) Ask the patient to state today's date—**CORRECT: assessment is the first step in planning care**

98 A 40-year-old woman visits the clinic with complaints of right calf tenderness and pain. It would be MOST important for the nurse to ask which of the following questions?

REWORDED QUESTION: What is a predisposing factor to developing DVT?

STRATEGY: Determine why you would ask each question.

NEEDED INFO: Thrombophlebitis (phlebitis, phlebothrombosis, or deep vein thrombosis [DVT]): clot formation in a vein secondary to inflammation of vein or partial vein obstruction. Risk factors: history of varicose veins, hypercoagulation, cardiovascular disease, pregnancy, oral contraceptives, immobility, recent surgery or injury.

CATEGORY: Assessment/Physiological Integrity

(1) "Do you exercise excessively?"—*could cause shin splints*

(2) "Have you had any fractures in the last year?"—*not relevant to client's complaints*

(3) "What type of birth control do you use?"—**CORRECT: increased risk of DVT with oral contraceptives**

(4) "Are you under a lot of stress?"—*should be concerned about possibility of DVT*

99

A mother calls the well-baby clinic to report that her 4-month-old son has an upper respiratory infection (URI) with a temperature of 104° F (40° C). The infant is scheduled to receive his DPT and TOPV immunizations later that day. The mother asks the nurse if she should bring him in for his scheduled immunizations. Which of the following responses by the nurse would be MOST appropriate?

REWORDED QUESTION: Is a URI and elevated temp contraindication for routine immunization?

STRATEGY: Picture the patient as described.

NEEDED INFO: URI: acute rhinitis (cold), pharyngitis, tonsillitis. Nursing responsibilities: liquid to soft diet, cool mist vaporizer, analgesics, antipyretics, antibiotics. Contraindications for immunizations: moderate to severe febrile illness, severe anaphylactic reaction from previous immunization, congenital disorders of immune system, immunosuppressive therapy, anaphylactic egg hypersensitivity for MMR and OPV.

CATEGORY: Implementation/Safe and Effective Care

(1) "Keep him at home. We'll give him a double dose next time."—*immunization not given, schedule resumed when infant well*

(2) "Bring him in. His illness will not interfere with his immunizations."—*febrile illness contraindication for all immunizations*

(3) "Keep him at home until his temperature and infection resolve."—**CORRECT: immunization contraindicated during infectious or inflammatory state, pre-existing symptoms could mask adverse or allergic reaction**

(4) "Bring him in. We'll give some antibiotics with the immunizations."—*involves giving immunization with febrile illness*

100

The nurse in the postpartum unit cares for a 27-year-old woman who delivered her first child the previous day. During her assessment of the patient, the nurse notes multiple varicosities on the patient's lower extremities. The nurse should:

REWORDED QUESTION: What is the BEST way to prevent thrombophlebitis?

STRATEGY: Focus in on the keyword of the question: "BEST."

NEEDED INFO: High risk of developing thrombophlebitis during pregnancy and immediate postpartum period. Thrombophlebitis: inflammation of vein associated with formation of a thrombus or blood clot. Other risk factors: prolonged immobility, use of oral contraceptives, sepsis, smoking, dehydration, and CHF. S/S: pain in the calf, localized edema of one extremity, positive Homan's sign (pain in calf when foot is dorsiflexed). Treatment: bed rest and elevation of extremity, anticoagulant (heparin).

CATEGORY: Planning/Health Promotion and Maintenance

(1) teach the patient to rest in bed when the baby sleeps—*not preventive; bed rest can cause thrombophlebitis*

(2) encourage early and frequent ambulation—**CORRECT: facilitates emptying of blood vessels in lower extremities**

(3) apply warm soaks for 20 minutes every four hours—*not a preventive measure but an intervention used to treat; must be ordered by physician; can be intermittent or continuous*

(4) perform passive range of motion exercises three times daily—*early ambulation more effective; passive ROM retains joint function, maintains circulation; passive exercises: no assistance from patient*

101

A 26-year-old man fractures his left femur in a bicycle accident. A cast is applied. Which of the following exercises would be MOST beneficial for this patient?

REWORDED QUESTION: What exercise is BEST for a patient in a cast?

STRATEGY: Picture the patient as described. Imagine patient performing each type of exercise.

NEEDED INFO: Fracture: break in continuity of bone. Complications: hemorrhage (bone vascular), shock, fat embolism (long bones), sepsis, peripheral nerve damage, delayed union, nonunion. Treatment: reduction (closed or open), immobilization (cast, traction, splints, internal and external fixation). Cast allows early mobility. Nursing responsibilities: teach isometric exercises.

CATEGORY: Planning/Physiological Integrity

(1) Passive exercise of the affected limb—*nurse moves extremity; unable to do*

(2) Quadriceps setting of the affected limb—**CORRECT: isometric exercise: contraction of muscle without movement of joint; maintains strength**

(3) Active ROM exercises of the unaffected limb—*not best*

(4) Passive exercise of the upper extremities—*need strengthening, not passive exercises*

102

The nurse plans care for a patient receiving electroconvulsive treatments (ECT). Immediately following a treatment, the nurse should take which of the following actions?

REWORDED QUESTION: What should you do right after a patient has ECT?

STRATEGY: Picture the patient as described in the question.

NEEDED INFO: ECT: stimulation of convulsions similar to grand mal seizures as treatment for depression. Requires 6–12 treatments. Preparation: NPO 4 hrs, informed consent, void, remove jewelry, atropine 30 min before to reduce secretions. During: short acting IV anesthesia and muscle relaxant, O_2, suction available. After: confusion and memory loss for recent events, stay with patient and orient, check vital signs.

CATEGORY: Implementation/Psychosocial Integrity

(1) Orient the patient to time and place—**CORRECT: short-term memory loss common side effect**

(2) Talk about events prior to the patient's hospitalization—*long-term memory not affected*

(3) Restrict fluid intake and encourage the patient to ambulate—*should encourage fluids, rest*

(4) Initiate comfort measures to relieve vertigo—*dizziness not common side effect*

103

A patient is to receive 35 mg/hr of intravenous aminophylline. The nurse mixes 350 mg of aminophylline in 500 cc D_5W. At what rate should this solution be infused?

REWORDED QUESTION: What is the IV flow rate?

STRATEGY: Set up a ratio and solve for *x*. If you miss this, review your nursing math.

NEEDED INFO: Formula: med on hand over volume on hand = desired med over *x*. Solve for *x*.

CATEGORY: Implementation/Physiological Integrity

(1) 20 cc/hr—*incorrect*

(2) 35 cc/hr—*incorrect*

(3) 50 cc/hr—**CORRECT: 350mg/500cc = 35mg/*x*, 350*x* = 17,500, *x* = 50**

(4) 70 cc/hr—*incorrect*

104

The nurse prepares an adult client for instillation of ear drops. The nurse should use which of the following methods to administer the ear drops?

REWORDED QUESTION: How are ear drops given?

STRATEGY: Picture yourself doing the procedure. Picture an arrow pointing upward for a "tall" adult to straighten ear canal.

NEEDED INFO: Pull earlobe up and back for adult. Pull earlobe down and back for child.

CATEGORY: Implementation/Safe and Effective Care

(1) Cool the solution for better adsorption. Drop the medication directly into the auditory canal—*stimulates acoustic nerve reflex, cause: N + V*

(2) Warm the solution. Flush the medication rapidly into the ear—*cause pressure against tympanic membrane, possible rupture*

(3) Warm the solution. Drop the medication along the side of the ear canal—**CORRECT: prevents acoustic nerve reflex and dizziness; will not damage tympanic membrane**

(4) Warm the solution to 40°C. Drop the medication slowly into the ear canal—*too hot, 35–37° C*

105

A 52-year-old man is receiving intravenous cimetidine (Tagamet). After 20 minutes of the infusion, the patient complains of a headache and dizziness. Which of the following actions should the nurse take FIRST?

REWORDED QUESTION: What should you do in this situation? Is the patient showing side effects of the medication?

STRATEGY: Always do what is safest for the patient. Be skeptical of passing the responsibility to other health care professionals. The exam wants to know what YOU are going to do.

NEEDED INFO: Cimetidine (Tagamet): antiulcer medication inhibits the action of histamine at the receptor sites and decreases the secretion of gastric acid. Side effects: mental confusion, dizziness, HA, diarrhea. If given IV may cause bradycardia, circulatory overload (infuse over 30 min). Take with meals or at hs.

CATEGORY: Implementation/Physiological Integrity

(1) Stop the infusion—**CORRECT: safest action**
(2) Call the physician—*not first action; don't pass the buck*
(3) Take vital signs—*not first action*
(4) Call the pharmacist—*not first action; don't pass the buck*

106

A 26-year-old man comes to the emergency room with complaints of nausea, vomiting, and abdominal pain. He is a type I diabetic (IDDM). Four days earlier, he reduced his insulin dose when flu symptoms prevented him from eating. The nurse performs an assessment of the patient that reveals poor skin turgor, dry mucous membranes, and fruity breath odor. The nurse should be alert for which of the following problems?

REWORDED QUESTION: What do these symptoms indicate?

NEEDED INFO: Diabetes mellitus: disorder of carbohydrate metabolism: insufficient insulin to meet metabolic needs. Type I (juvenile): insulin dependent, prone to ketoacidosis. Type II (adult onset): controlled by diet and oral agents, non ketosis prone. In ketoacidosis the body becomes dehydrated from osmotic diuresis. The fruity breath odor develops from acetone, a component of ketone bodies. Rate and depth of resp increase (Kussmaul) in attempt to blow off excess carbonic acid. Difference between ketoacidosis and HHNK—lack of ketonuria.

CATEGORY: Planning/Physiological Integrity

(1) Hypoglycemia—*cause: too much insulin; blood sugar below 60 mg; s/s: tachycardia, perspiration, confusion, lethargy, numbness lips, anxiety, hunger*
(2) Viral illness—*not best answer*
(3) Ketoacidosis—**CORRECT: cause: insufficient insulin; s/s: polyuria, polydipsia, N + V, dry mucous membranes, weight loss, abdominal pain, hypotension, shock, coma**
(4) Hyperglycemic hyperosmolar nonketotic coma—*(HHNK) extreme hyperglycemia (800–2,000 mg/dL) with absence of acidosis; some insulin production so don't mobilize fats for energy or form ketones; usually seen in type II; cause: infections, stress, meds (steroids, thiazide diuretics), TPN; s/s: polyphagia, polyuria, polydipsia, glycosuria, dehydration, abdominal discomfort, hyperpyrexia, changes in LOC, hypotension, shock; treatment: fluid replacement (2L 0.45% NaCl over 2 hrs), K^+, Na^+, Cl^-, phosphates, insulin given IV*

107

A 45-year-old homeless man is hospitalized with tuberculosis. The physician's orders include isoniazid (INH) and pyridoxine (vitamin B_6). The patient asks why he is receiving pyridoxine. The nurse's response should be based on the knowledge that pyridoxine:

REWORDED QUESTION: Why is vitamin B_6 given to patient together with INH?

NEEDED INFO: INH: primary antitubercular agent, used as preventative for those exposed to TB. Side effects: hemolytic anemia, peripheral neuropathy, hepatitis. Nursing responsibilities: monitor liver function, teach patient symptoms of hepatitis (anorexia, fatigue, jaundice, dark urine), take with food.

CATEGORY: Analysis/Physiological Integrity

(1) increases INH absorption—*no effect*
(2) prevents the development of tolerance to INH—*tolerance does not develop*
(3) decreases the severity of INH side effects: *no effect, aluminum-containing antacids and laxatives may decrease the effectiveness and the amount absorbed, give INH 1 hour before administering antacids or laxative*
(4) prevents INH-associated neuritis—**CORRECT: most common untoward effect, frequently seen in malnourished infants, alcoholics, and diabetic patients**

108

An 11-year-old boy is admitted to the hospital for evaluation for a kidney transplant. During the initial assessment, the nurse learns that the patient received hemodialysis for three years due to renal failure. The nurse knows that his illness can interfere with this patient's achievement of

REWORDED QUESTION: What developmental stage is altered in a patient due to this chronic disease?

STRATEGY: Picture the person described in the question. Think about his activities and interests. This helps eliminate incorrect answer choices. An 11-year-old is usually in grade school thinking about homework, doing chores at home.

NEEDED INFO: Eric Erikson developed a theory of the stages of personality development that progressed in predictable stages from birth to death. Other stages: autonomy versus shame and doubt (task of 1–3 yrs); initiative versus guilt (task of 3–6 yrs).

CATEGORY: Analysis/Health Promotion and Maintenance

(1) intimacy—*young adult: 20–40 yrs; achieving sexual and loving relationship with another; alternative: isolation*

(2) trust—*infancy; results from consistent care by a loving caretaker; teaches that basic needs will be met; alternative: mistrust*

(3) industry—**CORRECT: 6–12 yrs; aspires to be the best; learns social skills, how to finish tasks; sensitive about school expectations; may be impaired due to absences from school, growth retardation, and emotional difficulties**

(4) identity—*adolescence; peer groups important; used to define identity, establish body image, form new relationships; alternative: role diffusion*

109 The nurse assesses a patient with a history of Addison's disease who has received steroid therapy for several years. The nurse could expect the patient to exhibit which of the following changes in appearance?

REWORDED QUESTION: What changes are seen in a patient after taking steroids long term?

STRATEGY: All the options in an answer choice must be correct for the option to be right.

NEEDED INFO: Meds: cortisone and hydrocortisone usually given in divided doses: 2/3 in morning and 1/3 in late afternoon with food to decrease GI irritation. Teach to report s/s of excessive drug therapy (rapid weight gain, round face, fluid retention).

CATEGORY: Assessment/Physiological Integrity

(1) Buffalo hump, girdle-obesity, gaunt facial appearance—*hump and girdle-obesity true; gaunt face seen with lack of steroids*

(2) Tanning of the skin, discoloration of the mucous membranes, alopecia, weight loss—*tanning and weight loss seen with lack of steroids; rest not seen*

(3) Emaciation, nervousness, breast engorgement, hirsutism—*nothing to do with steroids; hirsutism: excessive growth of hair*

(4) Truncal obesity, purple striations on the skin, moon-face—**CORRECT: due to excess glucocorticoids**

110 Haloperidol (Haldol) 5 mg tid is ordered for a patient with schizophrenia. Two days later, the patient complains of "tight jaws and a stiff neck." The nurse should recognize that these complaints are:

REWORDED QUESTION: Why does the patient taking Haldol have these symptoms?

NEEDED INFO: Haldol is a med used in the treatment of psychotic disorders. High incidence of extrapyramidal reactions: pseudoparkinsonism (rigidity and tremors), akathisia (motor restlessness), dystonia (involuntary jerking, uncoordinated body movements), tardive dyskinesia (abnormal movements of lips, jaws, tongue). Schizophrenia: retreat from reality, flat affect, suspiciousness, hallucinations, delusions, loose associations, psychomotor retardation or hyperactivity, regression. Nursing responsibilities: maintain safety, meet physical needs, decrease sensory stimuli. Treatment: antipsychotic meds, individual therapy.

CATEGORY: Analysis/Psychosocial Integrity

(1) common side effects of antipsychotic medications that will diminish over time—*gets worse, untreated, life threatening*

(2) early symptoms of extrapyramidal reactions to the medication—**CORRECT: dystonic reaction, airway may become obstructed**

(3) psychosomatic complaints resulting from a delusional system—*not accurate*

(4) permanent side effects of Haldol—*reversible when treated with IV Benadryl*

111 The nurse is caring for a woman who states she was beaten and sexually assaulted by a male friend. What should the nurse do first?

REWORDED QUESTION: What is the most important initial nursing action to take with an sexual assault victim?

STRATEGY: Discriminate between what is appropriate and inappropriate nursing behavior.

NEEDED INFO: Nursing care for crime victims must address both physical and emotional needs. The nurse must be cautious not to disturb or eliminate any evidence until the victim has been examined by a physician. The nurse must document all evidence found during the nursing assessment. After the client has been examined and a course of action determined, the nurse can begin to address the expressed needs of the client, such as contacting legal counsel or the chaplain.

CATEGORY: Implementation/Psychosocial Integrity

(1) Encourage the client to call her family lawyer—*not the first action the nurse should take with this client*

(2) Ask for a psychiatry consult—*nurse should not initiate a psychiatry consult*

(3) Stay with the client during the physical exam— **CORRECT: provide consistent emotional and physical support for the client**

(4) Wash and dress the client's wounds before the physical exam—*contraindicated; eradicates potential evidence*

112 The nurse cares for a 65-year-old woman following surgery for removal of a cataract in her right eye. The patient complaints of severe eye pain in her right eye. The nurse knows this symptom:

REWORDED QUESTION: Is pain after surgery for a cataract normal?

NEEDED INFO: Cataract: change in the transparency of crystalline lens of eye. Causes: aging, trauma, congenital, systemic disease. S/S: blurred vision, decrease in color perception, photophobia. Treated by removal of lens under local anesthesia with sedation. Intraocular lens implantation, eyeglasses, or contact lenses after surgery. Complications: glaucoma, infection, bleeding, retinal detachment.

CATEGORY: Analysis/Physiological Integrity

(1) is expected and should administer analgesic to the patient—*mild discomfort treated with analgesics*

(2) is expected and should maintain the patient on bed rest—*activity restrictions: no coughing, bending at waist, vomiting, sneezing, lifting more than 15 lbs, squeezing eyelid, straining at stool, lying on affected side; these increase intraocular pressure*

(3) is unexpected and may signify a detached retina—*lens was removed during surgery*

(4) is unexpected and may signify hemorrhage— **CORRECT: ruptured blood vessel or suture causing hemorrhage or increased intraocular pressure; notify physician if restless, increased pulse, drainage on dressing**

113 A patient returns to his room following a lower GI series. When he is assessed by the nurse, he complains of weakness. Which of the following nursing diagnoses should receive priority in planning his care?

REWORDED QUESTION: What is MOST important for a patient after a GI series?

STRATEGY: Establish priorities.

NEEDED INFO: Upper GI series (barium swallow): radiologic visualization of esophagus, stomach, duodenum, jejunum.

Lower GI series (barium enema): visualize colon. Prep for test: NPO 6–8 hrs, enemas, laxatives, fluid restriction. Post-test: laxatives to remove barium. Nursing responsibilities after test: check abdomen for distention, encourage fluids. Initially stool is white from barium. Should return to normal color in 72 hrs.

CATEGORY: Analysis/Physiological Integrity

(1) Alteration in sensation-perception, gustatory—*not highest priority; gustatory: pertaining to sense of taste*

(2) Constipation, colonic—*not highest priority*

(3) High risk for fluid-volume deficit—**CORRECT: prep for test: low-residue or clear liquid diet 2 days, NPO midnight, enemas, laxatives; post-test: laxatives to remove barium**

(4) Nutrition, less than body requirements—*not highest priority*

114 A patient hospitalized with a gastric ulcer is scheduled for discharge. The nurse teaches the patient about an antiulcer diet. Which of the following statements, if made by the patient, would indicate to the nurse that dietary teaching was successful?

REWORDED QUESTION: What statement is TRUE about an antiulcer diet?

NEEDED INFO: Gastric ulcers form within 1 inch of the pylorus of the stomach usually caused by break in mucosa. Onset 45–54 years old, men twice as often as women, pain increased by food, relieved by vomiting, hematemesis common. Treatment: antacids (Amphojel), H_2 receptor antagonists (Tagamet), anticholinergics (Bentyl), mucosal barrier fortifiers (Carafate).

CATEGORY: Evaluation/Physiological Integrity

(1) "I must eat bland foods to help my stomach heal."— *transitional diet used for severe inflammation; not speed healing*

(2) "I can eat most foods, as long as they don't bother my stomach."—**CORRECT: not severely restricted; small frequent feedings; avoid foods known to increase gastric acidity: coffee, alcohol, seasonings, milk**

(3) "I cannot eat fruits and vegetables because they cause too much gas."—*restricted only if they bother stomach*

(4) "I should eat a low-fiber diet to delay gastric emptying."—*used with acute diverticulitis, ulcerative colitis; foods with fiber: cereals, whole grains products, fruits, vegetables*

115 A 6-year-old boy is returned to his room following a tonsillectomy. He remains sleepy from the anesthesia but is easily awakened. The nurse should place the child in which of the following positions?

REWORDED QUESTION: What is the best position after tonsillectomy to help with drainage of oral secretions?

STRATEGY: Picture the patient as described.

CATEGORY: Implementation/Safe and Effective Care

(1) Sims'—*on side with top knee flexed and thigh drawn up to chest and lower knee less sharply flexed: used for vaginal or rectal examination*
(2) Side-lying—**CORRECT: most effective to facilitate drainage of secretions from the mouth and pharynx; reduces possibility of airway obstruction**
(3) Supine—*increased risk for aspiration, would not facilitate drainage of oral secretions*
(4) Prone—*risk for airway obstruction and aspiration, unable to observe the child for signs of bleeding such as increased swallowing*

116 A 22-year-old woman is preparing to take her one-day-old infant home from the hospital. The nurse discusses the test for phenylketonuria (PKU) with the mother. The nurse's teaching should be based on an understanding that the test is MOST reliable

REWORDED QUESTION: When is the PKU test is MOST reliable?

STRATEGY: Focus on the key words in the question. Think about what you know about the PKU test.

NEEDED INFO: PKU: genetic disorder caused by a deficiency in liver enzyme phenylalanine hydroxylase. Body can't metabolize essential amino acid phenylalanine, allows phenyl acids to accumulate in the blood. If not recognized, resultant high levels of phenyl ketone in the brain cause mental retardation. Guthrie test: screening for PKU. Treatment: dietary restriction of foods containing phenylalanine. Blood levels of phenylalanine monitored to evaluate the effectiveness of the dietary restrictions.

CATEGORY: Analysis/Health Promotion and Maintenance

(1) after a source of protein has been ingested—**CORRECT: recommended to be performed before newborns leave hospital; if initial blood sample is obtained within first 24 hrs recommended to be repeated at 3 wks**

(2) after the meconium has been excreted—*no relationship; dark green tarry stool passed within first 48 hrs of birth*
(3) after the danger of hyperbilirubinemia has passed—*no relationship; excessive accumulation of bilirubin in blood; s/s: jaundice (yellow discoloration of skin); common finding in newborn; not cause for concern*
(4) after the effects of delivery have subsided—*no relationship*

117 A 54-year-old man is being treated for Addison's disease. The physician orders cortisone 25 mg PO daily. The nurse should explain to the patient that adjustment of the dosage may be required in which of the following situations?

REWORDED QUESTION: What adjustment of the medication is needed and when?

NEEDED INFO: Hormonal replacement: given in divided doses (2/3 in am, 1/3 in pm), take with meals, don't skip doses if ill. Teach: s/s of overdosage (Cushing's syndrome: rapid weight gain, round face, fluid retention); s/s of early adrenal insufficiency (fatigue, weakness, joint pain, fever, anorexia, dizziness).

CATEGORY: Evaluation/Physiological Integrity

(1) Dosage is increased when the blood glucose level increases—*not accurate*
(2) Dosage is decreased when dietary intake is increased—*no relationship*
(3) Dosage is decreased when infection stimulates endogenous steroid secretion—*endogenous (within organism); patient with Addison's insufficient supply*
(4) Dosage is increased relative to an increase in the level of stress—**CORRECT: take with food to decrease GI upset**

118 A 48-year-old woman is hospitalized with a diagnosis of bipolar disorder. While she is in the patient activities room on the psychiatric unit, she flirts with male patients and disrupts unit activities. Which of the following approaches would be MOST appropriate for the nurse to take at this time?

REWORDED QUESTION: How should you deal with a patient with bipolar disorder who is disruptive?

NEEDED INFO: Nursing responsibilities: accompany patient to room when hyperactivity escalates, set limits, remain nonjudgmental.

CATEGORY: Planning/Psychosocial Integrity

(1) Set limits on the patient's behavior and remind her of the rules—*too confrontational*

(2) Distract the patient and escort her back to her room—**CORRECT: patients are easily distracted, nonthreatening action**

(3) Instruct the other patients to ignore this patient's behavior—*does not ensure safety*

(4) Tell the patient that she is behaving inappropriately and send her to her room—*too confrontational, may agitate*

119

A 33-year-old man is brought to the emergency room bleeding profusely from a stab wound in the left chest area. The nurse's assessment reveals a blood pressure of 80/50, pulse of 110, and respiratory rate of 28. The nurse should expect which of the following potential problems?

REWORDED QUESTION: What type of shock is described?

STRATEGY: Form a mental image of the person described.

NEEDED INFO: Symptoms of hypovolemic shock: tachycardia, reduced output, irritability. Treatment: O_2, IV fluids to restore volume, Adrenaline, Apresoline. Nursing responsibilities: check airway, vital signs, insert IV, check blood gases, CVP measurements, insert catheter, hourly I + O, position flat with legs elevated, keep warm.

CATEGORY: Planning/Physiological Integrity

(1) Hypovolemic shock—**CORRECT: loss of circulating volume**

(2) Cardiogenic shock—*decrease in cardiac output; cause: cardiac dysfunction, MI, CHF*

(3) Neurogenic shock—*increase in vascular bed; cause: spinal anesthesia, spinal cord injury*

(4) Septic shock—*decreased cardiac output, hypotension; cause: gram+ or gram– bacteria*

120

A 42-year-old man is admitted to the hospital for surgical repair of a detached retina in the right eye. In planning care for this patient postoperatively, the nurse should

REWORDED QUESTION: What should you do after surgery for detached retina?

STRATEGY: Picture the patient as described.

NEEDED INFO: Detached retina: separation of retina from pigmented epithelium. S/S: curtain falling across field of vision, black spots, flashes of light, sudden onset. Treatment: surgical repair (photocoagulation, electrodiathermy, cryosurgery, scleral buckling). Complications: infection, redetachment, increased intraocular pressure. Nursing responsibilities postop: check eye patch for drainage, position with detached area dependent; no rapid eye movement (reading, sewing); no coughing, vomiting, sneezing.

CATEGORY: Planning/Physiological Integrity

(1) encourage self-care activities—*activity restrictions depend on location and size of tear*

(2) maintain patches over both eyes.—*only affected eye covered*

(3) limit movements of his eyes—**CORRECT: bed rest with eye patch or shield**

(4) caution him against excessive talking—*no restriction*

121

The nurse cares for a patient receiving full strength Ensure by tube feeding. The nurse knows that the MOST common complication of a tube feeding is

REWORDED QUESTION: What is a common complication of a tube feeding?

NEEDED INFO: Tube feedings are used with patients unable to tolerate the oral route but have a functioning GI tract. May be given by intermittent or continuous infusion. Elevate head of bed 30–45°. Give at room temp. Check for placement and residual before feeding or every 4–8 hrs (should be less than 50% of previous hour's intake). Replace residual to prevent fluid and electrolyte imbalances unless it appears abnormal (coffee ground–like material). Don't hang solution more than 6 hrs. Flush tubing with 20–30 cc water every 4 hrs. Change feeding set every 24 hrs. Ensure: balanced compete food product/supplement containing intact protein.

CATEGORY: Evaluation/Physiological Integrity

(1) edema—*not frequently seen; if present physician change formula to contain less Na^+*

(2) diarrhea—**CORRECT: intolerance to solution, rate; give slowly; other symptoms of intolerance: N+V, aspiration, glycosuria, diaphoresis**

(3) hypokalemia—*normal potassium 3.5–5.0 mEq/L; not commonly seen; common causes: diuretics, diarrhea, GI drainage*

(4) vomiting—*can happen with rapid increase in rate; give feeding slowly*

122 A 6-week-old infant is brought to the hospital for treatment of pyloric stenosis. The nurse enters the following nursing diagnosis on the infant's care plan: "fluid volume deficit related to vomiting." Which of the following assessments supports this diagnosis?

REWORDED QUESTION: What would indicate volume deficit?

NEEDED INFO: Pyloric stenosis: obstruction of the sphincter between stomach and duodenum. Onset: within 2 months of birth. S/S: vomiting that becomes projectile. Treatment: surgery. Nursing responsibilities: small frequent feedings with glucose water or electrolyte solutions 4–6 hrs postop. Small frequent feedings with formula 24 hrs postop.

CATEGORY: Analysis/Physiological Integrity

(1) The infant eagerly accepts feedings—*may vomit after eating*
(2) The infant vomited once since admission—*don't assume will continue to vomit*
(3) The infant's skin is warm and moist—*normal; would be cool and dry with fluid volume deficit*
(4) The infant's anterior fontanelle is depressed— **CORRECT: indicates dehydration**

123 A 68-year-old woman is diagnosed with thrombocytopenia due to acute lymphocytic leukemia. She is admitted to the hospital for treatment. The nurse should assign the patient

REWORDED QUESTION: What are the needs of a patient with acute lymphocytic leukemia and thrombocytopenia?

NEEDED INFO: Lymphocytic leukemia, disease characterized by proliferation of immature WBCs. Immature cells unable to fight infection as competently as mature white cells. Treatment: chemotherapy, antibiotics, blood transfusions, bone marrow transplantation. Nursing responsibilities: private room, no raw fruits or vegs, small frequent meals, O_2, good skin care.

CATEGORY: Planning/Safe and Effective Care

(1) to a private room so she will not infect other patients and health care workers—*poses little or no threat*
(2) to a private room so she will not be infected by other patients and health care workers—**CORRECT: protects patient from exogenous bacteria, risk for developing infection from others due to depressed WBC count, alters ability to fight infection**

(3) to a semi-private room so she will have stimulation during her hospitalization—*should be placed in a room alone*
(4) to a semi-private room so she will have the opportunity to express her feelings about her illness—*ensure that patient is provided with opportunities to express feelings about illness*

124 A 28-year-old woman comes to the clinic because she thinks she is pregnant. Tests are performed and the pregnancy is confirmed. The patient's last menstrual period began on September 8 and lasted for 6 days. The nurse calculates that her expected date of confinement (EDC) is

REWORDED QUESTION: How do you calculate the EDC?

STRATEGY: Perform the calculation required and check for math errors!

NEEDED INFO: EDC or estimated date of delivery (EDD): calculated according to Nägele's rule (first day of the last normal menstrual period –3 months and +7 days and 1 year). Assumes that every woman has a 28 day cycle and pregnancy occurred on fourteenth day. Most women deliver within a period extending from 7 days before to 7 days after the EDC.

CATEGORY: Implementation/Health Promotion and Maintenance

(1) May 15—*too early*
(2) June 15—**CORRECT September 8–3 months = June 8 + 7 days = June 15 of next year**
(3) June 21—*EDC is calculated from first, not last day, of last normal menstrual period*
(4) July 8—*not accurate*

125 A 2-month-old infant is brought to the pediatrician's office for a well-baby visit. During the examination, congenital subluxation of the left hip is suspected. The nurse knows that symptoms of congenital hip dislocation include

REWORDED QUESTION: What will you see with congenital hip dislocation?

STRATEGY: Form a mental image of the deformity.

NEEDED INFO: Subluxation: most common type of congenital hip dislocation. Head of femur remains in contact with acetabulum but is partially displaced. Diagnosed in infant less than 4 weeks old S/S: unlevel gluteal folds, limited abduction of hip, shortened femur affected side, Ortolani's sign (click).

Treatment: abduction splint, hip spica cast, Bryant's traction, open reduction.

CATEGORY: Assessment/Health Promotion and Maintenance

(1) lengthening of the limb on the affected side—*inaccurate*
(2) deformities of the foot and ankle—*inaccurate*
(3) asymmetry of the gluteal and thigh folds—
CORRECT: restricted movement on affected side
(4) plantar flexion of the foot—*seen with clubfoot*

126 After two weeks of receiving lithium therapy, a patient in the psychiatric unit becomes depressed. Which of the following evaluations of the patient's behavior by the nurse would be MOST accurate?

REWORDED QUESTION: Is the depression normal, or something to be concerned about?

CATEGORY: Evaluation/Psychosocial Integrity

(1) The treatment plan is not effective; the patient requires a larger dose of lithium—*not accurate*
(2) This is a normal response to lithium therapy; the patient should continue with the current treatment plan—*does not address safety needs*
(3) This is a normal response to lithium therapy; the patient should be monitored for suicidal behavior—
CORRECT: delay of 1–3 wks before med benefits seen
(4) The treatment plan is not effective; the patient requires an antidepressant—*normal response*

127 A 67-year-old woman is admitted for treatment of pulmonary edema. During the admission interview, she states she has a six-year history of congestive heart failure (CHF). The nurse performs an initial assessment. When the nurse auscultates the breath sounds, the nurse should expect to hear

REWORDED QUESTION: What will you hear when listening to the breath sounds for a patient with CHF?

STRATEGY: Picture the situation as described.

NEEDED INFO: Use diaphragm of stethoscope to listen to breath sounds. Normal breath sounds: (1) vesicular: low-pitched, swishing sounds heard at bases of lungs, (2) bronchial: loud, high-pitched, hollow sounds heard over large tracheal airways during expiration, (3) bronchovesicular: breeze sound heard over central large airways.

CATEGORY: Assessment/Physiological Integrity

(1) crackling—**CORRECT: rales; air passes over fluid; heard during inspiration; found with pulmonary edema, pneumonia**
(2) wheezing—*passage of air through narrowed airway; heard during inspiration and expiration; found with asthma*
(3) whistling—*noisy resp; air through obstructed larynx*
(4) absent breath sounds—*pneumothorax; collapse of lung*

128 A 63-year-old man is diagnosed with cancer of the larynx and comes to the hospital for a total laryngectomy. When admitting this patient, how should the nurse assess laryngeal nerve function?

REWORDED QUESTION: How do you assess normal functioning of laryngeal nerve? What functions are controlled by laryngeal nerve?

NEEDED INFO: Risk factors: smoking, chronic bronchitis, polluted air, abuse alcohol. S/S: chronic hoarseness, lump in neck, difficulty swallowing, persistent sore throat. Treatment: radiation therapy, surgical removal. Total laryngectomy: loss of voice. Nursing responsibilities postop: position semi- to high-Fowler's, care for cuffed tracheostomy tube, chest physiotherapy, assess drainage on dressing or Hemovac container. Teach use of artificial larynx or esophageal speech.

CATEGORY: Assessment/Physiological Integrity

(1) Assess the extent of neck edema—*not accurate*
(2) Check his ability to swallow—**CORRECT**
(3) Observe for excessive drooling—*seen with facial paralysis, Bell's palsy*
(4) Tap the side of his neck gently and observe for facial twitching—*Chvostek's sign: test for hypocalcemia and tetany, tap over facial nerve on side of face, if mouth twitches, indicates tetany*

129 The nurse supervises care at an adult day-care center. Four meal choices are available to the residents. The nurse should ensure that a resident on a low-cholesterol diet receives which of the following meals?

REWORDED QUESTION: What should a patient on a low-cholesterol diet eat?

NEEDED INFO: Low-cholesterol diet should reduce total fat to 20–25% of total calories and reduce the ingestion of saturated fat. Carbohydrates (especially complex carbohydrates) should be 55–60% of calories. High-cholesterol foods: eggs, dairy products, meat, fish, shellfish, poultry.

CATEGORY: Implementation/Physiological Integrity

(1) Egg custard, boiled liver—*high amounts of cholesterol*
(2) Fried chicken, potatoes—*avoid fried foods*
(3) Hamburger, french fries—*avoid fried foods*
(4) Grilled flounder, green beans—**CORRECT: fish instead of meat, increase vegetables**

130

The nurse cares for a patient with a possible bowel obstruction. A nasogastric tube is to be inserted. Before inserting the tube, the nurse explains its purpose to the patient. Which of the following explanations, if made by the nurse, is MOST accurate?

REWORDED QUESTION: What is the purpose of an NG tube?

NEEDED INFO: Gastric tubes can also be used for tube feedings. Decompression relieves pressure caused by GI contents and gases that remain in stomach due to obstruction.

CATEGORY: Implementation/Physiological Integrity

(1) "It empties the stomach of fluids and gas."—**CORRECT: used for decompression, gavage, lavage, gastric analysis**
(2) "It prevents spasms of the sphincter of Oddi."—*controls release of pancreatic juices and bile into duodenum*
(3) "It prevents air from forming in the small and large intestine."—*goes only to duodenum*
(4) "It removes bile from the gall bladder."—*action of T-tube*

131

A 25-year-old man is being treated in the burn unit for second- and third-degree burns over 45% of his body. The physician's orders include the application of silver sulfadiazine (Silvadene cream). The BEST way to apply this medication is to use a sterile

REWORDED QUESTION: How should Silvadene cream be applied to a burn?

NEEDED INFO: Application should be 1/16" thickness using sterile application technique that is nontraumatic to burn. Side effects: neutropenia, check renal function.

CATEGORY: Implementation/Physiological Integrity

(1) 4 × 4 soaked in saline—*should be applied to a clean, dry surface*

(2) tongue depressor—*can cause trauma to damaged tissues*
(3) cotton-tipped applicator—*not practical due to size of applicators, can cause trauma to damaged tissues*
(4) gloved hand—**CORRECT: causes least amount of trauma to tissues, will maintain sterile technique while decreasing chance of breaking blisters**

132

The nurse teaches a 20-year-old primigravida how to measure the frequency of uterine contractions. The nurse should explain to the patient that the frequency of uterine contractions is determined

REWORDED QUESTION: How do you determine the frequency of uterine contractions?

NEEDED INFO: There must be at least 3 contractions to establish frequently.

CATEGORY: Implementation/Health Promotion and Maintenance

(1) from the beginning of one contraction to the end of the next contraction—*not accurate*
(2) from the beginning of one contraction to the end of the same contraction—*defines duration*
(3) by the number of contractions that occur within a given period of time—**CORRECT**
(4) by the strength of the contraction at its peak—*describes intensity*

133

The nurse performs teaching with a 49-year-old woman receiving estrogen replacement therapy. Which of the following statements, if made by the nurse to the woman, indicates that the nurse is aware of the possible complications of estrogen therapy?

REWORDED QUESTION: What complications are seen with the use of estrogen therapy?

NEEDED INFO: Estrogen therapy predisposes to cancer of reproductive organs. Other side effects are nausea, skin rashes, pruritis, breast secretion, and thromboembolic disorders. Used cautiously with family history of breast or genital tract cancer.

CATEGORY: Implementation/Health Promotion and Maintenance

(1) "Take an analgesic before you take estrogen, since estrogen may cause discomfort."—*not accurate; may cause nausea, weight gain, lethargy*

(2) "Make sure you keep your clinic appointments, especially your gynecologic checkup."—**CORRECT: have check-up q 6 months**

(3) "Limit your fluid intake since estrogen promotes the retention of fluids."—*causes fluid retention and edema; monitor weight; restrict Na⁺ intake; don't limit fluids*

(4) "Increase roughage in your diet to avoid constipation."—*not best*

134 Several days after being admitted for depression, a man is observed sitting alone in the patient's dining room. The nurse notes that the patient has not finished his meal. Which of the following nursing measures would be MOST appropriate?

REWORDED QUESTION: How would you meet this patient's needs?

NEEDED INFO: Symptoms of depression: withdrawn, regressive behavior, psychomotor retardation.

CATEGORY: Planning/Psychosocial Integrity

(1) Allow the patient to eat in his room until he becomes more comfortable eating with other patients—*social isolation, reinforces depression*

(2) Ask the patient's family to bring foods that he likes to eat—*does not address problem*

(3) Order small frequent meals and sit with the patient while he eats in the dining room—**CORRECT: diminished appetite, prevents social isolation**

(4) Do not focus on eating behaviors since his appetite will improve over time—*does not meet nutritional needs*

135 A 21-year-old woman is being treated for injuries sustained in an automobile accident. The patient has a central venous pressure (CVP) line in place. The nurse recognizes that CVP measurement reflects

REWORDED QUESTION: What does CVP measure?

NEEDED INFO: CVP: central venous line placed in superior vena cava. To obtain a reading: patient placed supine, 0 on manometer placed at level of right atrium (midaxillary line at 4th intercostal space), turn stopcock to allow manometer to fill with fluid, turn to allow fluid to go into patient. Fluid will fluctuate with resp. When stabilizes take reading at highest level of fluctuation. Normal: 4–10cm/H_2O. Elevated: hypervolemia, CHF, pericarditis. Low: hypovolemia.

CATEGORY: Analysis/Physiological Integrity

(1) cardiac output—*Swan-Gantz line*
(2) pressure in the left ventricle—*Swan-Gantz line*
(3) pressure in the right atrium—**CORRECT: determined by blood vol, vascular tone, action of right side of heart**
(4) pressure in the pulmonary artery—*Swan-Gantz line: 4 lumen balloon-tipped, flow-directed catheter*

136 A mother brings her 4-year-old daughter to the pediatrician for treatment of chronic otitis media. The mother asks the nurse how she can prevent her child from getting ear infections so often. The nurse's response should be based on an understanding that the recurrence of otitis media can be decreased by

REWORDED QUESTION: What will prevent the development of otitis media? What causes otitis media?

NEEDED INFO: Otitis media: frequently follows respiratory infection. Reduce occurrences: holding child upright for feedings, encourage gentle nose blowing, teach modified Valsava maneuver (pinch nose, close lips and force air up through eustachian tubes), blow up balloons or chew gum, eliminate tobacco smoke or known allergens.

CATEGORY: Analysis/Health Promotion and Maintenance

(1) covering the child's ears while bathing—*not prevent*
(2) treating upper respiratory infections quickly—**CORRECT: respiratory fluids are a medium for bacteria; antihistamines used**
(3) administering nose drops at bedtime—*not prevent*
(4) isolating her child from other children—*too extreme a measure*

137 A patient receives 10 units of NPH insulin every morning at 8 A.M. At 4 P.M., the nurse observes that the patient is diaphoretic and slightly confused. The FIRST action the nurse should take is to

REWORDED QUESTION: What is the cause of these symptoms? What is the FIRST thing you should do?

NEEDED INFO: NPH insulin: intermediate acting preparation: onset 1–4 hrs, peak 2–15 hrs, duration 12–28 hrs. S/S hypoglycemia: confusion, tremors, hypotension, cool clammy skin, diaphoresis. Treatment: if conscious, liquids containing sugar; dextrose 50% IV if unconscious; patient education.

CATEGORY: Planning/Physiological Integrity

(1) check vital signs—*not first action; should recognize s/s hypoglycemia*

(2) check urine for glucose and ketones—*indicates only hyperglycemia, no information about hypoglycemia; should recognize s/s hypoglycemia*

(3) give 6 oz of skim milk—**CORRECT: s/s of hypoglycemia; give fast acting sugar and protein; recheck blood sugar in 15 min**

(4) call the physician—*not necessary; don't pass the buck*

138

Prior to the patient undergoing a scheduled intravenous pyelogram (IVP), the nurse reviews the patient's health history. It would be important for the nurse to obtain the answer to which of the following questions?

REWORDED QUESTION: What do you need to know before an IVP?

NEEDED INFO: IVP: radiopaque dye injected into the body and is filtered through the kidneys and excreted by the urinary tract. Visualizes kidneys, ureters, and bladder. Preparation: NPO midnight, cathartics evening before test. Injection of dye causes flushing of face, nausea, salty taste in mouth.

CATEGORY: Assessment/Physiological Integrity

(1) Does the patient have difficulty voiding?—*not most important*

(2) Does the patient have any allergies to shellfish or iodine?—**CORRECT: anaphylactic reaction; itching, hives, wheezing; treatment: antihistamines, O$_2$, CPR, epinephrine, vasopressor**

(3) Does the patient have a history of constipation?—*not essential info*

(4) Does the patient have frequent headaches?—*not most important*

139

A 6-year-old girl with chickenpox (varicella) is brought by her parents to the physician for evaluation. The nurse knows the rash characteristic of chickenpox can be described as

REWORDED QUESTION: What does the rash from chickenpox look like?

STRATEGY: Form a mental image of patient with characteristic rash.

NEEDED INFO: Chickenpox transmission: direct contact, droplet. Incubation period: 13–17 days. Treatment: Zovirax,

Benadryl and/or calamine lotion for itching, good skin care to prevent secondary infection, bathe daily, change clothes and linens, strict isolation in hospital, at home isolate until vesicles have dried (usually 1 week after onset), short fingernails, avoid use of aspirin due to Reye's syndrome. Measles transmission: direct contact, droplets. Incubation period: 10–20 days. Symptoms: fever, cough, conjunctivitis, erythematous maculopapular rash on face. Treatment: bed rest, antipyretics, antibiotics to prevent secondary infection. Isolate till fifth day of rash, cool mist vaporizer, good skin care, dim lights.

CATEGORY: Assessment/Health Promotion and Maintenance

(1) maculopapular—**CORRECT: prodromal stage: slight fever, malaise and anorexia, maculopapular rash, becomes vesicular: fluid filled, vesicles form crusts, or scabs, communicable from 1 day before eruption of lesions (during prodromal stage) up to 6 days after first crop of vesicles appear and crusts form**

(2) small irregular red spots with minute bluish-white centers—*Koplik spots: prodromal stage of measles, first seen on buccal mocosa 2 days before rash*

(3) round or oval erythematous scaling patches—*psoriasis: treatment: exposure to sunlight/ultraviolet light, topical corticosteroids, coal tar derivates*

(4) petechiae—*pinpoint, nonraised, perfectly round purplish red spots caused by intradermal or submucosal hemorrhage, seen in severe sepsis with disseminated intravascular coagulation (DIC), Rocky Mountain spotted fever, and subacute bacterial endocarditis (SBE)*

140

A 17-year-old primigravida at 28 weeks gestation, takes a three-hour glucose tolerance test. The results indicate a fasting blood sugar of 100 mg/dL and a two hour post-load blood sugar of 300 mg/dL. Which of the following nursing diagnoses should be considered the HIGHEST priority at this time?

REWORDED QUESTION: What is MOST important for newly diagnosed patient with GDM?

STRATEGY: Use Maslow's hierarchy of needs to establish priorities. Remember to first meet physical needs before addressing other concerns.

NEEDED INFO: GDM: carbohydrate intolerance that occurs during pregnancy in women with no prior history of diabetes. May exhibit the classic symptoms of diabetes: polyuria (excessive urination), polydipsia (excessive thirst), and polyphagia (hunger). Half the women are asymptomatic. Diagnosed: 3-hr glucose tolerance test (GTT) (administer a high glucose load to fasting pt; blood glucose levels are measured fasting, and at 1-hr intervals for 3 hrs; test is pos if 2 or more of the blood sugars are elevated). Normal: fasting, 60–110 mg/dL, 1 hr—190, 2 hrs—165, 3 hrs—145.

CATEGORY: Analysis/Physiological Integrity

(1) Potential impaired family coping related to diagnosis of gestational diabetes mellitus (GDM)—*not highest priority; psychosocial need*

(2) Potential noncompliance related to lack of knowledge or lack of adequate support system—**CORRECT: patient may not be able to meet physical needs because of lack of knowledge**

(3) Potential for altered parenting related to disappointment—*psychosocial need; not highest priority*

(4) Ineffective family coping related to anticipatory grieving—*psychosocial need*

141

The nurse cares for a 45-year-old man admitted for a possible herniated intervertebral disk. Ibuprofen (Motrin), propoxyphene hydrochloride (Darvon), and cyclobenzaprine hydrochloride (Flexeril) are ordered PRN. Several hours after admission, the patient complains of pain. Which of the following actions should the nurse do FIRST?

REWORDED QUESTION: What should you do first?

STRATEGY: Set priorities. Compare the answers to the steps in the nursing process.

NEEDED INFO: Herniated disk: knifelike pain aggravated by sneezing, coughing, straining.

CATEGORY: Planning/Physiological Integrity

(1) Administer ibuprofen (Motrin)—*implementation; not first step*

(2) Call the physician to determine which medication should be given—*assess before implement*

(3) Gather more information from the patient about the complaint—**CORRECT: assess; first step in nursing process**

(4) Allow the patient some time to rest and see if the pain subsides—*implementation; not first step*

142

When planning care for a 56-year-old man hospitalized with depression, the nurse includes measures to increase his self-esteem. Which of the following actions should the nurse take to meet this goal?

REWORDED QUESTION: How do you increase the self-esteem of a depressed patient?

NEEDED INFO: Increase self esteem: warm, supportive environment, consistent daily care.

CATEGORY: Implementation/Psychosocial Integrity

(1) Encourage him to accept leadership responsibilities in milieu activities—*too demanding*

(2) Set simple, realistic goals with him to help him experience success—**CORRECT: sense of accomplishment**

(3) Help him to accept his illness and the adjustments that are required—*does not help feelings of hopelessness*

(4) Assure him that when he is discharged, he will be able to resume his previous activities—*false reassurance*

143

The nurse finds a visitor unconscious on the floor of a patient's room during visiting hours at the hospital. Which of the following nursing assessments is consistent with cardiopulmonary arrest?

REWORDED QUESTION: What are the signs of cardiopulmonary arrest?

STRATEGY: Think about the steps you would take to evaluate an unconscious patient.

NEEDED INFO: Cardiopulmonary arrest: heart, circulation and respirations cease. CPR: (1) determine unresponsiveness, (2) open airway (head tip-chin lift maneuver or jaw thrust), (3) determine breathlessness (look, listen, feel), (4) perform rescue breathing (2 slow breaths, chest rise 1–2 inches), (5) determine pulselessness (check carotid pulse 5–10 sec), (6) provide circulation (chest compressions 1.5–2 inches).

CATEGORY: Assessment/Physiological Integrity

(1) Absent pulse, fixed dilated pupils—*not accurate*

(2) Absent respirations, fixed dilated pupils—*not accurate*

(3) Absent pulse and respirations—**CORRECT: no palpable pulse; no breath sounds; ashen color**

(4) Thready pulse and pupillary changes—*not accurate*

144

A 68-year-old man is transferred to an extended care facility following a cerebrovascular accident (CVA). The patient has right-sided paralysis and has been experiencing dysphagia. The nurse observes an aide prepare the patient to eat lunch. Which of the following situations would require an intervention by the nurse?

REWORDED QUESTION: What option is WRONG?

STRATEGY: This is a NEGATIVE question. Make sure you know if you are looking for a correct situation, or a problematic situation.

NEEDED INFO: Dysphagia: difficulty swallowing. Provide support if necessary for the head, have the patient upright, feed the patient slowly in small amounts, place food on unaffected side of mouth. Maintain upright position for 30–45 minutes after eating. Good oral care after eating.

CATEGORY: Evaluation/Physiological Integrity

(1) The patient is in bed in high Fowler's position—*correct positioning, or may sit in chair*
(2) The patient's head and neck are positioned slightly forward—*correct positioning; helps patient chew and swallow*
(3) The aide puts the food in the back of his mouth on the unaffected side—*helps patient handle food*
(4) The aide waters down the pudding to help the patient swallow—**CORRECT: requires intervention, usually able to better handle soft or semisoft foods; difficulty with liquids**

145

The home care nurse plans care for a patient with pernicious anemia. A monthly intramuscular injection is ordered for the patient. The nurse knows that the best muscle to administer an intramuscular injection in an adult is the

REWORDED QUESTION: Where should you give an IM injection in an adult?

NEEDED INFO: Pernicious anemia: lack of intrinsic factor from stomach leading to decreased absorption of vitamin B_{12}. S/S: low hemoglobin and hematocrit. Diagnosed: Shillings test (measures absorption of orally administered radioactive B_{12} by amount of radioactive B_{12} excreted in urine in 24 hrs). Treatment: lifelong B_{12} injections, iron supplements. Factors to consider when selecting site for injection: amount of muscle mass and condition, amount and character of med, type of med, frequency of injections.

CATEGORY: Implementation/Physiological Integrity

(1) gluteus maximus—*possible injury to sciatic nerve*
(2) deltoid—*not well developed in some adults, especially elderly; possible injury to brachial artery; can only use for small amount of med*
(3) vastus lateralis—**CORRECT: no major nerves or blood vessels; to locate, palpate greater trochanter and knee joint; divide distance between them into quadrants; inject into middle of upper quadrant**
(4) dorsogluteal—*possible injury to sciatic nerve*

146

A 56-year-old man comes to the emergency room complaining of nausea, vomiting and severe right upper quadrant pain. His temperature is 101.3° F (38.5° C) and an abdominal X-ray reveals an enlarged gall bladder. He is given a diagnosis of acute cholecystitis and is scheduled for surgery. After administering an analgesic to the patient, the nurse recognizes that which of the following actions is a priority?

REWORDED QUESTION: What should you do after giving an analgesic to the patient?

STRATEGY: Establish priorities. Remember Maslow's hierarchy of needs. Meet physical needs first.

NEEDED INFO: S/S: pain in upper midline area radiating around to back, jaundice, N + V, flatulence, bloating, belching, intolerance to fatty foods. Treatment: cholecystectomy (removal of gallbladder). Postop: T-tube inserted for drainage from bile duct. Complications: hemorrhage, pneumonia, thrombophlebitis, urinary retention, ileus. Preop nursing responsibilities: Demerol for pain (morphine contraindicated; causes spasms for sphincter of Oddi), nitroglycerine to relax smooth muscle, NG tube for decompression, IVs. Postop nursing responsibilities: change position every 2 hrs, check breath sounds and vital signs every 4 hrs, I + O, antiembolitic stockings.

CATEGORY: Planning/Physiological Integrity

(1) Assessing the patient's need for dietary teaching—*not highest priority*
(2) Assessing the patient's fluid and electrolyte status—**CORRECT: hypokalemia and hypomagnesemia common**
(3) Examining the patient's health history for allergies to antibiotics—*not highest priority*
(4) Determining whether the patient has signed consent for surgery—*not highest priority*

147

A mother with four children calls the clinic for advice on how to care for her oldest child, who has developed chickenpox. Which of the following statements, if made by the mother, indicates a need for further teaching?

REWORDED QUESTION: What teaching is necessary for parent of child with chickenpox?

STRATEGY: Be careful! This is a NEGATIVE question. You are looking for INCORRECT info.

NEEDED INFO: Teaching: calamine lotion for itching, good skin care to prevent secondary infection, bathe daily, change clothes and linens, isolate until vesicles have dried (usually 1 week after onset), short finger nails, avoid use of aspirin due to Reye's syndrome.

CATEGORY: Evaluation/Safe and Effective Care

(1) "I should keep my child home from school until the vesicles are crusted."—*correct information, chickenpox transmitted by direct contact with droplets of infected person, communicable period: 2 days before rash until vesicles crusted (scabbed), then child may interact with siblings and others*

(2) "I can use calamine lotion if needed."—*correct information, used to treat itching*

(3) "I should remove the crusts so the skin can heal."—**CORRECT: indicates need for further teaching. Good skin care important, crusts usually not removed, can cause scarring**

(4) "I can use mittens if scratching becomes a problem."—*rash itches, mittens used to prevent scratching*

148

A 23-year-old woman comes the clinic at 32 weeks gestation. A diagnosis of pregnancy induced hypertension (PIH) is made. The nurse performs teaching. Which of the following statements, if made by the patient, indicates to the nurse that further teaching is required?

REWORDED QUESTION: What is NOT ACCURATE about the care of a woman with PIH?

STRATEGY: This is a NEGATIVE question. It can be reworded to say, "All of the following are true EXCEPT."

NEEDED INFO: Pregnancy induced hypertension (PIH), preeclampsia, toxemia: development of hypertension (increase 30 mmHg systolic or 15 mmHg diastolic) with proteinuria and/or edema (dependent or facial) after 20 weeks gestation. Risk factors: parity (first-time mothers), age (younger than 20 or older than 35), geographic location (southern or western U.S.), multifetal gestation, hydatidiform mole, hypertension, and diabetes. Prevention: early prenatal care, identify high risk patients, recognize s/s early; bed rest lying on L side, daily weights. Treatment: urine checks for proteinuria; diet (increased protein and decreased Na$^+$). Can develop into eclampsia (convulsions or coma).

CATEGORY: Evaluation/Health Promotion and Maintenance

(1) "Lying in bed on my left side is likely to increase my urinary output."—*true; bed rest promotes good perfusion of blood to uterus; decreases BP and promotes diuresis*

(2) "If the bed rest works, I may lose a pound or two in the next few days."—*true; causes diuresis; results in reduction of retained fluids; instruct to monitor weight daily and notify physician if notices abrupt increase even after resting in bed for 12 hrs*

(3) "I should be sure to maintain a diet that has a good amount of protein."—*true; replaces protein lost in urine; increases plasma colloid osmotic pressure; avoid salty foods; avoid alcohol; drink 8 glasses of water daily; eat foods high in roughage*

(4) "I will have to keep my room darkened and not watch much television."—**CORRECT: incorrect info, not necessary; diversional activities helpful**

149

The nurse evaluates the care provided to a 42-year-old man hospitalized for treatment of adrenal crisis. Which of the following changes would indicate to the nurse that the patient is responding favorably to medical and nursing treatment?

REWORDED QUESTION: What shows a positive response to treatment for adrenal crisis?

NEEDED INFO: In adrenal crisis the required adrenal hormones exceed the supply available. Usually precipitated by stress, surgery, trauma, or infection. S/S: hypotension, cool pale skin, increased urinary output, dehydration.

CATEGORY: Evaluation/Physiological Integrity

(1) The patient's urinary output has increased—*indicates continuing lack of hormones; will decrease with treatment*

(2) The patient's blood pressure has increased—**CORRECT: hypotension s/s of adrenal insufficiency; without treatment Na$^+$ level falls resulting in volume depletion and hypotension; K$^+$ rises resulting in cardiac dysrhythmias**

(3) The patient has lost weight—*indicates continuing loss of water and continuing lack of hormones*

(4) The patient's peripheral edema has decreased—*edema not seen with adrenal crises*

150 After completing an assessment, the nurse determines that a 45-year-old woman is exhibiting early symptoms of a dystonic reaction related to the use of an antipsychotic medication. Which of the following actions by the nurse would be MOST appropriate?

REWORDED QUESTION: What is the first thing you do for a patient with a dystonic reaction?

STRATEGY: Set priorities. Remember Maslow's hierarchy of needs.

NEEDED INFO: Dystonic reaction: muscle tightness in throat, neck, tongue, mouth, eyes, neck and back; difficulty talking and swallowing. Treatment: IM or IV Benadryl or Cogentin.

CATEGORY: Implementation/Psychosocial Integrity

(1) Reality test with the patient and assure her that her physical symptoms are not real—*real symptoms, not delusions*

(2) Teach the patient about common side effects of antipsychotic medications—*physical needs highest priority*

(3) Explain to the patient that there is no treatment that will relieve these symptoms—*Benadryl used IM or IV*

(4) Notify the physician and obtain an order for IM Benadryl—**CORRECT: emergency situation, can occlude airway**

151 The physician orders heparin for a 46-year-old woman. In order to evaluate the effectiveness of the patient's heparin therapy, the nurse should monitor which of the following laboratory values?

REWORDED QUESTION: What blood work is done to monitor heparin therapy?

NEEDED INFO: Heparin: anticoagulant. Side effects: hemorrhage, thrombocytopenia. Antidote: Protamine sulfate. When given SQ, inject slowly; leave needle in place 10 seconds, then withdraw; don't massage site; rotate sites. Nursing responsibilities: check for bleeding gums, bruises, nosebleeds, petechiae, melena, tarry stools, hematuria; use electric razor and soft toothbrush.

CATEGORY: Assessment/Physiological Integrity

(1) Platelet count—*evaluates platelet production; not altered*

(2) Clotting time—**CORRECT: or partial thromboplastin time (PTT); 1.5–2 × control, clotting time 2–3 × control**

(3) Bleeding time—*duration of bleeding after small puncture wound; detects platelet and vascular problems; not altered*

(4) Prothrombin time—*PT used to monitor Coumadin therapy*

152 A 50-year-old woman comes to the clinic for evaluation of acute onset of seizures. A thorough history and physical examination is performed. The nurse would expect which of the following diagnostic tests to be performed FIRST?

REWORDED QUESTION: What test is used to diagnose seizure disorders?

NEEDED INFO: EEG: recording of electrical activity of brain. Electrodes attached to scalp, waveforms recorded. Checked relaxing, hyperventilating, sleeping, with lights flickering. Prep: kept awake night before, shampoo hair. Stimulants (tea, coffee, alcohol, cola, cigarettes), antidepressants, tranquilizers, anticonvulsants withheld 24–48 hours before test. After test, seizure precautions and wash hair. Seizure: uncontrolled discharge of electrical activity from brain.

CATEGORY: Planning/Physiological Integrity

(1) Magnetic resonance imaging (MRI)—*uses magnetic fields to get detailed pictures; prep: remove jewelry, metal objects, lie still, may feel claustrophobic*

(2) Cerebral angiography—*dye injected into catheter in femoral artery, X rays taken; prep: check sensitivity to dye, post test: pressure on insertion site*

(3) Electroencephalogram (EEG)—**CORRECT**

(4) Electromyogram (EMG)—*evaluates activity of muscles; electrodes placed in nerves, sm amt. electricity applied*

153 The nurse performs dietary teaching with a patient on a low-protein diet. The nurse would know that teaching had been successful if the patient identified which of the following meals as LOWEST in protein?

REWORDED QUESTION: Which foods are the LOWEST in protein?

NEEDED INFO: Avoid high-protein foods: eggs, milk products, meat, beans, nuts, cereals.

CATEGORY: Evaluation/Physiological Integrity

(1) Cranberries and broiled chicken—**CORRECT: cranberries no protein, chicken 7 gm/oz**

(2) Tomatoes and flounder—*tomato 2 gm/oz, flounder 8 gm/oz*

(3) Broccoli and veal—*broccoli 2 gm/oz, veal 7 gm/oz*

(4) Spinach and tofu—*spinach 2 gm/serving, tofu 7 gm/oz*

154

A patient has a vagotomy with antrectomy to treat a duodenal ulcer. Postoperatively, the patient develops dumping syndrome. Which of the following statements, if made by the patient, should indicate to the nurse that further dietary teaching is necessary?

REWORDED QUESTION: What is CONTRAINDICATED for the patient with dumping syndrome?

STRATEGY: Be careful! You are looking for INCORRECT information.

NEEDED INFO: Antrectomy: surgery to reduce acid-secreting portions of stomach. Delays or eliminates gastric phase of digestion. Dumping syndrome occurs in patients after a gastric resection. It occurs after eating and is related to the reduced capacity of the stomach. Undigested food is dumped into the jejunum resulting in distention, cramping, pain, diarrhea 15–30 min after eating. Subsides in 6–12 months. S/S 5–30 min after eating: vertigo, tachycardia, syncope, diarrhea, nausea. Treatment: sedatives, antispasmodics, high-protein, high-fat, low-carbohydrate, dry diet. Eat in semirecumbent position, lying down after eating.

CATEGORY: Evaluation/Physiological Integrity

(1) "I should eat bread with each meal."—**CORRECT: incorrect info; should decrease intake of carbohydrates**

(2) "I should eat smaller meals more frequently."—*true; 5–6 small meals*

(3) "I should lie down after eating."—*true; delays gastric emptying time*

(4) "I should avoid drinking fluids with my meals."—*true; no fluids 1 hr before, with, or 2 hrs after meal*

155

A 25-year-old man is admitted to the hospital with a diagnosis of acquired immune deficiency syndrome (AIDS). He is being treated for pneumocystis carinii pneumonia. The nurse evaluates the care provided to this patient by other members of the health care team. The nurse should intervene in which of the following situations?

REWORDED QUESTION: Which situation describes an unsafe or inappropriate practice?

STRATEGY: Picture each situation as described in the question.

CATEGORY: Evaluation/Safe and Effective Care

(1) A housekeeper cleans up spilled blood with a bleach solution—*appropriate activity, solution of 1:10 sodium hypochlorite, or bleach with water, kills AIDS virus*

(2) A nursing student takes the patient's blood pressure wearing a mask and gloves—**CORRECT: inappropriate practice; mask and gloves necessary only when possibility of contact with blood and body fluids; when taking a BP very low risk for contact with blood and body fluids, behavior insensitive to patient's feelings, does not promote trust**

(3) A technician wears gloves to perform a venipuncture—*safe practice, barrier precaution used to prevent skin and mucous-membrane exposure if contact with blood or other body fluids of any patient anticipated*

(4) A nurse attendant allows visitors to enter his room without masks—*appropriate activity: visitors do not need masks, PCP parasite found in lungs of healthy people, thought to cause subclinical pulmonary infection worldwide, only dangerous to immunosuppressed patients; sick people not permitted to visit patient*

156

An 18-year-old woman comes to the physician's office for a routine prenatal checkup at 34 weeks gestation. Abdominal palpation reveals the fetal position as right occipital anterior (ROA). At which of the following sites would the nurse expect to find the fetal heart tone?

REWORDED QUESTION: The fetus is ROA. Where should the nurse listen for the FHT?

STRATEGY: Picture the situation described. It may be helpful for you to draw this out so that you can imagine where the heartbeat would be found.

NEEDED INFO: Describing fetal position: practice of defining position of baby relative to mother's pelvis. The point of maximum intensity (PMI) of the fetus: point on mother's abdomen where FHT is the loudest, usually over the fetal back. Divide mother's pelvis into 4 parts or quadrants: right and left anterior (front), and right and left posterior (back). Abbreviated: R and L for right and left, and A and P for anterior and posterior. The head, particularly the occiput, is the most common presenting part, and is abbreviated O. LOA is most common fetal presentation and FHT heard on left side.

In a vertex presentation, FHT is heard below the umbilicus. In a breech presentation, FHT is heard above umbilicus.

CATEGORY: Assessment/Health Promotion and Maintenance

(1) Below the umbilicus, on the mother's left—*found on right not left side*

(2) Below the umbilicus, on the mother's right side—**CORRECT: occiput and back are pressing against right side of mother's abdomen; FHT would be heard below umbilicus on right side**

(3) Above the umbilicus, on the mother's left side—*found in breech presentation*

(4) Above the umbilicus, on the mother's right side—*found in breech presentation*

157 A 20-year-old man is admitted to the hospital with complaints of seizures and a high fever. A brain scan is ordered. Before the scan, the patient asks the nurse what position he will be in while the procedure is being done. Which of the following statements, if made by the nurse, is MOST accurate?

REWORDED QUESTION: What is the proper position for a brain scan?

NEEDED INFO: Brain scan: measures amount of uptake by the brain of radioactive isotopes. Damaged tissue absorbs more than normal tissue. Nursing care before: withhold meds (antihypertensives, vasoconstrictors, vasodilators for 24 hrs). During the test patient will need to change position while pictures of the brain are taken. Test is painless. After test, force fluids to promote excretion of isotopes. Urine doesn't need special handling.

CATEGORY: Implementation/Physiological Integrity

(1) "You will be in a side-lying position, with the foot of the bed elevated."—*incorrect*

(2) "You will be in a Fowler's position, with your knees flexed."—*incorrect*

(3) "You will be lying supine with a small pillow under your head."—**CORRECT**

(4) "You will be in Trendelenburg's position, with your head elevated by two pillows."—*incorrect*

158 A 28-year-old man is admitted to the psychiatric hospital with a diagnosis of obsessive-compulsive disorder. He is unable to stay employed because his ritualistic behavior causes him to be late for work. Which of the follow-

ing interpretations of the patient's behavior, by the nurse, is MOST accurate?

REWORDED QUESTION: Why does the patient perform ritualistic behavior?

NEEDED INFO: Obsession: recurrent or persistent thought, image, or impulse. Compulsion: repetitive, purposeful or intentional behavior performed in a stereotypical manner. Nursing responsibilities: accept ritualistic behavior, structure environment, meet physical needs, minimize choices. Anafranil: tricyclic antidepressant. Side effects: dizziness, libido change, nervousness, dry mouth, sweating, urine retention, constipation, photosensitivity.

CATEGORY: Analysis/Psychosocial Integrity

(1) He is responding to auditory hallucinations and trying to gain control over his behavior—*hallucinations: false sensory perceptions in the absence of external stimuli, associated with schizophrenia*

(2) He is fulfilling an unconscious desire to punish himself—*not accurate*

(3) He is attempting to reduce anxiety by taking control of the environment—**CORRECT: unconscious attempt to reduce anxiety**

(4) He is malingering in order to avoid responsibilities at work—*conscious feigning of illness to promote secondary gain, conscious effort to manipulate*

159 A 58-year-old man, diagnosed with chronic lymphocytic leukemia, is admitted to the hospital for treatment of hemolytic anemia. Which of the following measures, if incorporated into the nursing care plan, would BEST address the patient's needs?

REWORDED QUESTION: What should you do for a patient with anemia?

STRATEGY: Although the patient has leukemia, he is admitted with anemia. You must focus on the anemia.

NEEDED INFO: Lymphocytic leukemia: characterized by proliferation of lymphocytes. S/S: fatigue, weakness, HA, easy bruising, bleeding gums, epistaxis, fever, generalized pain. Diagnostic tests: CBC, bone marrow aspiration, lumbar puncture, X-rays, lymph node biopsy. Treatment: total body irradiation or radiation to spleen, chemotherapy. Nursing responsibilities: low-bacteria diet (no raw fruits or vegetables), institute bleeding precautions (soft toothbrush, don't floss, no injections, no aspirin, pad bed rails, use air mattress, use paper tape), antiemetics, comfort measures. Hemolytic anemia s/s: jaundice, splenomegaly, hepatomegaly, fatigue, weakness. Treatment: O_2, blood transfusions, corticosteroids.

CATEGORY: Planning/Physiological Integrity

(1) Encourage activities with other patients in the day room—*does not meet need for rest*

(2) Isolate him from visitors and patients to avoid infection—*no info given about WBC or reverse isolation; on reverse isolation if neutrophil count is less than 500/mm³*

(3) Provide a diet high in vitamin C—*needed for wound healing and resistance to infection; not best choice*

(4) Provide a quiet environment to promote adequate rest—**CORRECT: primary problem activity intolerance due to fatigue**

160 The nurse plans morning care for a 69-year-old man hospitalized after a cerebrovascular accident (CVA) resulting in left-sided paralysis and homonymous hemianopia. During morning care, the nurse should

REWORDED QUESTION: What should you do for A.M. care for this patient?

NEEDED INFO: Homonymous hemianopia: blindness in half of each visual field caused by damage to brain. Patient cannot see past midline toward the side opposite the lesion without turning the head toward that side. Approach patient from side that is not visually impaired. Reduce noise and complexity of decision making.

CATEGORY: Implementation/Physiological Integrity

(1) provide care from the patient's right side—**CORRECT: approach from side with intact vision**

(2) speak loudly and distinctly when talking with the patient—*no hearing loss*

(3) reduce the level of lighting in the patient's room to prevent glare—*increase light to assist with vision*

(4) provide all of the patient's care to reduce his energy expenditure—*encourage independence*

161 The nurse prepares for the admission of a client with a perforated duodenal ulcer. Which of the following should the nurse expect to observe as the primary initial symptom?

REWORDED QUESTION: What symptom is seen FIRST with a perforated abdominal ulcer?

NEEDED INFO: Perforation of ulcer: medical emergency. Gastroduodenal contents empty into peritoneal cavity resulting in peritonitis, paralytic ileus, septicemia and shock. S/S: sudden, sharp pain; abdomen becomes tender, rigid. Treatment: fluids, electrolytes, antibiotics, NG suction, vagotomy, hemigastrectomy. S/S of duodenal ulcer: 25–30 years old, male-female 4:1, blood type O, pain 2–3 hrs after meal and hs, food intake relieves pain. Treatment: small frequent feedings; avoid coffee, alcohol, seasonings; antacids (Maalox) 1 hr before or after meals; anticholinergics (Probanthine), take 30 minutes before meals; histamine receptor site antagonists (Tagamet), take with meals.

CATEGORY: Assessment/Physiological Integrity

(1) Fever—*later with peritonitis (s/s: pain, N + V, rigid abdomen, low-grade fever, absent bowel sounds, shallow respirations)*

(2) Pain—**CORRECT: sudden, sharp, begins mid-epigastric; boardlike abdomen**

(3) Dizziness—*later with shock (s/s: hypotension, tachycardia, tachypnea, decreased urinary output, decreased LOC)*

(4) Vomiting—*seen with peritonitis*

162 A 3-week-old boy is admitted with a diagnosis of pyloric stenosis. The mother tells the nurse that this is her first child and asks if there is anything she can do to prevent this from happening to her next child. Which of the following statements, if made by the nurse, BEST addresses her concern?

REWORDED QUESTION: What should you say to the mother about the possibility of this happening in the future?

STRATEGY: Remember your therapeutic communication techniques.

CATEGORY: Implementation/Psychosocial Integrity

(1) "This type of thing generally happens to first children"—*inaccurate*

(2) "When you have your second child at least you'll know what signs to look for"—*invalidates concerns*

(3) "This is a structural problem; it is not a reflection of your parenting skills"—**CORRECT: provides acknowledgment; contains facts**

(4) "This is an inherited condition; it is not your fault"—*does not acknowledge feelings*

163 The nurse in a well-child clinic assesses a 4-year-old girl and observes multiple bruises on her back and buttocks. The parents state they don't know how the girl sustained the injury. The nurse should

REWORDED QUESTION: What is the nurse's responsibility when abuse is suspected?

NEEDED INFO: Symptoms of abuse: bruises, burns, fractures, genital lacerations, incompatibility of injury and history, disturbed parent/child interaction, signs of emotional neglect. Nursing responsibilities: nonjudgmental approach with parents; by law it is necessary to report suspected abuse; education and support for parents and child.

CATEGORY: Planning/Psychosocial Integrity

(1) confront the parents about the suspected abuse—*would create distance and alienation between parents and health care team, need to develop relationship of trust*

(2) report the suspected child abuse to the appropriate authority—**CORRECT: must report all suspected cases to appropriate agency/authority; failure to report is considered professional negligence**

(3) refer the family to social services for counseling—*not the appropriate intervention*

(4) document the suspicions about child abuse in the child's medical record—*must do more than document*

164 The nurse is caring for a Rh negative mother who has delivered an Rh positive child. The mother states, "The doctor told me about RhoGAM, but I'm still a little confused." Which of the following responses, if made by the nurse, is MOST appropriate?

REWORDED QUESTION: What is RhoGAM and why is it used?

NEEDED INFO: RhoGAM: given to unsensitized Rh⁻ mother after delivery or abortion of an Rh⁺ infant or fetus to prevent development of sensitization. Rh⁻ mother produces antibodies in response to the Rh⁺ RBCs of fetus. If occurs during pregnancy, fetus is affected. If occurs during delivery, later pregnancies may be affected. An indirect Coombs' test is performed on the mother during pregnancy, and a direct Coombs' test is done on cord blood after delivery. If both are negative and the neonate is Rh⁺, the mother is given RhoGAM to prevent sensitization. RhoGAM is usually given to unsensitized mothers within 72 hrs of delivery, but may be effective when given 3–4 weeks after delivery. To be effective RhoGAM must be given after the first delivery and repeated after each subsequent delivery. RhoGAM is ineffective against Rh⁺ antibodies that are already present in the maternal circulation. The administration of RhoGAM at 26–28 weeks gestation is also recommended.

CATEGORY: Implementation/Health Promotion and Maintenance

(1) "RhoGAM is given to your child to prevent the development of antibodies."—*not given to neonate*

(2) "RhoGAM is given to your child to supply the necessary antibodies."—*not given to neonate*

(3) "RhoGAM is given to you to prevent the formation of antibodies."—**CORRECT: prevents maternal circulation from developing antibodies**

(4) "RhoGAM is given to you to encourage the production of antibodies."—*not accurate; given to discourage antibody production*

165 The nurse performs patient teaching with a 45-year-old woman with osteoarthritis. The patient asks what she can do to effectively decrease pain and stiffness in her joints before beginning her daily routine. The nurse should instruct the patient to

REWORDED QUESTION: What should the patient with osteoarthritis do first thing in the morning?

CATEGORY: Implementation/Physiological Integrity

(1) perform isometric exercises for 10 minutes—*done to preserve muscle strength; tighten muscle, hold for few seconds, then relax without moving joint*

(2) do range-of-motion exercises then apply ointment to her joints—*done after ointment applied; ROM does not reduce pain*

(3) take a warm bath and rest for a few minutes—**CORRECT: heat reduces pain, spasms, stiffness in joints**

(4) stretch all muscles groups—*would be painful*

166 When caring for a patient with anorexia nervosa, which of the following observations indicate to the nurse that the patient's condition is improving?

REWORDED QUESTION: How would you know if the patient with anorexia nervosa is getting better?

STRATEGY: Objective criteria is better than subjective criteria in evaluation.

NEEDED INFO: Nursing responsibilities: monitor weight, intake, vital signs, implement behavioral modification, support efforts to take responsibility for self, explore sexuality issues.

CATEGORY: Evaluation/Psychosocial Integrity

(1) The patient eats all the food on her meal tray—*could meet goal without eating all food on tray*
(2) The patient asks friends to bring her special foods—*cause: not loss of appetite but distorted body image*
(3) The patient weighs herself daily—*uses to deal with anxiety*
(4) The patient's weight has increased—**CORRECT: best objective evidence**

167 A 44-year-old man returns to his room following a cardiac catheterization. Which of the following assessments, if made by the nurse, would justify calling the physician?

REWORDED QUESTION: What is the most serious complication that can occur after a cardiac catheterization? How would you know it occurred?

NEEDED INFO: Cardiac catheterization prep: may feel palpitations as catheter is passed and feelings of heat and desire to cough as dye is injected (check allergies to iodine and shellfish). Obtain consent. No solid food for 6–8 hours or liquids 4 hours before test. Mark peripheral pulses. Post-test: check vital signs every 30 min for 2 hours. Keep extremity of insertion site straight 4–6 hours. If femoral artery used bed rest 6–12 hours with bed flat. Check pressure dressing for drainage. Check pulses, color, warmth, sensation every 30 minutes. Monitor cardiac rhythm. Encourage fluids.

CATEGORY: Evaluation/Physiological Integrity

(1) Pain at the site of the catheter insertion—*expected; pain med given*
(2) Absence of a pulse distal to the catheter insertion site—**CORRECT: decrease in blood supply; report change in sensation, color, pulses to physician immediately**
(3) Drainage on the dressing covering the catheter insertion site—*some expected; pressure dressing applied; may have sandbag applied 4–6 hours*
(4) Redness at the catheter insertion site—*some expected*

168 An 8-year-old boy is seen in a clinic for treatment of Attention Deficit Disorder (ADD). Medication has been prescribed for the child along with family counseling. The nurse teaches the parents about the medication and discusses parenting strategies. Which of the following statements, if made by the parents, would indicate that further teaching is necessary?

REWORDED QUESTION: What information is WRONG for child with ADD?

STRATEGY: Be careful! You are looking for incorrect info.

NEEDED INFO: ADD: developmentally inappropriate inattention, impulsivity, hyperactivity. Treatment: medication (Ritalin), family counseling, remedial eduction, environmental manipulation (decrease external stimuli), psychotherapy.

CATEGORY: Evaluation/Psychosocial Integrity

(1) "We will give the medication at night so it doesn't decrease his appetite."—**CORRECT: incorrect info; stimulants (Ritalin) used; side effects: insomnia, palpitations, growth suppression, nervousness, decreased appetite; give 6 hrs before bedtime**
(2) "We will provide a regular routine for sleeping, eating, working, and playing"—*true*
(3) "We will establish firm, but reasonable limits on his behavior"—*true*
(4) "We will reduce distractions and external stimuli to help him concentrate"—*true*

169 A client has been taking Amphojel daily for three weeks. The nurse should be alert for which of the following side effects?

REWORDED QUESTION: What is a side effect of Amphojel?

NEEDED INFO: Aluminum hydroxide (Amphojel): antacid that reduces the total amount of acid in the GI tract and elevates the gastric pH level. May cause hypophosphatemia. Shake suspension well and give with milk or water.

CATEGORY: Assessment/Physiological Integrity

(1) Nausea—*not common*
(2) Hypercalcemia—*seen with Calcium-containing antacids (Tums); normal Ca 8.5–10.5 mg/dL*
(3) Constipation—**CORRECT: may need laxatives or stool softeners**
(4) Anorexia—*not common*

170 The nurse cares for a 38-year-old man after an appendectomy. The patient continues to complain of discomfort to the nurse shortly after receiving an analgesic. Which of the following measures, if taken by the nurse, would be MOST appropriate?

REWORDED QUESTION: What should you do after giving the analgesic?

NEEDED INFO: Appendicitis s/s: abdominal pain at McBurney's point (midway between right iliac crest and umbilicus), vomiting, anorexia, low-grade fever, leukocytosis (WBCs 10,000–15,000). Treatment: surgery. Nursing responsibilities preop: IVs, I + O, NG tube, antibiotics, no laxatives or cathartics. Postop: monitor vital signs, I + O, check LOC, IVs, wound care.

CATEGORY: Implementation/Physiological Integrity

(1) Notify the physician—*not necessary*
(2) Place him in Fowler's position—**CORRECT: relieve pressure on abdomen; HOB elevated 45–60°**
(3) Massage his abdomen—*would increase pain*
(4) Provide him with reading material—*not best*

171

A 68-year-old man returns to his room following a transurethral resection of the prostate (TURP) for benign prostatic hypertrophy (BPH). Which of the following would cause the nurse to suspect postoperative hemorrhage?

REWORDED QUESTION: What are the signs of postop hemorrhage?

STRATEGY: The entire answer choice must be correct for the answer to be correct. Read each one carefully.

NEEDED INFO: Symptoms of hemorrhage: restlessness, dizziness, pallor, cool, clammy skin, dyspnea, rapid thready pulse, fall in BP, decrease in level of consciousness. Treatment: elevate legs 45°, knees straight, trunk flat, head slightly elevated, IV fluids (Ringer's lactate, normal saline, D_5W, dextran), packed cells, vasoactive meds (Levophed, Nipride).

CATEGORY: Assessment/Physiological Integrity

(1) Decreased blood pressure, increased pulse, increased respirations—**CORRECT: caused by decreased blood volume, as intravascular volume decreases and BP falls, heart rate increases in attempt to maintain cardiac output, resp increase in attempt to increase oxygenation**
(2) Fluctuating blood pressure, decreased pulse, rapid respirations—*pulse rate will increase, not decrease*
(3) Increased blood pressure, bounding pulse, irregular respirations—*BP drops, pulse increases to compensate for decreased cardiac output*
(4) Increased blood pressure, irregular pulse, shallow respirations—*BP drops, heart rate increases to maintain cardiac output*

172

A 22-year-old woman is admitted to the hospital and delivers a healthy 7 lb, 2 oz girl. The mother decides to bottle-feed her infant. Which of the following statements, if made by the mother after a teaching session, indicates to the nurse that the patient needs further instruction?

REWORDED QUESTION: What statement contains INCORRECT info?

STRATEGY: Remember, you're looking for the statement that is incorrect and indicates the need for further teaching.

NEEDED INFO: Treatment of engorgement in non–breast feeding mother: tight binder, ice packs and mild analgesics. Care of breasts for breast feeding mothers: wash breast daily with plain water, prepare nipples by exposing to air and sun, wear loose clothing. Redness and swelling indicates infection.

CATEGORY: Evaluation/Health Promotion and Maintenance

(1) "I'll pump my breasts and use warm packs to relieve breast pain."—**CORRECT: incorrect info; stimulates hormonal responses; increases production of milk causing engorgement; stimulation of breast tissue by pumping of breasts, sucking of infant, running warm water over breasts is avoided**
(2) "I'll use a tight bra and ice packs to relieve engorgement discomfort."—*true; wear tight bra that supports breasts for 72 hrs after delivery; ice packs help relieve discomfort*
(3) "I'll take the medication prescribed by the doctor for pain."—*true; mild analgesics prescribed*
(4) "I'll take the pills ordered by my doctor to help stop the production of milk."—*true; bromocriptine (Parlodel) prescribed to prevent lactation; prevents secretion of prolactin; should be taken 2x/day for 14 days; may have rebound engorgement when med is withdrawn; other meds used: estrogenous (Tace or Deladumone), used less frequently due to high incidence of thrombus formation*

173

The nurse performs teaching with a 52-year-old man undergoing a paracentesis for treatment of cirrhosis. The patient asks what position he will be in for the procedure. The nurse's reply should be based on an understanding that the MOST appropriate position for the patient is:

REWORDED QUESTION: What is the correct position for a paracentesis?

NEEDED INFO: Paracentesis: removal of fluid from abdominal or peritoneal cavity. Can be used for diagnostic purposes, to remove ascitic fluid, to prepare for peritoneal dialysis. Preparation: have patient void, take vital signs, weigh patient, measure abdominal girth. During procedure: check vital signs every 15 min. Measure and document amount of drainage (2–3 L can be removed), characteristics. After procedure: apply pressure dressing, check for leakage. Bed rest till vital signs stable. Complications: hypovolemia and shock. Cirrhosis: degenerative liver disease; tissue is replaced by scar tissue. Causes: alcoholism, hepatic inflammation or necrosis, chronic bilary obstruction. S/S: ascites, lower leg edema, jaundice, esophageal varices, hemorrhoids, bleeding tendencies, pruritis, dark urine, clay-colored stools. Nursing responsibilities: high-protein, high carbohydrate, low Na^+ diet, good skin care, promote rest, reduce exposure to infection.

CATEGORY: Analysis/Physiological Integrity

(1) sitting with his lower extremities well supported— **CORRECT: Fowler's position or sitting on side of bed with feet on stool; easy access to abdominal area; allows intestines to float to prevent laceration**
(2) side-lying with a pillow between his knees—*not accurate*
(3) prone, with his head turned to the left side—*not accurate*
(4) dorsal-recumbent with a pillow at the back of his head—*not accurate*

174 A man calls the Suicide Prevention Hotline and states that he is going to kill himself. Which of the following questions should the nurse ask FIRST?

REWORDED QUESTION: What is MOST important to know about a patient who has threatened to kill himself?

NEEDED INFO: Signs of suicide: symptoms of depression, patient gives away possessions, gets finances in order, has a means, makes direct or indirect statements, leaves notes, increase in energy. Predisposing factors: male over age 50, age 15–19, poor social attachments, patients with previous attempts, patients with auditory hallucinations, overwhelming precipitating events (terminal disease, death or loss of loved one, failure at school, job).

CATEGORY: Assessment/Psychosocial Integrity

(1) "What has happened to cause you to want to end your life?"—*does not determine immediate need for safety*
(2) "How have you planned to kill yourself?"— **CORRECT: lets you prioritize interventions to assure safety**

(3) "When did you start to feel as though you wanted to die?"—*does not determine immediate need for safety*
(4) "Do you want me to prevent you from killing yourself?"—*yes/no question, closed*

175 A 45-year-old man is admitted for treatment of congestive heart failure (CHF). The physician orders an IV of 125 cc of normal saline per hour and central venous pressure (CVP) readings every 4 hours. Sixteen hours after admission, the patient's CVP reading is 3 cm/H_2O. Which of the following evaluations of the patient's fluid status, if made by the nurse, would be MOST accurate?

REWORDED QUESTION: What does this CVP reading indicate?

NEEDED INFO: CVP: central venous line placed in superior vena cava. To obtain a reading: patient placed supine, 0 on manometer placed at level of right atrium (midaxillary line at fourth intercostal space), turn stopcock to allow manometer to fill with fluid, turn to allow fluid to go into patient. Fluid will fluctuate with resp. When stabilized, take reading at highest level of fluctuation. Normal: 4–10 cm/H_2O. Elevated: hypervolemia, CHF, pericarditis. Low: hypovolemia.

CATEGORY: Evaluation/Physiological Integrity

(1) The patient has received enough fluid—*inaccurate*
(2) The patient's fluid status remains unaltered—*nothing to compare to*
(3) The patient has received too much fluid—*inaccurate*
(4) The patient needs more fluid—**CORRECT: normal 4–10 cm/H_2O; indicates hypovolemia**

176 An agitated 20-year-old patient throws a chair across the dayroom on the psychiatry floor and threatens the other patients with physical harm. The nurse's initial action should be to

REWORDED QUESTION: What is the nurse's first action?

STRATEGY: Use Maslow. Safety first—the patient must be removed from the situation.

NEEDED INFO: The nurse can initiate seclusion procedures in an escalating situation per hospital policy. The principle of seclusion is containment, to avoid injury, and to prevent anticipated violence. Violence must be prevented to ensure the safety of other patients and staff.

CATEGORY: Implementation/Psychosocial Integrity

(1) tell the patient that his wife will be called to the hospital —*calling wife will not solve the immediate problem and may complicate the situation*

(2) ask the patient why he is so angry—*asking patient for causes of anger is inappropriate when the patient's behavior is escalating*

(3) remove the other patients from the dayroom—*allowing patient to determine disposition of other patients gives patient control over staff and other patients*

(4) assemble staff and put the patient in preventive seclusion—**CORRECT: seclusion may be used alone or in conjunction with medication to de-escalate a potentially dangerous situation; nurse can initiate and terminate patient seclusion based on established protocols**

177 The nurse is caring for a depressed 40-year-old male patient who spends most of the day sitting at a window, and is about to implement a physical activity plan for him. The nurse knows that the purpose of this plan is to:

REWORDED QUESTION: What is the purpose of the different plans typically implemented for patients with mental illness?

STRATEGY: Consider the rationales for plans typically used for patients with mental illness.

NEEDED INFO: Physical and mental health are linked. A level of fitness enhances a sense of mental well-being. Withdrawn patients have decreased motivation to exercise. Physical exercise can also distract patients from stressful thoughts, and helps patients focus on things other than themselves.

CATEGORY: Planning/Psychosocial Integrity

(1) help the patient understand the problems creating the depression—*purpose of physical activity is not to provide insight into one's problems*

(2) reduce the patient's risk for obesity and diabetes—*this would not necessarily reduce the risk for obesity and diabetes*

(3) transform self-destructive impulses into positive behaviors—*physical activity may channel energy differently, but does not guarantee to change self-destructiveness*

(4) encourage socialization and improve self-esteem—**CORRECT: purpose of physical activity is to promote focused socialization with patients and staff and to increase a sense of self-esteem**

178 The nurse is caring for a patient with bipolar disorder. Which behavior, if demonstrated by the patient, would indicate to the nurse that a manic episode is subsiding?

REWORDED QUESTION: What indicates normalizing behavior?

STRATEGY: Think about the behaviors that indicate mania.

NEEDED INFO: Manic patients may tease, talk, and joke excessively. They usually cannot sit to eat and may need to carry fluids and food around in order to eat. Manic patients often try to take a leadership position in an environment, and try to engage others.

CATEGORY: Assessment/Psychosocial Integrity

(1) The patient tells several jokes at a group meeting—*reflects an elated mood and no real participation in the meeting; manic patients may tease, talk, and joke excessively*

(2) The patient sits and talks with other patients at mealtimes—**CORRECT: manic patients have difficulty socializing because of flight of ideas and intrusiveness; usually cannot sit to eat and will carry fluids and food around**

(3) The patient begins to write a book about his life—*manic patients often write voluminously; may help to express feelings, but does not reflect improvement, especially if thoughts are grandiose*

(4) The patient initiates an effort to start a radio station on the unit—*manic patients often try to take a leadership position in an environment and try to recruit others*

179 A patient hospitalized for treatment of delusions tells the nurse that he is really the head of the hospital system and that his cover is being a patient to get information on patient abuse. The nurse's initial response should be:

REWORDED QUESTION: How would you handle a patient with delusions?

STRATEGY: Know when further assessment is needed and what the appropriate communication techniques are to use with delusional patients.

NEEDED INFO: The initial approach to delusions is to clarify meanings. After clarification, the delusions should not be discussed as this could reinforce them. Arguing with a patient about delusions may also reinforce them. Delusions that entail injury or death should be addressed immediately, and patient protections put into place.

CATEGORY: Assessment/Psychosocial Integrity

(1) "Tell me what you mean about being head of the hospital system and getting patient abuse information."— **CORRECT: initial approach is to further assess by clarifying the meaning of the delusion to the patient**

(2) "I think you should share this story with the other patients at dinnertime and see what they say."—*could cause disruption among other patients and embarrass the patient*

(3) "You are not the head of the hospital system, you are an accountant under treatment for a mental disorder."—*arguing with patient about delusion is ineffective and inappropriate and may strengthen the patient's belief in it*

(4) "It worries me when you say these things; it means you are not responding to the medication."—*nurse is communicating disappointment to the patient and treating the delusion as though it were a behavior under the client's control*

180 The nurse is caring for a patient in labor. The nurse palpates a firm, round form in the uterine fundus, small parts on the woman's right side, and a long, smooth, curved section on the left side. Based on these findings, the nurse should anticipate auscultating the fetal heart in which of the following locations?

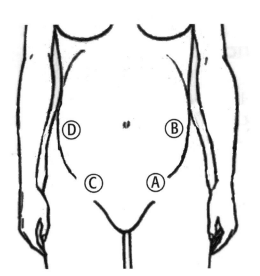

REWORDED QUESTION: If a fetus is LOA, where should the nurse listen for the fetal heart tone?

STRATEGY: Examine the diagram carefully. Know the woman's right from left.

NEEDED INFO: Fetal reference point: Vertex presentation—dependent upon degree of flexion of fetal head on chest; full flexion/occiput (O), full extension chin (M), moderate extension (military) brow (B). Breech presentation—sacrum (S). Shoulder presentation—scapula (SC). Maternal pelvis is designated per her right/left and anterior/posterior. Position = relationship of fetal reference point to mother's pelvis; expressed as standard 3-letter abbreviation: LOA (left occiput anterior) (most common), LOP (left occiput posterior), ROA (right occiput anterior), ROP (right occiput posterior), LOT (left occiput transverse), ROT (right occiput transverse).

CATEGORY: Planning/Health Promotion and Maintenance

(1) A—**CORRECT: point of maximum intensity for fetal heart with fetus in LOA position**

(2) B—*PMI location for fetus in LOP position*

(3) C—*PMI location for fetus in ROA position*

(4) D—*PMI location for fetus in ROP position*

PART THREE

APPENDIXES

APPENDIX A

Chart of
Critical Thinking Paths

The chart on the reverse side of this page is reprinted from chapter 3. Tear out this page and use the chart to practice using this book's strategies when answering practice NCLEX-style questions.

Critical Thinking Paths to Correct Answers on the NCLEX

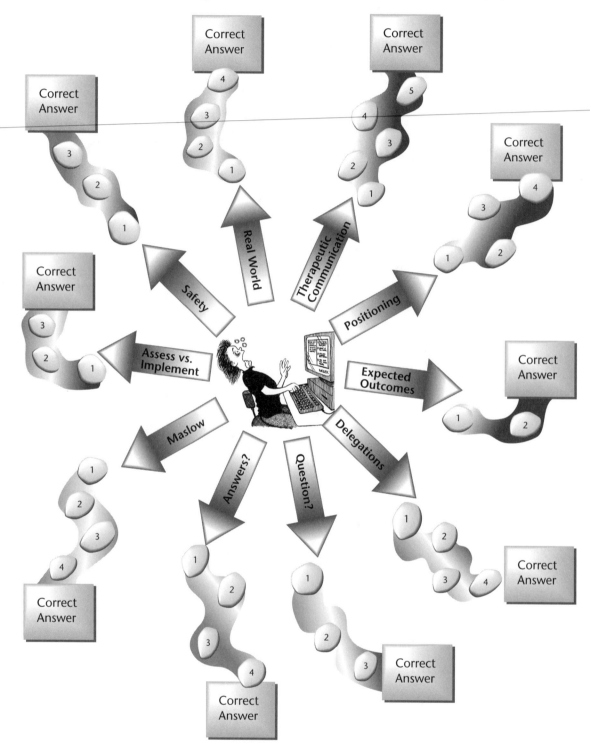

KAPLAN

APPENDIX B

NCLEX Terminology

TERM	DEFINITION
abduction	to move away from the midline
abraded	scraped
acetonuria	acetone in the urine
adduction	to move toward the midline
afebrile	without fever
albuminuria	albumin in the urine
ambulatory	walking
amenorrhea	absence of menstruation
amnesia	loss of or defective memory
ankyloses	stiff joint
anorexia	loss of appetite
anuria	total suppression of urination
apnea	short periods when breathing has ceased
arthritis	inflammation of joint
asphyxia	suffocation
atrophy	wasting

auscultation, auscultate	to listen for sounds
bradycardia	heartbeat fewer than 60 beats per minute
choluria	bile in the urine
Cheyenne-Stokes respirations	increasing dyspnea with periods of apnea
clonic tremor	shaking with intervals of rest
conjunctivitis	inflammation of conjunctiva
coryza	watery drainage from nose
cyanotic	bluish in color due to poor oxygenation
defecation	bowel movement
dental caries	decay of the teeth
dentures	false teeth
diarrhea	excessive or frequent defecation
diplopia	double vision
distended	appears swollen
diuresis	large amount of urine voided
dorsal recumbent	lying on back, knees flexed and apart
dysmenorrhea	painful menstruation
dyspnea	difficulty breathing
dysrhythmia, arrhythmia	abnormal heartbeat
dysuria	painful urination
edematous	puffy, swollen
emaciated	thin, underweight
emetic	agent given to produce vomiting
enuresis	bed-wetting
epistaxis	nosebleed
eructation	belching

erythema	redness
eupnea	normal breathing
excoriation	raw surface
exophthalmos	abnormal protrusion of eyeball
extension	to straighten
fatigued	tired
feigned	pretended
fetid	foul
fixed	motionless
flaccid	soft, flabby
flatus, flatulence	gas in the digestive tract
flexion	bending
flushed	pink or hot
Fowler's position	semierect, knees flexed, head of bed elevated 45–60°
gavage	forced feeding through a tube passed into the stomach
glossy	shiny
glycosuria	glucose in the urine
gustatory	dealing with taste
heliotherapy	using sunlight as a therapeutic agent
hematemesis	blood in vomitus
hematuria	blood in the urine
hemiplegia	paralysis of one side of the body
hemoglubinuria	hemoglobin in the urine
hemoptysis	spitting of blood
horizontal	flat

hydrotherapy	using water as a therapeutic agent
hypernea	rapid breathing
hypertonic	concentration greater than body fluids
hypotonic	concentration less than body fluids
infrequent	not often
insomnia	inability to sleep
instillation	pouring into a body cavity
intermittent	starting and stopping, not continuous
intradermal	within or through the skin
intramuscular	within or through the muscle
intraspinal	within or through the spinal canal
intravenous	within or through the vein
involuntary, incontinent	unable to control bladder or bowels
isotonic	having the same tonicity or concentration as body fluids
jackknife position	prone with hips over break in table and feet below level of head
jaundice	yellow color
knee-chest position	in face-down position resting on knees and chest
kyphosis	hump back, concavity of spine
labored	difficult, requires an effort
lacerated	torn, broken
lateral position	on the side, knees flexed
lithotomy position	on back, buttocks near edge of table, knees well flexed and separated
locia	drainage from the vagina after delivery
lordosis	sway-back, convexity of spine

manipulation, manipulate	to handle
menopause	cessation of menstruation
menorrhagia	profuse menstruation
metrorrhagia	variable amount of uterine bleeding occurring frequently but at irregular intervals
moist	wet
monoplegia	paralysis of one limb
mucopurulent	drainage containing mucus and pus
mydriasis	dilation of pupil
myopia	near-sightedness
myosis	contraction of pupil
nausea	desire to vomit
necrosis	death of tissue
nocturia	frequently voiding at night
obese	overweight
objective	able to document by other than observation
oliguria	scant urination, less than 400 ml per 24 hrs
orthopnea	inability to breathe or difficulty breathing lying down
palliative	offering temporary relief
pallor	white
palpation, palpate	to feel with hands or fingers
paraplegia	paralysis of legs
paroxysm	spasms or convulsive seizure
paroxysmal	coming in seizures

pediculi, pediculosis	lice
percussion, percuss	to strike
persistent	lasting over a long time
petechia	small rupture of blood vessels
photophobia	sensitive to light
photosensitivity	skin reaction caused by exposure to sunlight
pigmented	containing color
polyuria	increased amount of voiding
profuse, copious	large amount
projectile	ejected or projected some distance
pronation	to turn downward
prone	on abdomen, face turned to one side
prophylactic	preventative
protruding	extends outward
pruritus	itching
ptosis	drooping eyelid
purulent	drainage containing pus
pyrexia	elevated temperature
pyuria	pus in the urine
radiating	spreads to distant areas
radiotherapy	using X ray or radium as a therapeutic agent
rales, crackles	abnormal breath sounds
rapid	quickly
rotation	to move in circular pattern
sanguineous	bloody drainage

scanty	small amount
semi-Fowler's position	semi-erect, head of bed elevated 30–45°
serous	drainage of lymphatic fluid
Sim's position	on left side, left arm behind back, left leg slightly flexed, right leg slightly flexed
sprain	wrenching of joint
stertorous	snoring
stethoscope	instrument used for auscultation
strabismus	squinting
stuporous	partial unconsciousness
subcutaneous	under the skin
subjective	observed
sudden onset	started all at once
superficial	on the surface only
supination	to turn upward
suppurating	discharging pus
syncope	fainting
syndrome	group of symptoms
tachycardia	fast heartbeat, greater than 100 beats per minute
tenacious	tough and sticky
thready	barely perceptible
tonic tremor	continuous shaking
Trendelenburg position	flat on back with pelvis higher than head, foot of bed elevated six inches
tympanic	filled with gas
urticaria	hives or wheals, eruption on skin or mucous membranes

vertigo	dizziness
vesicle	fluid-filled blister
visual acuity	sharpness of vision
void, micturate	to urinate or pass urine

APPENDIX C

Common Medical Abbreviations

TERM	DEFINITION
ABC	airway, breathing, circulation
abd.	abdomen
ABG	arterial blood gas
ABO	system of classifying blood groups
ac	before meals
ACE	angiotensin converting enzyme
ACS	acute compartment syndrome
ACTH	adrenocorticotrophic hormone
ADH	antidiuretic hormone
ADL	activities of daily living
ad lib	freely, as desired
AFP	alpha-fetoprotein
AIDS	acquired immunodeficiency syndrome
AKA	above the knee amputation
ALL	acute lymphocytic leukemia
ALS	amyotrophic lateral sclerosis
ALT	alkaline phosphatase (formerly SGPT)
AMI	antibody-mediated immunity
AML	acute myelogenous leukemia

amt.	amount
ANA	antinuclear antibody
ANS	autonomic nervous system
AP	anteroposterior
A&P	anterior and posterior
APC	atrial premature contraction
aq.	water
ARDS	adult respiratory distress syndrome
ASD	atrial septal defect
ASHD	atherosclerotic heart disease
AST	aspartate aminotransferase (formerly SGOT)
ATP	adenosine triphosphate
AV	atrioventricular
BCG	Bacille Calmette-Guerin
bid	two times a day
BKA	below the knee amputation
BLS	basic life support
BMR	basal metabolic rate
BP	blood pressure
BPH	benign prostatic hypertrophy
bpm	beats per minute
BPR	bathroom privileges
BSA	body surface area
BUN	blood, urea, nitrogen
C	centigrade, Celsius
$\bar{c}$	with
Ca	calcium
CA	cancer

CABG	coronary artery bypass graft
CAD	coronary artery disease
CAPD	continuous ambulatory peritoneal dialysis
caps	capsules
CBC	complete blood count
CC	chief complaint
cc	cubic centimeter
CCU	coronary care unit, critical care unit
CDC	Centers for Disease Control and Prevention
CHF	congestive heart failure
CK	creatine kinase
Cl	chloride
CLL	chronic lymphocytic leukemia
cm	centimeter
CMV	cytomegalovirus infection
CNS	central nervous system
CO	carbon monoxide, cardiac output
CO_2	carbon dioxide
comp	compound
cont	continuous
COPD	chronic obstructive pulmonary disease
CP	cerebral palsy
CPAP	continuous positive airway pressure
CPK	creatine phosphokinase
CPR	cardiopulmonary resuscitation
CRP	C-reactive protein
C&S	culture and sensitivity
CSF	cerebrospinal fluid

CT	computerized tomography
CTD	connective tissue disease
CTS	carpal tunnel syndrome
cu	cubic
CVA	cerebrovascular accident or costovertebral angle
CVC	central venous catheter
CVP	central venous pressure
DC	discontinue
D&C	dilation and curettage
DIC	disseminated intravascular coagulation
DIFF	differential blood count
dil.	dilute
DJD	degenerative joint disease
DKA	diabetic ketoacidosis
dL	deciliter (100 ml)
DM	diabetes mellitus
DNA	deoxyribonucleic acid
DNR	do not resuscitate
DO	doctor of osteopathy
DOE	dyspnea on exertion
DPT	vaccine for diphtheria, pertussis, tetanus
Dr.	doctor
DVT	deep vein thrombosis
D/W	dextrose in water
Dx	diagnosis
ECF	extracellular fluid
ECG or EKG	electrocardiogram
ECT	electroconvulsive therapy

ED	emergency department
EEG	electroencephalogram
EMD	electromechanical dissociation
EMG	electromyography
ENT	ear, nose, and throat
ESR	erythrocyte sedimentation rate
ESRD	end stage renal disease
ET	endotracheal tube
F	Fahrenheit
FBD	fibrocystic breast disease
FBS	fasting blood sugar
FDA	Food and Drug Administration
FFP	fresh frozen plasma
fl	fluid
4 × 4	piece of gauze 4" by 4" used for dressings
FSH	follicle-stimulating hormone
ft	foot, feet (unit of measure)
FUO	fever of undetermined origin
g, gm	gram
GB	gall bladder
GFR	glomerular filtration rate
GH	growth hormone
GI	gastrointestinal
gr	grain
GSC	Glasgow coma scale
gtts	drops
GU	genitourinary
GYN	gynecological

h or hrs	hour or hours
(H)	hypodermically
Hb or Hgb	hemoglobin
HCG	human chorionic gonadotropin
HCO_3^-	bicarbonate
Hct	hematocrit
HD	hemodialysis
HDL	high-density lipoproteins
Hg	mercury
Hgb	hemoglobin
HGH	human growth hormone
HHNC	hyperglycemia hyperosmolar nonketotic coma
HIV	human immunodeficiency virus
HLA	human leukocyte antigen
HR	heart rate
hr	hour
hs	at bedtime, hour of sleep
HSV	herpes simplex virus
HTN	hypertension
H_2O	water
Hx	history
Hz	hertz (cycles/second)
IAPB	intra-aortic balloon pump
IBBP	intermittent positive pressure breathing
IBS	irritable bowel syndrome
ICF	intracellular fluid
ICP	increased intracranial pressure
ICS	intercostal space

ICU	intensive care unit
IDDM	insulin dependent diabetes mellitus
IgA	immunoglobulin A
IM	intramuscular
I&O	intake and output
IOP	increased intraocular pressure
IPG	impedance plethysmogram
IPPB	intermittent positive-pressure breathing
IU, iu	international unit
IUD	intrauterine device
IV	intravenous
IVC	intraventricular catheter
IVP	intravenous pyelogram
JRA	juvenile rheumatoid arthritis
K^+	potassium
kcal	kilocalorie (food calorie)
kg	kilogram
KO, KVO	keep vein open
KS	Kaposi's sarcoma
KUB	kidneys, ureters, bladder
L, l	liter
lab	laboratory
lb.	pound
LBBB	left bundle branch block
LDH	lactate dehydrogenase
LDL	low-density lipoproteins
LE	lupus erythematosus
LH	luteinizing hormone

liq	liquid
LLQ	left lower quadrant
LOC	level of consciousness
LP	lumbar puncture
LPN, LVN	licensed practical or vocational nurse
Lt, lt	left
LTC	long term care
LUQ	left upper quadrant
LV	left ventricle
m	minum, meter, micron
MAO	monoamine oxidase inhibitors
MAST	military antishock trousers
mcg	microgram
MCH	mean corpuscular hemoglobin
MCV	mean corpuscular volume
MD	muscular dystrophy, medical doctor
MDI	metered dose inhaler
mEq	milliequivalent
mg	milligram
Mg	magnesium
MG	myasthenia gravis
MI	myocardial infarction
ml	milliliter
mm	millimeter
MMR	vaccine for measles, mumps, rubella
MRI	magnetic resonance imaging
MS	multiple sclerosis, morphine sulfate
N	nitrogen, normal (strength of solution)

NIDDM	non-insulin dependent diabetes mellitus
Na^+	sodium
NaCl	sodium chloride
NADA	North American Nursing Diagnosis Association
NG	nasogastric
NGT	nasogastric tube
NLN	National League for Nursing
noc	at night
NPO	nothing by mouth
NS	normal saline
NSAIDS	nonsteroidal anti-inflammatory drugs
NSNA	National Student Nurses' Association
NST	non-stress test
O_2	oxygen
OB-GYN	obstetrics and gynecology
OCT	oxytocin challenge test
OD, od	right eye
OOB	out of bed
OPC	outpatient clinic
OR	operating room
OS, os	left eye
$\overline{os}$	by mouth
OSHA	Occupational Safety and Health Administration
OTC	over the counter (drug that can be obtained without a prescription)
OU, ou	both eyes
oz	ounce
$\overline{p}$	with

P	pulse, pressure, phosphorus
PA Chest	posterior-anterior chest x-ray
PAC	premature atrial complexes
$PaCO_2$	partial pressure of carbon dioxide in arterial blood
PaO_2	partial pressure of oxygen in arterial blood
PAD	peripheral artery disease
Pap	Papanicolaou smear
pc	after meals
PCA	patient controlled analgesia
PCO_2	partial pressure of carbon dioxide
PCP	Pneumocystis carinii pneumonia
PD	peritoneal dialysis
PE	pulmonary embolism
PEEP	positive end-expiratory pressure
PERRLA	pupils equal, round, react to light and accommodation
PET	postural emission tomography
PFT	pulmonary function tests
pH	hydrogen ion concentration
PID	pelvic inflammatory disease
PKD	polycystic disease
PKU	phenylketonuria
PMS	premenstrual syndrome
PND	paroxysmal nocturnal dyspnea
PO, po	by mouth
PO_2	partial pressure of oxygen
PPD	positive purified protein derivative (of tuberculin)
PPN	partial parenteral nutrition

PRN, prn	as needed, whenever necessary
pro time	prothrombin time
PSA	prostate-specific antigen
psi	pounds per square inch
PSP	phenol-sulfonphthalein
PT	physical therapy, prothrombin time
PTCA	percutaneous transluminal coronary angioplasty
PTH	parathyroid hormone
PTT	partial thromboplastin time
PUD	peptic ulcer disease
PVC	premature ventricular contraction
q	every
QA	quality assurance
qh	every hour
q 2 h	every two hours
q 4 h	every four hours
qid	four times a day
qs	quantity sufficient
R	rectal temperature, respirations, roentgen
RA	rheumatoid arthritis
RAI	radioactive iodine
RAIU	radioactive iodine uptake
RAS	reticular activating system
RBBB	right bundle branch block
RBC	red blood cell or count
RCA	right coronary artery
RDA	recommended dietary allowance
resp	respirations

RF	rheumatic fever, rheumatoid factor
Rh	antigen on blood cell indicated by + or −
RIND	reversible ischemic neurologic deficit
RLQ	right lower quadrant
RN	registered nurse
RNA	ribonucleic acid
R/O, r/o	rule out, to exclude
ROM	range of motion (of joint)
Rt, rt	right
RUQ	right upper quadrant
Rx	prescription
$\bar{s}$	without
S. or Sig.	(Signa) to write on label
SA	sinoatrial node
SaO2	systemic arterial oxygen saturation (%)
sat sol	saturated solution
SBE	subacute bacterial endocarditis
SC, sc	subcutaneous
SDA	same day admission
SDS	same day surgery
sed rate	sedimentation rate
SGOT	serum glutamic-oxaloacetic transaminase (see AST)
SGPT	serum glutamic-pyruvic transaminase (see ALT)
SI	International System of Units
SIADH	syndrome of inappropriate antidiuretic hormone
SIDS	sudden infant death syndrome
SL	sublingual
SLE	systemic lupus erythematosus

SOB	short of breath
sol	solution
SMBG	self-monitoring blood glucose
SMR	submucous resection
sp gr	specific gravity
spec.	specimen
SQ	subcutaneous
$\overline{ss}$	one half
SS	soap suds
SSKI	saturated solution of potassium iodide
stat	immediately
STD	sexually transmitted disease
sx	symptoms
Syr.	syrup
T	temperature, thoracic to be followed by the number designating specific thoracic vertebra
T&A	tonsillectomy and adenoidectomy
tabs	tablets
TB	tuberculosis
T&C	type and crossmatch
TED	antiembolitic stockings
temp	temperature
TENS	transcutaneous electrical nerve stimulation
TIA	transient ischemic attack
TIBC	total iron binding capacity
tid	three times a day
tinct, or tr.	tincture
TMJ	temporomandibular joint

t-pa, TPA	tissue plasminogen activator
TPN	total parenteral nutrition
TPR	temperature, pulse, respiration
TQM	total quality management
TSE	testicular self-examination
TSH	thyroid-stimulating hormone
tsp	teaspoon
TSS	toxic shock syndrome
TURP	transuretheral prostatectomy
U	units
UA	urinalysis
ung	ointment
URI	upper respiratory tract infection
UTI	urinary tract infection
VAD	venous access device
VDRL	Veneral Disease Research laboratory (test for syphilis)
VF, Vfib	ventricular fibrillation
VPC	ventricular premature complexes
VS, vs	vital signs
VSD	ventricular septal defect
VT	ventricular tachycardia
WBC	white blood cell or count
WHO	World Health Organization
wt	weight

APPENDIX D

State Licensing Requirements*

Alabama

Board of Nursing
RSA Plaza, Suite 250
770 Washington Avenue
Montgomery, AL 36130-3900
Phone: (334) 242-4060
Fax: (334) 242-4360
www.abn.state.al.us/

Temporary Permit: 90 days from date of graduation; three months if by endorsement; $50

State Board Fee: $85

Additional State Endorsement: $85

NCLEX Test Fee: $200

Re-Examination Limitations: Every 91 days

License Renewal: December 31, every even year; $60

CEU Requirements: 24 contact hours per biennial renewal period. Nurses licensed by exam are exempt from CE requirements for the first renewal after initial licensure.

Alaska

Board of Nursing
Dept. of Community and Economic Development
Division of Occupational Licensing
P.O. Box 110806
Juneau, AK 99811-0806
Phone: (907) 465-2544 (last names A–K);
           (907) 465-2648 (last names L–Z)
Fax: (907) 465-2974
www.dced.state.ak.us/occ/pnur.htm

Temporary Permit: Four months by exam or by endorsement; $50

State Board Fee: $215 permanent license fee; $50 application fee

Additional State Endorsement: $215 permanent license fee; $50 application fee

NCLEX Test Fee: $200

Re-Examination Limitations: Every 91 days. Must pass within 5 years, then retake with remediation.

License Renewal: November 30, every even year; $105

CEU Requirements: Two of the three required for renewal: (1) 30 contact hours of CE, (2) 30 hours of professional nursing activities, (3) 320 hours of nursing employment

*The information in this section is up-to-date at the time of publication. However, state licensing requirements may change after this book is published. Contact your state licensure board for the latest information.

Arizona

Board of Nursing
1651 E. Morten Avenue, Suite 210
Phoenix, AZ 85020-4613
Phone: (602) 331-8111
Fax: (602) 906-9365
www.azboardofnursing.org

Temporary Permit: Four months pending results of fingerprint check, must have already passed the exam; $25

State Board Fee: $220, plus $36 fingerprint fee

Additional State Endorsement: $150, plus $36 fingerprint fee

NCLEX Test Fee: $200

Re-Examination Limitations: Every 91 days

License Renewal: June 30, every four years; $120

CEU Requirements: None

Arkansas

State Board of Nursing
University Tower Building
1123 South University, Suite 800
Little Rock, AR 72204-1619
Phone: (501) 686-2700
Fax: (501) 686-2714
www.accessarkansas.org/nurse/

Temporary Permit: Up to 90 days if by endorsement and advanced practice; $20

State Board Fee: $55

Additional State Endorsement: $85

NCLEX Test Fee: $200

Re-Examination Limitations: Every 91 days

License Renewal: Birthday, every two years; $55

CEU Requirements: For license renewal between 7/1/03 and 6/30/04: 8 contact hours. After 7/1/04: 15 contact hours.

California

Board of Registered Nursing
400 R Street, Suite 4030
P.O. Box 944210
Sacramento, CA 94244-2100
Phone: (916) 322-3350
Fax: (916) 327-4402
www.rn.ca.gov/

Temporary Permit: Interim license pending results of first exam; six months if by endorsement; $30

State Board Fee: $75 application fee, plus $32 fingerprint fee

Additional State Endorsement: $50, plus $56 fingerprint fee

NCLEX Test Fee: $200

Re-Examination Limitations: Every 91 days

License Renewal: Last day of the month following birth month, every two years; $80

CEU Requirements: 30 contact hours every two years. Nurses licensed by exam are exempt from CE requirements for the first renewal after initial licensure.

Colorado

Board of Nursing
1560 Broadway, Suite 880
Denver, CO 80202
Phone: (303) 894-2430
Fax: (303) 894-2821
www.dora.state.co.us/nursing/

Temporary Permit: 90 days; four months if by endorsement. Fee is included in application fee.

State Board Fee: $65 initial exam; $35 retake fee

Additional State Endorsement: $60

NCLEX Test Fee: $200

Re-Examination Limitations: Every 91 days

License Renewal: September 30, every two years; $100

CEU Requirements: None

Connecticut

Board of Examiners for Nursing
Department of Public Health
RN Licensure
410 Capitol Avenue, MS 12 APP
P.O. Box 340308
Hartford, CT 06134-0308
Phone: (860) 509-7573
Fax: (860) 509-7553
www.state.ct.us/dph/

Temporary Permit: 90 days from completion of nursing program. Temporary permit also available for endorsement applicants, valid for 120 days, non-renewable; must hold valid license in another state. Fee is included in application fee.

State Board Fee: $90

Additional State Endorsement: $90

NCLEX Test Fee: $200

Re-Examination Limitations: Every 91 days, no more than four times in one year

License Renewal: Last day of birth month, every year; $50

CEU Requirements: None

Delaware

Division of Professional Regulation
Board of Nursing
861 Silver Lake Boulevard
Cannon Building, Suite 203
P.O. Box 1401
Dover, DE 19903
Phone: (302) 739-4522
Fax: (302) 739-2711
www.state.de.us/license/index.htm

Temporary Permit: 90 days by endorsement or pending results of first exam. Fee is included in licensure fee.

State Board Fee: $74; $10 re-examination fee

Additional State Endorsement: $84

NCLEX Test Fee: $200

Re-Examination Limitations: Every 91 days

License Renewal: February 28, May 31, and September 30, every odd year; $74

CEU Requirements: 30 contact hours every two years. Nurses licensed by exam are exempt from CE requirements for the first renewal after initial licensure. Minimum practice requirement of 1,000 hours in five years or 400 hours in two years.

District of Columbia

Board of Nursing
Department of Health
825 N. Capitol Street, N.E., Room 2224
Washington, DC 20002
Phone: (202) 442-9200
Fax: (202) 442-9431

Temporary Permit: None

State Board Fee: $75 license fee; $25 application fee

Additional State Endorsement: $75 license fee; $50 application fee

NCLEX Test Fee: $200

Re-Examination Limitations: Every 91 days

License Renewal: June 30, every two years, $48

CEU Requirements: Applicants for reinstatement of a license must submit 12 contact hours for each year after 6/30/90 that the applicant was not licensed, up to maximum of 24 contact hours.

Florida

Board of Nursing
4052 Bald Cypress Way, BIN C02
Tallahassee, FL 32399
Phone: (904) 858-6940
Fax: (904) 858-6964
www.doh.state.fl.us/mqa/

Temporary Permit: 90 days pending results of first exam; 60 days if by endorsement. Fee is included in licensure fee.

State Board Fee: $180 initial exam; $95 retake fee

Additional State Endorsement: $203

NCLEX Test Fee: $200

Re-Examination Limitations: Every 91 days; remedial training program is required after three attempts

License Renewal: Every odd year; $65

CEU Requirements: 25 contact hours every two years. One credit per month. Proof of training in HIV and domestic violence by a provider approved by the state of Florida.

Georgia

Board of Nursing
237 Coliseum Drive
Macon, GA 31217-3858
Phone: (478) 207-1640
Fax: (478) 207-1660
www.sos.state.ga.us/plb/rn/

Temporary Permit: Six months if by endorsement. Fee is included in application fee.

State Board Fee: $40

Additional State Endorsement: $60

NCLEX Test Fee: $200, plus $9.25 when registering by telephone

Re-Examination Limitations: Every 91 days, three years maximum

License Renewal: January 31, every even year. $40 if paid before November 30, $60 after November 30.

CEU Requirements: None

Hawaii

DCCA—PVL
Board of Nursing
P.O. Box 3469
Honolulu, HI 96801
Phone: (808) 586-3000
Fax: (808) 586-2689
www.state.hi.us/dcca/pvl/areas_nurse.html

Temporary Permit: No temporary permits

State Board Fee: $40

Additional State Endorsement: $95 or $140, depending on the year license is issued. Noted on application information sheet.

NCLEX Test Fee: $200

Re-Examination Limitations: Every 91 days

License Renewal: June 30, every odd year. $90

CEU Requirements: None

Idaho

Board of Nursing
(street address) 280 North 8th Street, Suite 210
(mailing address) P.O. Box 83720
Boise, ID 83720-0061
Phone: (208) 334-3110
Fax: (208) 334-3262
www.state.id.us/ibn/ibnhome.htm

Temporary Permit: 90 days if by endorsement, $15

State Board Fee: $75

Additional State Endorsement: $90

NCLEX Test Fee: $200

Re-Examination Limitations: Every 91 days

License Renewal: August 31, every odd year; $45

CEU Requirements: None

Illinois

Department of Professional Regulation
320 W. Washington Street, 3rd floor
Springfield, IL 62786
Phone: (217) 785-0800
Fax: (217) 782-7645
www.dpr.state.il.us/

Temporary Permit: Three-month approval letter

State Board Fee: $50

Additional State Endorsement: $50

NCLEX Test Fee: $200

Re-Examination Limitations: Three years from first writing to board

License Renewal: May 31, every even year; $40

CEU Requirements: None

Indiana

State Board of Nursing
Health Professions Bureau
402 W. Washington Street, Room 041
Indianapolis, IN 46204
Phone: (317) 234-2043
Fax: (317) 233-4236
www.state.in.us/hpb/boards/isbn

Temporary Permit: 90 days if by endorsement, $10. No graduate nurse status.

State Board Fee: $30

Additional State Endorsement: $30 in, $10 out

NCLEX Test Fee: $200

Re-Examination Limitations: Every 91 days, no maximum limit

License Renewal: October 31, every odd year; $20

CEU Requirements: None

Iowa

Board of Nursing
Riverpoint Business Park
400 SW 8th Street, Suite B
Des Moines, IA 50309-4685
Phone: (515) 281-3255
Fax: (515) 281-4825
www.state.ia.us/government/nursing/

Temporary Permit: 30 days if by endorsement. Fee is included in application fee.

State Board Fee: $75

Additional State Endorsement: $78; license by endorsement $101

NCLEX Test Fee: $200

Re-Examination Limitations: Every 91 days

License Renewal: Month of birth, every three years; $81

CEU Requirements: 45 contact hours or 4.5 CEUs every three years

Kansas

State Board of Nursing
Landon State Office Building
900 SW Jackson, Suite 551-S
Topeka, KS 66612-1230
Phone: (785) 296-4929
Fax: (785) 296-3929
www.ksbn.org

Temporary Permit: Pending results of first exam, or no longer than 90 days from graduation; 120 days if by endorsement. Fee is included in application fee.

State Board Fee: $75

Additional State Endorsement: $75

NCLEX Test Fee: $200

Re-Examination Limitations: Every 91 days, unlimited number of times; after two years the applicant must provide an approved study plan

License Renewal: Month of birth, every two years; $60

CEU Requirements: 30 contact hours every two years

Kentucky

Board of Nursing
312 Whittington Parkway, Suite 300
Louisville, KY 40222-5172
Phone: (502) 329-7000
Fax: (502) 329-7011
www.kbn.state.ky.us/

Temporary Permit: No temporary work permits are issued to new graduates

State Board Fee: $110

Additional State Endorsement: $120

NCLEX Test Fee: $200

Re-Examination Limitations: Every 91 days

License Renewal: October 31, every even year; $95 active, $65 inactive

CEU Requirements: 30 contact hours every two years; two of the 30 hours must be AIDS CE-approved by the Kentucky Cabinet for Health Services. A one-time, three-hour domestic violence requirement must be completed within three years of the date of initial licensing.

Louisiana

Board of Nursing
3510 North Causeway Boulevard, Suite 501
Metairie, LA 70002
Phone: (504) 838-5332
Fax: (504) 838-5349
www.lsbn.state.la.us/

Temporary Permit: Pending results of first exam; 90 days if by endorsement. Fee is included in application fee.

State Board Fee: $80

Additional State Endorsement: $100 in, plus $34 fingerprint fee

NCLEX Test Fee: $200

Re-Examination Limitations: Every 91 days, up to four times in four years

License Renewal: January 31, every year; $90

CEU Requirements: For all RNs: 5, 10, or 15 contact hours every year, based on employment

Maine

Board of Nursing
24 Stone Street
#158 State House Station
Augusta, ME 04333
Phone: (207) 287-1133
Fax: (207) 287-1149
www.state.me.us/nursingbd/

Temporary Permit: 90 days. Fee is included in application fee.

State Board Fee: $60

Additional State Endorsement: $60

NCLEX Test Fee: $200

Re-Examination Limitations: Every 91 days

License Renewal: Birthday, every two years; $40

CEU Requirements: None

Maryland

Board of Nursing
4140 Patterson Avenue
Baltimore, MD 21215
Phone: (410) 585-1900
Fax: (410) 358-3530
www.mbon.org

Temporary Permit: 90 days, not renewable; no graduate nurse status; $25

State Board Fee: $75

Additional State Endorsement: $75

NCLEX Test Fee: $200

Re-Examination Limitations: Every 91 days

License Renewal: 28th day of month of birth, every year; $45

CEU Requirements: None

Massachusetts

Division of Professional Licensure
Board of Registration in Nursing
239 Causeway Street
Boston, MA 02114
Phone: (617) 727-9961
Fax: (617) 727-1630
www.state.ma.us/reg/boards/rn/

Temporary Permit: Not granted

State Board Fee: $278 initial exam (includes test fee); $228 retake fee

Additional State Endorsement: $130

NCLEX Test Fee: $200, included in state board fee

Re-Examination Limitations: Every 91 days

License Renewal: Birthday, every even year; $40; $25 late fee

CEU Requirements: 15 contact hours every two years

Michigan

Michigan CIS
Board of Nursing
Ottawa Towers North
611 W. Ottawa, 4th floor
Lansing, MI 48933
Phone: (517) 373-9102
Fax: (517) 373-2179
www.cis.state.mi.us/bhser/genover.htm

Temporary Permit: No longer available

State Board Fee: $40

Additional State Endorsement: $40

NCLEX Test Fee: $200

Re-Examination Limitations: Every 91 days, up to six attempts within three years

License Renewal: March 31, every two years

CEU Requirements: 25 credits every two years

Minnesota

Board of Nursing
2829 University Avenue, SE #500
Minneapolis, MN 55414
Phone: (612) 617-2270
Fax: (612) 617-2190
www.nursingboard.state.mn.us/

Temporary Permit: 60 days, license by exam; $60. One year if by endorsement, no fee.

State Board Fee: $105 initial exam; $60 retake fee

Additional State Endorsement: $105

NCLEX Test Fee: $200

Re-Examination Limitations: Every 91 days, for a maximum of 4 times per year

License Renewal: Birth month, every two years; $85

CEU Requirements: 24 contact hours every two years

Mississippi

Board of Nursing
1935 Lakeland Drive, Suite B
Jackson, MS 39216-5014
Phone: (601) 987-4188
Fax: (601) 364-2352
www.msbn.state.ms.us/

Temporary Permit: 90 days by endorsement; $25

State Board Fee: $60

Additional State Endorsement: $60

NCLEX Test Fee: $200

Re-Examination Limitations: Every 91 days

License Renewal: December 31, every even year; $50

CEU Requirements: None

Missouri

Board of Nursing
P.O. Box 656
Jefferson City, MO 65102-0656
Phone: (573) 751-0681
Fax: (573) 751-0075
www.ecodev.state.mo.us/pr/nursing/

Temporary Permit: Six months. Fee is included in application fee.

State Board Fee: $67 initial exam; $40 retake fee

Additional State Endorsement: $77

NCLEX Test Fee: $200

Re-Examination Limitations: Every 91 days

License Renewal: April 30, every two years; $100

CEU Requirements: None

Montana

Department of Labor and Industry
Board of Nursing
301 South Park, 4th floor
P.O. Box 200513
Helena, MT 59620-0513
Phone: (406) 841-2340
Fax: (406) 841-2343
www.discoveringmontana.com/dli/bsd/

Temporary Permit: 90 days by endorsement or exam. Fee is included in application fee.

State Board Fee: $70

Additional State Endorsement: $70

NCLEX Test Fee: $200

Re-Examination Limitations: Every 91 days, up to attempts in three years. After failing twice, must ﾟnt a plan of study to the Board before next

retake. If one doesn't pass within three years, must take Nursing Program before sixth retake.

License Renewal: December 31, every year, $50

CEU Requirements: None

Nebraska

Department of HHS Regulation and Licensure
Nursing and Nursing Support Section
P.O. Box 94986
Lincoln, NE 68509-4925
Phone: (402) 471-4376
Fax: (402) 471-1066
www.hhs.state.ne.us/crl/nursing/Rn-Lpn/rn-lpn.htm

Temporary Permit: 60 days if by endorsement. Fee is included in licensing fee.

State Board Fee: $75 application fee

Additional State Endorsement: $75 application fee

NCLEX Test Fee: $200

Re-Examination Limitations: Every 91 days

License Renewal: October 31, every even year; $40

CEU Requirements: 20 contact hours every two years with 500 practice hours every five years, or a review course of study in previous five years, or new grads within two years

Nevada

Board of Nursing
P.O. Box 46886
Las Vegas, NV 89103
Phone: (888) 590-NSBN or (702) 486-5800
Fax: (702) 486-5803
www.nursingboard.state.nv.us/

Temporary Permit: Three months if by exam, not renewable. Four months if by endorsement, not renewable in 12-month period. Fee is included in application fee; $50 if not seeking permanent license.

State Board Fee: $100

Additional State Endorsement: $105

NCLEX Test Fee: $200

Re-Examination Limitations: Every 91 days, up to three times, then only with remediation

License Renewal: Birthday, every two years; $100

CEU Requirements: 30 contact hours every two years at renewal. New grads may be exempt from CE requirements for their first renewal period.

New Hampshire

Board of Nursing
78 Regional Drive, Building B
P.O. Box 3898
Concord, NH 03302-3898
Phone: (603) 271-2323
Fax: (603) 271-6605
www.state.nh.us/nursing/

Temporary Permit: Six months or until results of first exam are received and license is issued, $20

State Board Fee: $80

Additional State Endorsement: $70

NCLEX Test Fee: $200

Re-Examination Limitations: Every 91 days

License Renewal: Birthday, every two years; $60

CEU Requirements: 30 contact hours every two years at renewal

New Jersey

Board of Nursing
P.O. Box 45010
Newark, NJ 07101
Phone: (973) 504-6430
Fax: (973) 648-3481
www.state.nj.us/lps/ca/medical.htm

Temporary Permit: Graduate nurse status available

State Board Fee: $75

Additional State Endorsement: $75 application fee; $65 license certificate fee

NCLEX Test Fee: $200

Re-Examination Limitations: Every 91 days; only with remediation after three attempts; $75

License Renewal: December 31, every two years; $75

CEU Requirements: None

New Mexico

Board of Nursing
4206 Louisiana NE, Suite A
Albuquerque, NM 87109
Phone: (505) 841-8340
Fax: (505) 841-8347
www.state.nm.us/clients/nursing

Temporary Permit: 24 weeks from graduation if application process is completed within 12 weeks of graduation; six months if by endorsement. Fee is included in application fee; must have NM employment verified.

State Board Fee: $90 initial exam; $45 retake fee

Additional State Endorsement: $90

NCLEX Test Fee: $200

Re-Examination Limitations: Every 91 days; $45

License Renewal: Every two years from date of issue; $60

CEU Requirements: 30 contact hours every two years

New York

Board of Nursing
NYS Education Department
89 Washington Avenue, 2nd floor
Albany, NY 12234
Phone: (518) 474-3817, ext. 320
Fax: (518) 474-3706
www.op.nysed.gov/nurse.htm

Temporary Permit: Must have completed all other requirements for licensure except the licensing examination. Valid for one year from date of issue or until ten days after the applicant is notified of failure on the licensing examination, whichever occurs first; $35

State Board Fee: $135 (includes first license and 3-year registration)

Additional State Endorsement: $135

NCLEX Test Fee: $200

Re-Examination Limitations: Every 91 days

License Renewal: Every three years; $65

CEU Requirements: None

North Carolina

Board of Nursing
P.O. Box 2129
Raleigh, NC 27602
Phone: (919) 782-3211
Fax: (919) 781-9461
www.ncbon.com

Temporary Permit: None for new graduates. By endorsement: six months or until the endorsement is approved, whichever occurs first; not renewable. Fee is included in application fee.

State Board Fee: $50

Additional State Endorsement: $105

NCLEX Test Fee: $200

Re-Examination Limitations: Every 91 days

License Renewal: Month of birth, every two years; prorated

CEU Requirements: None

North Dakota

Board of Nursing
919 S. 7th Street, Suite 504
Bismarck, ND 58504-5881
Phone: (701) 328-9777
Fax: (701) 328-9785
www.ndbon.org

Temporary Permit: By endorsement: 90 days; fee is included in endorsement fee. By exam: 90 days after the date of issue or upon notification of exam results, whichever occurs first.

State Board Fee: $90

Additional State Endorsement: $90

NCLEX Test Fee: $200

Re-Examination Limitations: Every 91 days, up to five attempts in three years

License Renewal: Every two years; $70

CEU Requirements: Nursing practice for relicensure must meet or exceed 500 hours within preceding five years

Ohio

Board of Nursing
17 South High Street, Suite 400
Columbus, OH 43215-3413
Phone: (614) 466-3947
Fax: (614) 466-0388
www.state.oh.us/nur/

Temporary Permit: 120 days if by endorsement, not renewable. Fee is included in endorsement application fee.

State Board Fee: $50

Additional State Endorsement: $50

NCLEX Test Fee: $200

Re-Examination Limitations: Every 91 days

License Renewal: August 31, every odd year, $35

CEU Requirements: 24 hours in a 2-year period

Oklahoma

Board of Nursing
2915 N. Classen Boulevard, Suite 524
Oklahoma City, OK 73106
Phone: (405) 962-1800
Fax: (405) 962-1821

Temporary Permit: 90 days if by endorsement; fee is included in licensure by endorsement application fee

State Board Fee: $75

Additional State Endorsement: $75

NCLEX Test Fee: $200

Re-Examination Limitations: Every 91 days

License Renewal: Last day of birth month, every even year

CEU Requirements: Only for APNs applying for or renewing prescriptive authority

Oregon

Board of Nursing
800 NE Oregon Street, Suite 465
Portland, OR 97232-2162
Phone: (503) 731-4745
Fax: (503) 731-4755
www.osbn.state.or.us/

Temporary Permit: None

State Board Fee: $80

Additional State Endorsement: $115

NCLEX Test Fee: $200

Re-Examination Limitations: Every 91 days, up to three years from the date of graduation

License Renewal: Birthday, every two years; $65

CEU Requirements: None

Pennsylvania

Board of Nursing
P.O. Box 2649
Harrisburg, PA 17105-2649
Phone: (717) 783-7142
Fax: (717) 783-0822
www.dos.state.pa.us/bpoa/nurbd/mainpage.htm

Temporary Permit: 1 year maximum; examination results preempt permit, $35

State Board Fee: $35

Additional State Endorsement: $100

NCLEX Test Fee: $200

Re-Examination Limitations: Every 91 days

License Renewal: Renewal date by license number every two years; $45

CEU Requirements: None

Rhode Island

Board of Nurse Registration and Nursing Education
3 Capitol Hill, Room 105
Providence, RI 02908
Phone: (401) 222-5700
Fax: (401) 222-3352
www.health.state.ri.us/hsr/professions/nurses.htm

Temporary Permit: Pending results of first exam but no longer than 90 days after graduation; 90 days if by endorsement. Not renewable. No fee.

State Board Fee: $93.75

Additional State Endorsement: $93.75

NCLEX Test Fee: $200

Re-Examination Limitations: Every 91 days

License Renewal: March 1, every two years by license number; $62.50

CEU Requirements: None

South Carolina

Board of Nursing
P.O. Box 12367
Columbia, SC 29211
Phone: (803) 896-4550
Fax: (803) 896-4525
www.llr.state.sc.us/pol/nursing/

Temporary Permit: 90 days if by endorsement, $10

State Board Fee: $65

Additional State Endorsement: $75

NCLEX Test Fee: $200

Re-Examination Limitations: Every 91 days, up to four times in one year, then must remediate; $65

License Renewal: January 31, every year; $32

CEU Requirements: Minimum practice requirement of 960 hours in preceding five years

South Dakota

Board of Nursing
4300 S. Louise Avenue, Suite C-1
Sioux Falls, SD 57106-3124
Phone: (605) 362-2760
Fax: (605) 362-2768
www.state.sd.us/dcr/nursing/

Temporary Permit: 90 days from graduation pending results of first exam; 90 days if by endorsement; $25

State Board Fee: $75

Additional State Endorsement: $75

NCLEX Test Fee: $200

Re-Examination Limitations: Every 91 days, maximum of four times per year in three years postgraduation, then must requalify

License Renewal: Birthday, every two years; $65 (includes $10 for nurse education assistance loan fund)

CEU Requirements: Continuing employment 140 hours in one year or 480 hours in six years

Tennessee

Board of Nursing
425 Fifth Avenue North
Cordell Hull Building, First Floor
Nashville, TN 37247-1010
Phone: (615) 532-3202
Fax: (615) 741-7899
www.state.tn.us/health/

Temporary Permit: Six months if by endorsement; $25

State Board Fee: $115

Additional State Endorsement: $115

NCLEX Test Fee: $200

Re-Examination Limitations: Every 91 days, up to three years, then only with remediation

License Renewal: Last day of month of birth, every two years; $50

CEU Requirements: Continued practice requirement over a five-year period

Texas

Board of Nurse Examiners
P.O. Box 430
Austin, TX 78767
Phone: (512) 305-7400
Fax: (512) 305-7401
www.bne.state.tx.us/

Temporary Permit: By endorsement: 12 weeks, $100. By exam: 60 days or pending results of first exam.

State Board Fee: $65

Additional State Endorsement: $100 (includes temporary license)

NCLEX Test Fee: $200

Re-Examination Limitations: Every 91 days, up to three attempts within four years

License Renewal: Every even year for those born in even years, every odd year for those born in odd years (initial licensure period ranges from six months to 29 months depending on birth year); $42

CEU Requirements: 20 contact hours (2 CEUs) every two years. Nurses licensed by exam or by endorsement are exempt from CE requirements for the first renewal after initial licensure.

Utah

Board of Nursing
Division of Occupational and Professional Licensing
P.O. Box 146741
Salt Lake City, UT 84114-6741
Phone: (801) 530-6597
Fax: (801) 530-6511
www.commerce.utah.gov/opl/licensing/nurse.html

Temporary Permit: None

State Board Fee: $50

Additional State Endorsement: $50

NCLEX Test Fee: $200

Re-Examination Limitations: Every 91 days; those who fail to pass exam within two years after completing educational program must submit plan of action for approval before retaking

License Renewal: January 31, every odd year; $40

CEU Requirements: Must have practiced not less than 400 hours during two years preceding application for renewal, or have completed 30 contact hours, or have practiced not less than 200 hours and completed 15 contact hours during two years preceding application for renewal

Vermont

Board of Nursing
Office of the Secretary of State
109 State Street
Montpelier, VT 05609-1106
Phone: (802) 828-2396
Fax: (802) 828-2484
vtprofessionals.org/nurses/

Temporary Permit: 90 days if by endorsement; $25

State Board Fee: $60

Additional State Endorsement: $60

NCLEX Test Fee: $200

Re-Examination Limitations: Every 91 days; Board of Nursing approval is needed after two attempts

License Renewal: March 31, every odd year; $60

CEU Requirements: Minimum practice requirement of 960 hours in five years or 400 hours in two years

Virginia

Board of Nursing
6606 West Broad Street, 4th floor
Richmond, VA 23230-1717
Phone: (804) 662-9909
Fax: (804) 662-9512
www.dhp.state.va.us/nursing/

Temporary Permit: 90 days pending results of exam

State Board Fee: $105

Additional State Endorsement: $105

NCLEX Test Fee: $200

Re-Examination Limitations: Every 91 days

License Renewal: Last day of month of birth, every even year for those born in even years, every odd year for those born in odd years; $70

CEU Requirements: None

Washington

Nursing Care Quality Assurance Commission
1300 SE Quince Street
P.O. Box 47864
Olympia, Washington 98504-7864
Phone: (360) 236-4702
Fax: (360) 236-4738
www.doh.wa.gov/nursing/

Temporary Permit: None

State Board Fee: $65

Additional State Endorsement: $65

NCLEX Test Fee: $200

Re-Examination Limitations: Every 91 days, up to four times in two years, then must requalify

License Renewal: Birthday, every year; $50

CEU Requirements: Not mandatory

West Virginia

Board of Examiners for Registered Professional Nurses
101 Dee Drive
Charleston, WV 25311-1620
Phone: (304) 558-3596
Fax: (304) 558-3666
www.state.wv.us/nurses/rn/

Temporary Permit: 90 days pending results of first exam; 90 days if by endorsement; $10

State Board Fee: $51.50

Additional State Endorsement: $30

NCLEX Test Fee: $200

Re-Examination Limitations: Every 91 days; additional requirements are needed after two attempts

License Renewal: December 31, every year, $25

CEU Requirements: 30 contact hours every odd year. If initial licensure occurs during the first half of any 2-year reporting period: must complete 12 contact hours before the end of that reporting period. If initial licensure occurs during the second half of any 2-year reporting period: exempt from CE requirements for the entire reporting period.

Wisconsin

Bureau of Health Service Professions—RN
Department of Regulation and Licensing
1400 E. Washington Avenue
P.O. Box 8935
Madison, WI 53708-8935
Phone: (608) 266-0145
www.drl.state.wi.us/

Temporary Permit: Three months pending results of exam; three months if by endorsement; $10

State Board Fee: $53 initial credential fee; $15 examination contract fee

Additional State Endorsement: $66

NCLEX Test Fee: $200

Re-Examination Limitations: Every 91 days

License Renewal: February 28 or 29, every even year; $66

CEU Requirements: None

Wyoming

Board of Nursing
2020 Carey Avenue, Suite 110
Cheyenne, WY 82002
Phone: (307) 777-7601
Fax: (307) 777-3519
nursing.state.wy.us/

Temporary Permit: 90 days by endorsement or by exam. Fee is included in application fee.

State Board Fee: $130

Additional State Endorsement: $135

NCLEX Test Fee: $200

Re-Examination Limitations: Every 91 days, maximum of 10 times within 5 years of graduation

License Renewal: December 31, every even year; $110

CEU Requirements: Minimum practice requirement of 1,600 hours in five years or 500 hours in two years

APPENDIX E

User's Guide to the CD-ROM

Installation and Tech Support

If you're using **Windows® 3.1x**:
1. Insert the CD-ROM into your drive.
2. From the File menu of the Program Manager, run "d:\KapNCLEX.exe" (where "d" is the letter of your CD-ROM drive).
3. Follow the directions on the screen.

If you're using **Windows® 95/NT**:
1. Insert the CD-ROM into your drive.
2. Double-click on "My Computer," then on your CD-ROM drive icon, and then on "KapNCLEX.exe."
3. Follow the directions on the screen.

If you're using **Macintosh®**:
1. Insert the CD-ROM into your drive.
2. Double-click on the "Kaplan NCLEX Install" icon.
3. Follow the directions on the screen.

If you need further assistance with installation or have any other software questions, call Kaplan at (503) 968-4058, Monday–Friday 9 A.M. to 9 P.M. or Saturday–Sunday 9 A.M. to 8 P.M. (EST).

Logging In

1. Type in your **First Name** and **Last Name**. Use the **Tab** button to move between fields.

2. Your **School Identification Number** is **9999**. Enter this number in the **School ID** field.

3. Your **Student Enrollment Number** is 97NCDX5030. Enter this number in the appropriate place on the **Log In** screen. If you wish to review your results at a later date, enter this number on the **Review Log In** screen. Your **Alternate Enrollment Number** is 97NCDX5050.

Timing

You have three hours to complete the test of 180 questions. If you fail to complete the test in the allotted time, the test will continue, but this indicates that you need to work on your pacing.

Review Modes

Press one of the following key combinations to view your results immediately after completing the test:

Control + 1   to view your overall performance (number of questions correct, incorrect, etcetera)

Control + 2   to view your detailed graphical summary (breakdown of performance by content area)

Control + 3   to view the explanations to the questions

To return to a previously viewed review mode, press the appropriate **Control + <number>** combination.

To view your results at a later date, press **Control + 4** from the first field of the **Log In** screen before entering any information. Enter your enrollment number in the appropriate place on the **Review Log In** screen and then press **Return (Enter)**, followed by one of the **Control + <number>** combinations listed above.

Quitting

Press **Control + Alt + 0** to quit the program at any time, except while viewing the **Log In** screen.

Press **Control + 4** to quit the program from the **Log In** screen. Then press **Control + Alt + 0** when you see the **Review Log In** screen.

Press **Q** to quit in the middle of a test. Then press **Quit** when the dialog box appears. This returns you to the **Log In** screen. Press **Control + 4** to exit the **Log In** screen and then press **Control + Alt + 0**.

If you quit before completing the test, you can take the test once again at a later date using your **alternate enrollment number** or any other 10-digit number. You can use each number code only once.

Notes

Notes

Notes

Notes

How Did We Do? Grade Us.

Thank you for choosing a Kaplan book. Your comments and suggestions are very useful to us. Please answer the following questions to assist us in our continued development of high-quality resources to meet your needs.

The title of the Kaplan book I read was: _____

My name is: _____

My address is: _____

_____

My e-mail address is: _____

What overall grade would you give this book?   Ⓐ   Ⓑ   Ⓒ   Ⓓ   Ⓕ

How relevant was the information to your goals?   Ⓐ   Ⓑ   Ⓒ   Ⓓ   Ⓕ

How comprehensive was the information in this book?   Ⓐ   Ⓑ   Ⓒ   Ⓓ   Ⓕ

How accurate was the information in this book?   Ⓐ   Ⓑ   Ⓒ   Ⓓ   Ⓕ

How easy was the book to use?   Ⓐ   Ⓑ   Ⓒ   Ⓓ   Ⓕ

How appealing was the book's design?   Ⓐ   Ⓑ   Ⓒ   Ⓓ   Ⓕ

What were the book's strong points? _____

How could this book be improved? _____

Is there anything that we left out that you wanted to know more about?

Would you recommend this book to others?   ☐ YES   ☐ NO

Other comments: _____

_____

_____

Do we have permission to quote you?   ☐ YES   ☐ NO

Thank you for your help.
Please tear out this page and mail it to:

Managing Editor
Kaplan, Inc.
888 Seventh Avenue
New York, NY 10106

KAPLAN®

Thanks!

About Kaplan

KAPLAN TEST PREPARATION & ADMISSIONS

With 3,000 classroom locations throughout the U.S. and abroad, Kaplan has served more than three million students in its classes over the past 60-plus years. Kaplan's nationally-recognized programs for roughly 35 standardized tests include entrance exams for secondary school, college and graduate school as well as English language and professional licensing exams. Kaplan also offers private tutoring and one-on-one admissions guidance and is a leader in test prep for computerized exams. Kaplan is the first major player to provide online test prep to students across the globe, as well as admissions courses and other resources at **www.kaptest.com.**

SCORE! LEARNING, INC.

SCORE! Learning, Inc. is a national provider of customized learning programs for students. *SCORE!* Educational Centers help students in K-10 build confidence along with academic skills in a motivating, sports-oriented environment after school and on weekends. *SCORE!* Prep provides in-home, one-on-one tutoring for high school academic subjects and standardized tests. *SCORE!* Educational Centers and *SCORE!* Prep share a highly personalized approach, proven educational techniques, and the goal of cultivating a love of learning in children.

THE KAPLAN COLLEGES

The Kaplan Colleges system (**www.kaplancollege.edu**) is a collection of institutions offering an extensive array of online and traditional educational programs for working professionals who want to advance their careers. Learners will find programs leading to bachelor and associates degrees, certificates and diplomas in fields such as business, IT, paralegal studies, legal nurse consulting, criminal justice and financial planning. The Kaplan Colleges system includes Concord Law School (**www.concordlawschool.com**), the nation's only online law school, offering J.D., Executive J.D. and LL.M. degrees for working professionals, family caregivers, students in rural communities, and others whose circumstances prevent them from attending a fixed facility law school.

QUEST EDUCATION CORPORATION

Kaplan's Quest Education unit (**www.questeducation.com**) is a leading provider of post-secondary education. Quest offers bachelor and associate degrees and diploma programs designed to provide students with the skills necessary to qualify them for entry-level employment. Programs are primarily in the fields of healthcare, business, information technology, fashion and design.

KAPLAN PUBLISHING

Kaplan Publishing, in a joint venture with Simon & Schuster, publishes more than 150 titles on test preparation, admissions, education, career development, and life skills. Kaplan Publishing emerged as a leader in sales of books for statewide assessments with the publication of dozens of new state test titles. Books are offered in traditional paper form, pre-packaged with computer software, and now in e-book form.

KAPLAN INTERNATIONAL

Kaplan International (**www.kaptest.com**) provides students and professionals with intensive English instruction, university preparation, test preparation programs, housing and activities at 12 city and campus centers in the U.S. and Canada. Kaplan also has a strong presence overseas with 41 centers in 18 countries outside of the United States.

KAPLAN COMMUNITY OUTREACH

Kaplan Community Outreach provides educational resources and opportunities to thousands of economically disadvantaged students annually. Kaplan joins forces with numerous nonprofit groups, educational institutions, government agencies, and other grass-roots organizations on a variety of local and national support programs. These programs help students and professionals from a variety of backgrounds achieve their educational and career goals.

KAPLAN PROFESSIONAL

The Kaplan Professional companies (**www.kaplanprofessional.com**) provide licensing and continuing education, training, certification, professional development courses, and compliance tracking for securities, insurance, financial services, legal, IT, and real estate professionals and corporations. Offering an array of educational tools, from on-site training and classroom instruction to nearly 200 online courses and programs, Kaplan Professional serves professionals who must maintain licenses and comply with regulatory mandates despite busy travel schedules and work obligations.

- **Dearborn Financial Services** provides innovative education and compliance solutions to the financial services industry, including registration services, firm element needs analysis and training plan development, securities and insurance prelicensing training, continuing education, and compliance management services, in classes nationwide, online and via books and software.

- **Dearborn Trade Publishing** publishes approximately 250 titles specializing in finance, business management and real estate, plus well-read consumer real estate books to help homebuyers, sellers and real estate investors make informed decisions.

- **Dearborn Real Estate Education** is the leading real estate content provider for real estate schools and associations, offering practical prelicensing and continuing education training materials on appraisal, home inspection, property management, brokerage, ethics, law, sales approaches, and contracts, and an online real estate campus at **RECampus.com**.

- **Perfect Access Speer** is a leader in software education and consulting, bringing both traditional and e-learning solutions to its clients in the legal, financial, and professional services industries.

- **The Schweser Study Program** offers training tools for the Chartered Financial Analyst (CFA®) examination, with a comprehensive product line of study notes, audiotapes, videotapes, flashcards and live seminars that are developed and taught by a top-notch faculty.

- **Kaplan Professional Real Estate Schools** provide real estate licensing and continuing education programs through live classroom instruction, Internet-based learning, and correspondence courses, to help real estate professionals acquire the skills needed to meet state licensing and educational requirements.

- **Self Test Software** is a world leader in exam simulation software and preparation for technical certifications including Microsoft, Oracle, Cisco, Novell, Lotus, CIW and CompTIA, serving businesses and individuals seeking to attain vendor-sponsored certification.

- **Call Center Solutions** provides assessment and training services to the call center industry.

Want more information about our services, products or the nearest Kaplan center?

1 **Call our nationwide toll-free numbers:**

1-800-KAP-TEST for information on our test prep courses, private tutoring and admissions consulting

1-800-KAP-ITEM for information on our books and software

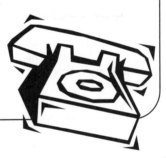

2 **Connect with us online:**

On the web, go to:

www.kaptest.com

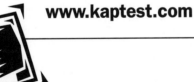

3 **Write to:**

Kaplan
888 Seventh Avenue
New York, NY 10106

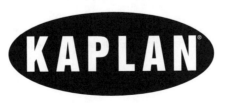

KAPLAN®

MINIMUM SYSTEM REQUIREMENTS

	Windows®	Macintosh®
Operating System:	Windows 3.1, Windows 95/NT	System 7.x or 8.x
CPU Type and Speed:	486SX, 50 Mhz	68040
Hard Drive Space:	8 MB	8 MB
Memory:	8 MB	8 MB
Graphics:	640 X 480 X 256	640 X 480 X 256
CD-ROM Speed:	2X	2X
Other:	Mouse	Mouse

Windows® 3.1x
After inserting the CD-ROM in your drive, run "d:\KapNCLEX.exe" (where "d" is the letter of your CD-ROM drive) from the File menu of the Program Manager. Follow the directions on the screen.

Windows® 95/NT
After inserting the CD-ROM in your drive, double-click on "My Computer," then on your CD-ROM drive icon, and then on "KapNCLEX.exe." Follow the directions on the screen.

Macintosh®
After inserting the CD-ROM in your drive, double-click on the "Kaplan NCLEX Install" icon. Follow the directions on the screen.

SOFTWARE LICENSE/DISCLAIMER OF WARRANTIES

1. ACCEPTANCE. By using this compact disc you hereby accept the terms and provisions of this license and agree to be bound hereby.

2. OWNERSHIP. The software contained on these compact discs, all content, related documentation and fonts (collectively, the "Software") are all proprietary copyrighted materials owned by Kaplan, Inc. ("Kaplan") or its licensors.

3. LICENSE. You are granted a limited license to use the Software. This License allows you to use the Software on a single computer only. You may not copy, distribute, modify, network, rent, lease, loan, or create derivative works based upon the Software in whole or in part. The Software is intended for personal usage only. Your rights to use the Software shall terminate immediately without notice upon your failure to comply with any of the terms hereof.

4. RESTRICTIONS. The Software contains copyrighted material, trade secrets, and other proprietary material. In order to protect them, and except as permitted by applicable legislation, you may not decompile, reverse engineer, disassemble or otherwise reduce the Software to human-perceivable form.

5. LIMITED WARRANTY; DISCLAIMER. Kaplan warrants the compact discs on which the Software is recorded to be free from defects in materials and workmanship under normal use for a period of ninety (90) days from the date of purchase as evidenced by a copy of the receipt. Kaplan's entire liability and your exclusive remedy will be replacement of the compact discs not meeting this warranty. The Software is provided "AS IS" and without warranty of any kind and Kaplan and Kaplan's licensors EXPRESSLY DISCLAIM ALL WARRANTIES, EXPRESS OR IMPLIED, INCLUDING THE IMPLIED WARRANTIES OF MERCHANTABILITY OR FITNESS FOR A PARTICULAR PURPOSE. FURTHERMORE, KAPLAN DOES NOT WARRANT THAT THE FUNCTIONS CONTAINED IN THE SOFTWARE WILL MEET YOUR REQUIREMENTS, OR THAT THE OPERATION OF THE SOFTWARE WILL BE UNINTERRUPTED OR ERROR-FREE, OR THAT DEFECTS IN THE SOFTWARE WILL BE CORRECTED. KAPLAN DOES NOT WARRANT OR MAKE ANY REPRESENTATIONS REGARDING THE USE OR THE RESULTS OF THE USE OF THE SOFTWARE IN TERMS OF THEIR CORRECTNESS, ACCURACY, RELIABILITY OR OTHERWISE. UNDER NO CIRCUMSTANCES, INCLUDING NEGLIGENCE, SHALL KAPLAN BE LIABLE FOR ANY DIRECT, INDIRECT, PUNITIVE, INCIDENTAL, SPECIAL OR CONSEQUENTIAL DAMAGES, INCLUDING, BUT NOT LIMITED TO, LOST PROFITS OR WAGES, IN CONNECTION WITH THE SOFTWARE EVEN IF KAPLAN HAS BEEN ADVISED OF THE POSSIBILITY OF SUCH DAMAGES. CERTAIN OF THE LIMITATIONS HEREIN PROVIDED MAY BE PRECLUDED BY LAW.

6. EXPORT LAW ASSURANCES. You agree and certify that you will not export the Software outside of the United States except as authorized and as permitted by the laws and regulations of the United States. If the Software has been rightfully obtained by you outside of the United States, you agree that you will not re-export the Software except as permitted by the laws and regulations of the United States and the laws and regulations of the jurisdiction in which you obtained the Software.

7. MISCELLANEOUS. This license represents the entire understanding of the parties, may only be modified in writing and shall be governed by the laws of the State of New York.